This book is dedicated to my husband and children

Other titles of interest

Visual Fields via the Visual Pathway
Fiona Rowe
ISBN: 978 1 4051 1525 4

Ophthalmology at a Glance
Jane Olver and Lorraine Cassidy
ISBN: 978 0 632 06473 1

Ophthalmic Nursing
Third Edition
Rosalind Stollery, Mary Shaw and Agnes Lee
ISBN: 978 1 4051 1105 8

ABC of Eyes
Fourth Edition
Peng Khaw, Andrew Elkington and Peter Shah
ISBN: 978 0 727 91659 4

Clinical Orthoptics

Second edition

Fiona Rowe
PhD, DBO, CGLI CertEd
Lecturer in Orthoptics, Division of Orthoptics, University of Liverpool and
*Honorary Research Vision Scientist, Department of Orthoptics and
Ophthalmology, Warrington Hospital, UK*

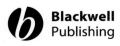
Blackwell
Publishing

© 1997, 2004 by Blackwell Publishing Ltd

Editorial offices:
Blackwell Publishing Ltd, 9600 Garsington Road, Oxford OX4 2DQ, UK
    Tel: +44 (0) 1865 776868
Blackwell Publishing Inc., 350 Main Street, Malden, MA 02148-5020, USA
    Tel: +1 781 388 8250
Blackwell Science Asia Pty Ltd, 550 Swanston Street, Carlton, Victoria 3053, Australia
    Tel: +61 (0)3 8359 1011

First edition published 1997 by Blackwell Science
Second edition published 2004 by Blackwell Publishing Ltd
3   2007

ISBN 978-1-4051-1342-7

Library of Congress Cataloging-in-Publication Data

Rowe, Fiona J.
    Clinical orthoptics / Fiona Rowe.—2nd ed.
    p. ; cm.
    Includes bibliographical references and index.
    ISBN 978-1-4051-1342-7 (pbk. : alk. paper)
    1. Orthoptics—Outlines, syllabi, etc.
    [DNLM: 1. Ocular Motility Disorders—Outlines. 2. Orthoptics—methods—Outlines. 3. Strabismus—Outlines. WW 18.2 R878c 2003] I. Title.

RE992.O7R686 2003
617.7'62—dc22
2004001029

A catalogue record for this title is available from the British Library

Set in 10/12.5 pt Palatino
by Graphicraft Limited, Hong Kong
Printed and bound in India by Replika Press Pvt. Ltd

For further information on Blackwell Publishing, visit our website:
www.blackwellpublishing.com

Contents

Preface

Clinical Orthoptics has become established as a basic reference text providing fundamental information on anatomy, innervation and orthoptic investigation, plus diagnosis and management of strabismus, ocular motility and related disturbances. As with the first edition the second edition is not designed to provide in-depth discussion of the content as it is recognised that this can be found in other excellent texts.

Following the revision of the content of the first edition, this second edition, in addition to many of the original illustrations, contains new figures, tables and flowcharts designed to enhance the written text. Reference and further reading lists for each chapter have been amended to include up-to-date literature.

The layout of many chapters has changed to incorporate more recent research and clinical findings. Section I concentrates on anatomy and innervation of extra-ocular muscles, including muscle pulley systems and associated cranial nerves. Ocular motility and orthoptic investigative techniques have been altered considerably to include more theoretical information but in a clinically applicable manner. Section II concentrates, as before, on concomitant strabismus and Section III on incomitant strabismus. There has been substantial revision of some chapters such as heterotropia and nystagmus. Section IV includes an updated list of abbreviations used in orthoptic practice and glossary of definitions but with new additions of diagnostic aids, diagnostic abbreviations and illustrative case reports.

ACKNOWLEDGEMENTS

Thanks are due to colleagues and undergraduate students at the University of Liverpool, the latter in particular whose comments and questions during teaching have provoked a revision of the delivery of content in this text. Special thanks are due to colleagues at Warrington Hospital for their unending support at all times. I am grateful to Addenbrooke's Hospital, Cambridge, for permission to use patient photographs and to the patients and parents for their consent to use these images. The glossary incorporates terminology from the British and Irish Orthoptic Society and thanks are due to the Society for permission to use the glossary terminology. Lastly, thanks to Caroline Connelly and the team at Blackwell Publishing for their input to this text.

Figures and tables

SECTION I

Chapter 1
Extraocular muscle anatomy and innervation

This chapter outlines the anatomy of the extraocular muscles and their innervation and associated cranial nerves (II, V, VII and VIII).

There are four recti and two oblique muscles attached to each eye. The recti muscles originate from the Annulus of Zinn which encircles the optic foramen and medial portion of the superior orbital fissure (Fig. 1.1). These muscles pass forward in the orbit and gradually diverge to form the orbital muscle cone. By means of a tendon, the muscles insert into the sclera anterior to the rotation centre of the globe (Fig. 1.2).

The extraocular muscles are striated muscles. They contain slow fibres, which produce a graded contracture on the exterior surface, and fast fibres which produce rapid movements on the interior surface adjacent to the globe. The slow fibres have a high content of mitochondria and oxidative enzymes. The fast fibres contain large amounts of glycogen and glycolytic enzymes and fewer oxidative enzymes than the slow fibres.

MUSCLE PULLEYS

There is stereotypic occurrence of connective tissue septa within the orbit and stereotypic organisation of connective tissue around the extra ocular muscles (Koornneef 1977, 1979). There is also stability of rectus

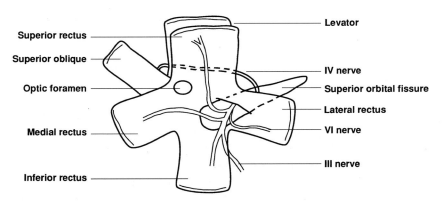

Figure 1.1   Orbital apex.

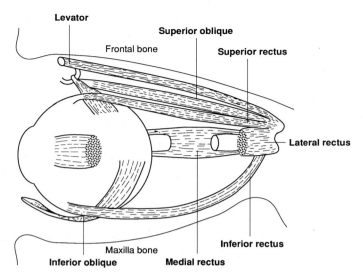

Figure 1.2 Extraocular muscles.

extraocular muscle belly paths throughout the range of eye movement and there is evidence for extraocular muscle path constraint by pulley attachment within the orbit (Miller 1989; Miller *et al.* 1993; Clark *et al.* 1999). High-resolution MRI has confirmed the presence of these attachments via connections that constrain the muscle paths during rotations of the globe (Demer *et al.* 1995; Clark *et al.* 1997). CT and MRI scans have shown that the paths of the rectus muscles remain fixed relative to the orbital wall during excursions of the globe and even after large surgical transpositions (Demer *et al.* 1996; Clark *et al.* 1999). It is only the anterior aspect of the muscle that moves with the globe relative to the orbit.

Histological studies have demonstrated that each rectus pulley consists of an encircling ring of collagen located near the globe equator in Tenon fascia attached to the orbital wall, adjacent extraocular muscles and equatorial Tenon fascia by slinglike bands which consist of densely woven collagen, elastin and smooth muscle (Demer *et al.* 1995; Porter *et al.* 1996). The global layer of each rectus extraocular muscle, containing about half of all extraocular muscle fibres, passes through the pulley and becomes continuous with the tendon to insert on the globe. The orbital layer containing the remaining half of the extraocular muscle fibres inserts on the pulley and not on the globe (Demer *et al.* 2000; Oh *et al.* 2001). The inferior oblique muscle also has a pulley which is mechanically attached to the inferior rectus pulley (Demer *et al.* 1999).

The general arrangement of orbital connective tissues is uniform throughout the range of human age from foetal life to the tenth decade. Such uniformity supports the concept that pulleys and orbital connective tissues are important for the mechanical generation and maintenance of ocular movements (Kono *et al.* 2002).

OCULAR MUSCLES

Medial rectus muscle

This muscle originates at the orbital apex from the medial portion of the Annulus of Zinn in close contact with the optic nerve. It courses forward for approximately 40 mm along the medial aspect of the globe and penetrates Tenon's capsule roughly 12 mm from the insertion. The last 5 mm of the muscle are in contact with the eye and the insertion is at 5.5 mm from the limbus with a width of 10.5 mm. The muscle is innervated by the inferior division of the III nerve which enters the muscle on its bulbar side. Its function is adduction of the eye (Fig. 1.3).

Lateral rectus muscle

This muscle arises by two heads from the upper and lower portions of the Annulus of Zinn where it bridges the superior orbital fissure. It courses forward for approximately 40 mm along the lateral aspect of the globe and crosses the inferior oblique insertion. It penetrates Tenon's capsule at roughly 15 mm from the insertion and the last 7–8 mm of the muscle is in contact with the eye. The insertion is at 7 mm from the limbus with a width of 9.5 mm. The muscle is innervated by the VI nerve which enters the muscle on its bulbar side. Its function is abduction of the eye (Fig. 1.4).

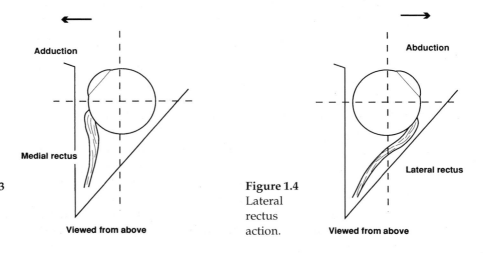

Figure 1.3 Medial rectus action.

Figure 1.4 Lateral rectus action.

Superior rectus muscle

This muscle arises from the superior portion of the Annulus of Zinn and courses forward for approximately 42 mm along the dorsal aspect of the globe, forming an angle of 23 degrees with the sagittal axis of the globe. Superiorly it is in close contact with the levator muscle. It penetrates Tenon's capsule at roughly 15 mm from the insertion and the last few millimetres of the muscle are in contact with the eye. The insertion is at 7.7 mm from the limbus with a width of 11 mm. The muscle is innervated by the superior division of the III nerve which enters the muscle on its bulbar side. Its functions are elevation, intorsion and adduction of the eye (Fig. 1.5).

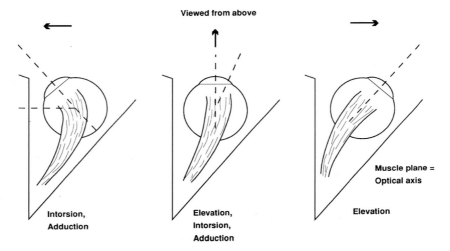

Figure 1.5   Superior rectus action. The course of the superior rectus is at an angle of 23 degrees to the medial wall of the orbit. Actions in adduction are principally intorsion and adduction; in the primary position, actions are elevation, intorsion and adduction; action in abduction is principally elevation.

Inferior rectus muscle

This muscle arises from the inferior portion of the Annulus of Zinn and courses forward for approximately 42 mm along the ventral aspect of the globe, forming an angle of 23 degrees with the sagittal axis. It penetrates Tenon's capsule roughly 15 mm from the insertion and the last few millimetres of the muscle are in contact with the eye as it arcs to insert at 6.5 mm from the limbus. Width of insertion is 10 mm. The muscle is innervated by the inferior division of the III nerve which

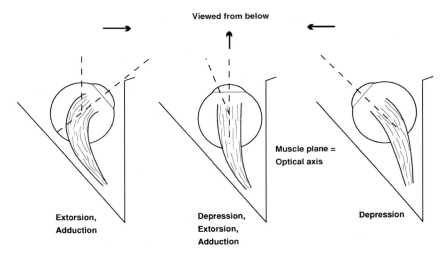

Figure 1.6 Inferior rectus action. The course of the inferior rectus is at an angle of 23 degrees to the medial wall of the orbit. In adduction, the actions are principally extorsion and adduction; in the primary position, actions are depression, extorsion and adduction; action in abduction is principally depression.

enters the muscle on its bulbar side. Its functions are depression, extorsion and adduction of the eye (Fig. 1.6).

Superior oblique muscle

This muscle originates from the orbital apex from the periosteum of the body of the sphenoid bone, medial and superior to the optic foramen. It courses forward for approximately 40 mm along the medial wall of the orbit to the trochlea (a V-shaped fibrocartilage which is attached to the frontal bone). The trochlear region is described by Helveston *et al.* (1982).

The muscle becomes tendonous roughly 10 mm posterior to the trochlea and is encased in a synovial sheath through the trochlea. From the trochlea, it courses posteriorly, laterally and downwards, forming an angle of 51 degrees with the visual axis of the eye in the primary position. It passes beneath the superior rectus and inserts on the upper temporal quadrant of the globe ventral to the superior rectus. Its insertion is fanned out in a curved line 10–12 mm in length. The muscle is innervated by the IV nerve which enters the muscle on its upper surface roughly 12 mm from its origin. Its functions are intorsion, depression and abduction of the eye (Fig. 1.7).

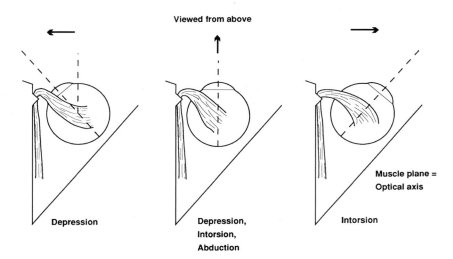

Figure 1.7   Superior oblique action. The course of the superior oblique tendon is at an angle of 51 degrees to the medial wall of the orbit. Action in adduction is depression; in the primary position, actions are depression, intorsion and abduction; in abduction, action is intorsion.

Inferior oblique muscle

This muscle arises from the floor of the orbit from the periosteum covering the anteromedial portion of the maxilla bone. It courses laterally and posteriorly for approximately 37 mm, forming an angle of 51 degrees with the visual axis. It penetrates Tenon's capsule near the posterior ventral surface of the inferior rectus, crosses the inferior rectus and curves upwards around the globe to insert under the lateral rectus just anterior to the macular area. The muscle is innervated by the inferior division of the III nerve which enters the muscle on its bulbar surface. Its functions are extorsion, elevation and abduction of the eye (Fig. 1.8).

Fig. 1.9 illustrates the muscle insertions in relation to the anterior segment of the eye. Fig. 1.10 illustrates the positions of main action of each extraocular muscle and Table 1.1 illustrates all primary, secondary and tertiary muscle actions.

Levator palpebrae superioris

This muscle originates from the undersurface of the lesser wing of sphenoid bone above and in front of the optic foramen by a short tendon which blends with the origin of the superior rectus. It runs forwards and changes directly from horizontal to vertical at the level of the equator of the globe. At approximately 10 mm above the superior margin of the tarsus, it divides into anterior and posterior lamellae. The anterior

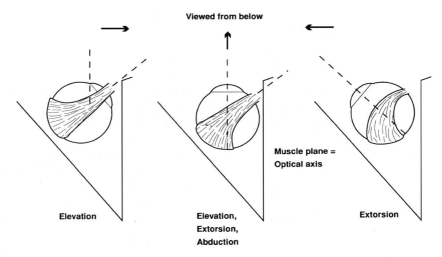

Figure 1.8 Inferior oblique action. The course of the inferior oblique is at an angle of 51 degrees to the medial wall of the orbit. Action in adduction is elevation; actions in the primary position are elevation, extorsion and abduction; in abduction, action is extorsion.

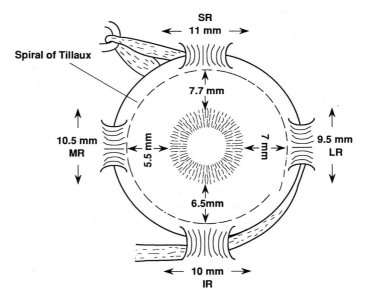

Figure 1.9 Extraocular muscle insertions. SR, superior rectus; MR, medial rectus; LR, lateral rectus; IR, inferior rectus.

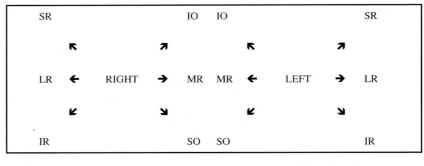

SR				IO	IO			SR
LR	←	RIGHT	→	MR	MR	←	LEFT	→	LR
IR				SO	SO			IR

SR	Superior rectus	IR	Inferior rectus	LR	Lateral rectus
MR	Medial rectus	IO	Inferior oblique	SO	Superior oblique

Figure 1.10   Cardinal positions of gaze – position of main action of extraocular muscles.

Table 1.1   Primary, secondary and tertiary muscle actions.

Muscle	Primary action	Secondary action	Tertiary action
Medial rectus	Adduction	—	—
Lateral rectus	Abduction	—	—
Superior rectus	Elevation, maximum in abduction	Intorsion, maximum in adduction	Adduction, maximum in adduction
Inferior rectus	Depression, maximum in abduction	Extorsion, maximum in adduction	Adduction, maximum in adduction
Superior oblique	Intorsion, maximum in abduction	Depression, maximum in adduction	Abduction, maximum in abduction
Inferior oblique	Extorsion, maximum in abduction	Elevation, maximum in adduction	Abduction, maximum in abduction

lamella forms the levator aponeurosis which is inserted into the lower third of the entire length of the anterior surface of the tarsus. Its fibres extend to the pretarsal portion of the orbit and skin. The posterior lamella forms Muller's muscle which is attached inferiorly to the superior margin of the tarsus.

INNERVATION

The extraocular muscles are innervated by the III, IV and VI nerves.

III nerve

The III nerve (third/oculomotor) supplies the superior rectus, inferior rectus, medial rectus, inferior oblique and levator muscles. Its visceral fibres innervate the ciliary muscle and sphincter pupillary muscle which synapse in the ciliary ganglion.

The nuclei are in the mesencephalon at the level of the superior colliculus. There is an elongated mass of cells which form the nuclei. Dorsal nucleus fibres pass to the ipsilateral inferior rectus, intermediate nucleus fibres pass to the ipsilateral inferior oblique, ventral nucleus fibres pass to the ipsilateral medial rectus, paramedian nucleus fibres pass to the contralateral superior rectus, central caudal nucleus fibres pass to both levator muscles and the anterior median/Edinger–Westphal nucleus contains the parasympathetic fibres. The nerve fibres emerge from the mesencephalon ventrally where they are closely associated with the posterior cerebellar and superior cerebral arteries. The nerve courses forward through the subarachnoid space to pierce the dura mater at the posterior clinoid process and enter the cavernous sinus.

IV nerve

The IV nerve (fourth/trochlear) supplies the superior oblique. The nucleus lies in the mesencephalon at the level of the inferior colliculus. The nerve fibres decussate and emerge from the brainstem dorsally. The nerves curve around the brainstem and course forward through the subarachnoid space to pierce the dura mater and enter the cavernous sinus.

VI nerve

The VI nerve (sixth/abducens) supplies the lateral rectus. The nucleus is situated in the pons in the floor of the IV ventricle near the midline, medial to the VIII nucleus and proximal to the paramedian pontine reticular formation. The medial longitudinal fasciculus lies medial to the nucleus. The nerve fibres emerge from the brainstem ventrally and course forward and laterally over the petrous tip of the temporal bone and under the petrosphenoid ligament. The nerve pierces the dura mater to enter the cavernous sinus.

Nerve pathways

The III, IV and VI nerves course forward together in the lateral aspect of the cavernous sinus, entering the orbit through the superior orbital fissure. The III and VI nerves enter within the muscle cone.

The III nerve divides into the superior and inferior divisions. The superior division enters the superior rectus on its bulbar surface and passes through the muscle to terminate in the levator muscle. The inferior branch supplies the medial rectus and inferior rectus and then passes beneath the optic nerve to the floor of the orbit and terminates in the inferior oblique. The terminal branch also sends a short branch to the ciliary ganglion. The VI nerve passes forward and laterally to enter the lateral rectus bulbar surface. The IV nerve enters through the superior orbital fissure laterally and superior to the Annulus of Zinn. It passes anteriorly and medially, crossing the III nerve, levator muscle and superior rectus, and enters the superior oblique on its orbital surface.

ASSOCIATED CRANIAL NERVES

Optic nerve

This nerve serves the sensory function of vision. Its pathway commences in the eye at the receptor cells in the retina. Retinal ganglion cells pass in nerve fibre bundles to the optic discs and pass from each eye to the intracranial cavity along the optic nerves. The optic nerves merge in the optic chiasm where there is crossing of nasal retinal fibres. Ipsilateral temporal and contralateral nasal fibres pass along the optic tracts to the lateral geniculate nuclei where the first synapse of nerve fibres occurs. The post-synaptic fibres then pass via the optic radiations to the visual cortex. The visual cortex (V1) occupies the calcarine sulcus in the occipital lobe and is the primary visual area.

V nerve

The V nerve (fifth/trigeminal) serves sensory and motor functions. The sensory nerve has three branches.

Sensory nerves

The **ophthalmic** division serves the sensory function to the lacrimal gland, conjunctiva, forehead, eyelids, anterior scalp and mucous membranes of the nose. The sensory fibres pass through the superior orbital fissure to the cavernous sinus and pass inferiorly to the trigeminal ganglion which is located under the cavernous sinus in Meckel's cave (a groove in the skull). Fibres pass from the ganglion posteriorly to the pons to the trigeminal nuclei.

The **maxillary** division serves the sensory function to the cheeks, upper gums and teeth, and lower eyelids. The sensory fibres pass through the foramen rotundum, underneath the cavernous sinus to the trigeminal ganglion and then on to the nuclei in the pons.

The **mandibular** division serves the sensory function to the teeth, gums of the lower jaw, pinna of ears, lower lip and tongue. The sensory fibres pass through the foramen ovale underneath the cavernous sinus to the trigeminal ganglion and then on to the nuclei in the pons.

Motor fibres

Motor fibres of the V nerve serve the muscles of mastication. The motor nuclei are located in the pons near the VII nerve nuclei and aqueduct. Nerve fibres leave ventrally and medially and pass anteriorly to the trigeminal ganglion, through the foramen ovale to the muscles of mastication.

VII nerve

The VII nerve (seventh/facial) serves sensory and motor functions.

Sensory fibres

Ganglion cells supply taste buds in the palate and tongue and sensory fibres are also present in the skin, in and around the external acoustic meatus. Fibres pass to the geniculate ganglion situated in the internal auditory meatus and pass back to the pons.

Motor fibres

The nuclei are located in the lateral part of the pons and fibres loop around the abducens nuclei, forming the facial colliculus, before leaving the pons ventrally. Fibres pass anteriorly and enter the internal auditory meatus. The nerve enters a narrow bony canal above the labyrinth and descends to the stylomastoid foramen where a branch supplies the stapedius muscle. It leaves the skull and supplies the facial muscles (frontal, zygomatic, buccal, mandibular marginal and cervical branches).

VIII nerve

The VIII nerve (eighth/auditory) serves the sensory function of hearing and balance.

Cochlear nerve (hearing)

Receptor cells are hair cells in the Organ of Corti. Fibres pass along the internal auditory meatus to the cisterna pontis, to the inferior cerebellar peduncle and to the cochlear vestibular nuclei in the pons.

Vestibular nerve (balance)

Receptor cells are hair cells in the utricles, saccules and semicircular canals. Fibres pass along the internal auditory meatus to the cisterna pontis and to the vestibular nuclei in the pons.

REFERENCES

Clark RA, Miller JM & Demer JL. (1997) Location and stability of rectus muscle pulleys. Muscle paths as function of gaze. *Investigative Ophthalmology and Visual Science*, 38: 227

Clark RA, Rosenbaum AL & Demer JL. (1999) Magnetic resonance imaging after surgical transposition defines the anteroposterior location of the rectus muscle paths. *Journal of American Association for Pediatric Ophthalmology and Strabismus*, 3: 9

Demer JL, Miller JM, Poukens V, Vinters HV & Glasgow BJ. (1995) Evidence for fibromuscular pulleys of the recti extraocular muscles. *Investigative Ophthalmology and Visual Science*, 36: 1125

Demer JL, Miller JM & Poukens V. (1996) Surgical implications of the rectus extraocular muscle pulleys. *Pediatric Ophthalmology and Strabismus*, 33: 208

Demer JL, Clark RA & Miller JL. (1999) Magnetic resonance imaging (MRI) of the functional anatomy of the inferior oblique (IO) muscle. (ARVO abstract.) *Investigative Ophthalmology and Visual Science*, 40(4): S772

Demer JL, Oh SY & Poukens V. (2000) Evidence for active control of rectus extraocular muscle pulleys. *Investigative Ophthalmology and Visual Science*, 41: 1280

Helveston EM, Merriam WW, Ellis FD, Shellhamer RH & Gosling CG. (1982) The trochlea: a study of the anatomy and physiology. *Ophthalmology*, 89: 124

Kono R, Poukens V & Demer JL. (2002) Quantitative analysis of the structure of the human extraocular muscle pulley system. *Investigative Ophthalmology and Visual Science*, 43: 2923

Koornneef L. (1977) New insights in the human orbital connective tissue; result of a new anatomical approach. *Archives of Ophthalmology*, 95: 1269

Koornneef L. (1979) Orbital septa: anatomy and function. *Ophthalmology*, 86: 876

Miller JM. (1989) Functional anatomy of normal human rectus muscles. *Vision Research*, 29: 223

Miller JM, Demer JL & Rosenbaum AL. (1993) Effect of transposition surgery on rectus muscle paths by magnetic resonance imaging. *Ophthalmology*, 100: 475

Oh SY, Poukens V & Demer JL. (2001) Quantitative analysis of extraocular muscle global and orbital layers in monkey and human. *Investigative Ophthalmology and Visual Science*, 42: 10

Porter JD, Poukens V, Baker RS & Demer JL. (1996) Structure–function correlations in the human medial rectus extraocular muscle pulleys. *Investigative Ophthalmology and Visual Science*, 37: 468

FURTHER READING

Apt L. (1980) An anatomical evaluation of rectus muscle insertions. *Transactions of the American Ophthalmological Society*, 78: 365

Bach-y-Rita P. (1967) Neurophysiology of extraocular muscle. *Investigative Ophthalmology*, 6: 229

Bjork A. (1952) Electrical activity of human extrinsic eye muscles. *Experientia*, 8: 226

Brandt DE & Leeson CR. (1966) Structural differences of fast and slow fibers in human extraocular muscle. *American Journal of Ophthalmology*, 62: 478

Duke-Elder S & Wybar KC. (1961) The anatomy of the visual system. In: *System of Ophthalmology, Volume 2*. Mosby-Year Book, St Louis

Howe L. (1902) Insertion of the ocular muscles. *Transactions of the American Ophthalmological Society*, 9: 668

Scobee RC. (1948) Anatomic factors in the etiology of strabismus. *American Journal of Ophthalmology*, 31: 781

Sevel P. (1986) The origins and insertions of the extraocular muscles: development, histologic features and clinical significance. *Transactions of the American Ophthalmological Society*, 84: 488

Souza-Dias C, Prieto-Diaz J & Uesegui CF. (1986) Topographical aspects of the insertions of the extraocular muscles. *Journal of Pediatric Ophthalmology and Strabismus*, 23: 183

Chapter 2
Binocular single vision

Binocular single vision is the ability to use both eyes simultaneously so that each eye contributes to a common single perception.

Normal binocular single vision occurs with bifoveal fixation and normal retinal correspondence in everyday sight. Abnormal binocular single vision occurs in the absence of bifoveal fixation usually with abnormal retinal correspondence in everyday sight.

CLASSIFICATION (WORTH)

Binocular single vision can be classified into three stages:

(1) simultaneous perception and superimposition
(2) fusion
(3) stereoscopic vision.

Simultaneous perception is the ability to perceive simultaneously two images, one formed on each retina. Superimposition is the simultaneous perception of the two images formed on corresponding areas, with the projection of these images to the same position in space. This may occur whether the correspondence is normal or abnormal. If fusion is absent two similar images are seen as separate but superimposed and no fusion range is demonstrable.

Fusion may be sensory or motor. Sensory fusion is the ability to perceive two similar images, one formed on each retina, and interpret them as one. Motor fusion is the ability to maintain sensory fusion through a range of vergence, which may be horizontal, vertical or cyclovergence. Stereoscopic vision is the perception of the relative depth of objects on the basis of binocular disparity.

DEVELOPMENT

The initial ocular position in the human neonate (Rethy 1969) is often one of divergence. In the early post-natal period divergence decreases towards a binocular coincidental position resulting in similar visual stimulation of each eye which in turn facilitates firing of binocular driven cells/neurons in the striate cortex (Hubel & Wiesel 1968) and once the straight position is attained, this is maintained preferentially.

Some sensory and motor binocular associations exist in the visual system of the newborn. The binocular reflexes relate to the development of binocular single vision on the basis of continued use of the visual system. Postural reflexes are inborn and must be present if binocular single vision is to develop.

(1) Static reflexes compensate for changes in position of the head relative to the body.
(2) Statokinetic reflexes compensate for changes in head position relative to space.

Fixation reflexes form the mechanism from which binocular vision develops.

(1) The fixation reflex achieves foveal fixation in either eye.
(2) The refixation reflex allows foveal refixation from target to target and maintenance of foveal fixation on a moving target.

Most neonates are capable of locating and briefly fixing a moving target and the eyes can move in a coarsely conjugate fashion. Thus the refixation reflex, although unstable, appears to be present at birth, despite the fact that in the first months of life, the fovea is still poorly differentiated.

(3) The conjugate fixation reflex, where the eyes learn to move together during versions, is the first reflex by which the eyes move binocularly.
(4) The disjugate fixation reflex allows binocular vision to be maintained through the range of vergence movements which follow changes of fixation distance.
(5) The corrective fusion reflex allows binocular vision to be maintained under conditions of stress such as overcoming prisms in clinical testing situations.
(6) Kinetic reflexes maintain binocular single vision through controlled accommodation and convergence.

The newborn does not converge the eyes, but the attempt to converge may be seen as early as one month after birth. By 5–6 weeks of age, the conjugate fixation reflex has developed and the two eyes will conjugately fix an object and follow it over a considerable range for at least a few seconds. By four months, saccades will occur. By six months, the conjugate movements of binocular vision become accurate and convergence is well developed. By 6–8 months, a fusional movement can be detected by placing a small prism over either eye.

RETINAL CORRESPONDENCE

This concerns the retinal areas of each eye which have the same visual direction during binocular vision.

Normal retinal correspondence

This is a binocular condition in which the fovea and areas on the nasal and temporal side of one retina correspond to and have respectively common visual directions with the fovea and temporal and nasal areas of the retina of the other eye. Normal retinal correspondence is the normal state in which the visual direction of each fovea is the same (Flom & Weymouth 1961; Flom & Kerr 1967) (Fig. 2.1).

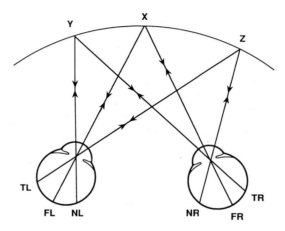

Figure 2.1   Projection in normal retinal correspondence with normal binocular single vision. Stimulation of corresponding points in both eyes results in localisation of the stimulus in the same direction in space. Both fovea, FL and FR, are corresponding points as are points on temporal and nasal retinas, TL and NR, NL and TR.

Abnormal retinal correspondence

This is a binocular condition in which there is a change in visual projection such that the fovea of the fixing eye has a common visual direction with an area other than the fovea of the deviating eye. The pairing of all retinal areas is similarly changed. The condition may occur whichever eye is used for fixation (Fig. 2.2).

Harmonious abnormal retinal correspondence is present where the angle of anomaly is equal to the objective angle and the subjective angle is zero. Unharmonious abnormal retinal correspondence is present where the angle of anomaly is different from the objective angle. The angle of anomaly is the difference between the objective and subjective angles of deviation. Abnormal retinal correspondence is present in constant manifest strabismus usually of a small angle less than 20 prism dioptres.

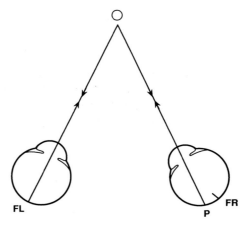

Figure 2.2   Projection in abnormal retinal correspondence with right esotropia. O is the fixation target. FL and FR are the fovea of both eyes and P is the pseudofovea of the right eye. FL and P are corresponding points as the right eye undergoes sensory adaptation with abnormal retinal correspondence. Stimulation of these corresponding points results in a single perception of the fixation target.

PHYSIOLOGY OF STEREOPSIS

The locus of all points in space that are imaged on corresponding retinal points is termed the *horopter*. Panum's space is a narrow band around the horopter within which object points give rise to binocular single vision. Objects are seen as single even though the object stimulates slightly disparate retinal elements.

Panum's area is the retinal area surrounding one corresponding retinal point within which disparity of correspondence may occur whilst maintaining binocular single vision. Binocular single vision is the result not of a rigid point to point correspondence but of a point to area relationship. The amount of foveal image disparity that permits fusion is small and disparity increases gradually from the fovea to the periphery. Panum's area is narrow at the fixation point and widens towards the periphery. The horizontal area at the fovea is approximately 6–10 minutes and this increases towards the periphery, measuring approximately 30–40 minutes at 12 degrees from the fovea. It may be larger than this as moving random-dot stereograms have shown fusion of disparities of 2–3 degrees (Hyson *et al.* 1983; Erkelens & Collewjin 1985; Piantanida 1986). Increases can be related to anatomical and physiological differences known to exist between the foveal cone system and the rod and cone system of the peripheral retina. The increase in Panum's area parallels the increase in size of the retinal receptive fields.

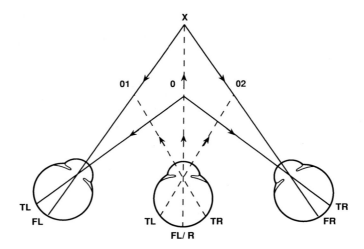

Figure 2.3   Projection in heteronymous diplopia. X is the fixation target which is seen as a single image by the corresponding fovea FL and FR. O is an object between the fixation target and the eyes which stimulates non-corresponding temporal retinal points, TL and TR, resulting in crossed physiological diplopia.

Physiological diplopia

This is a type of diplopia which exists in the presence of binocular vision. It consists of the appreciation that a near object appears double when a distant object is fixated (heteronymous or crossed diplopia) and a distant object appears double when a near object is fixated (homonymous or uncrossed diplopia) (Figs 2.3, 2.4).

All objects outside Panum's space give rise to physiological diplopia. Physiological diplopia indicates that the patient is capable of using both eyes and is not suppressing one eye.

Fixation disparity

Fixation disparity is a phenomenon which occurs in binocular single vision in which the image is seen singly despite a slight underconvergence or overconvergence of the visual axes; the fixation target is imaged on slightly disparate retinal points within Panum's area. There is an apparent displacement of uniocularly observed details of targets whose other details are fused binocularly.

The phenomenon can be demonstrated clinically when targets having mainly identical features but also certain dissimilar features are presented to the eyes. Fusion occurs for the identical features, but a displacement occurs for the dissimilar features in the direction of the projection of the existing heterophoria.

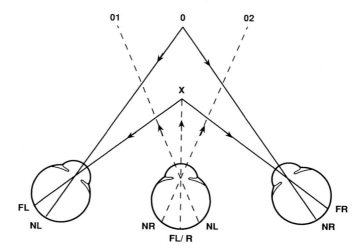

Figure 2.4   Projection in homonymous diplopia. X is the fixation target seen as a single image by the corresponding foveal points, FL and FR. O is an object further away than the fixation target which stimulates non-corresponding nasal retinal points, NL and NR, resulting in uncrossed physiological diplopia.

Fixation disparity may be involved in the maintenance of binocular single vision. Disparity of retinal images causes fusional movements. At the end of a fusional movement, not all the disparity is annulled; a small disparity remains which acts as an error signal. The residual fixation disparity may control the direction and strength of the innervation that maintains the new binocular position.

When visual objects are fused by being imaged on horizontally disparate points, within Panum's space, stereopsis results (Fig. 2.5). The greater the horizontal disparity, the greater the depth effect. A vertical disparity produces no stereoscopic effect.

Local stereopsis occurs where localised features of objects are extracted from a visual scene and assigned relative depth values, indicating that one feature is further away from another. Global stereopsis occurs where the perception of whole objects in stereoscopic depth is achieved.

Monocular clues are important in the estimation of the relative distance of visual objects and are active in monocular as well as binocular vision. These clues are the result of experience:

- **Motion parallax**: targets further away move more in the horizontal plane than nearer targets.
- **Linear perspective**: objects of the same size decrease in size the further away they are.
- **Overlapping contours**: overlap in images determines which is in front or behind the other.

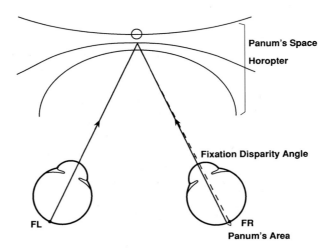

Figure 2.5   Projection in stereopsis. O is the fixation target which projects directly to the fovea of the left eye. This should also project directly to the right eye. However, due to slight under- or overconvergence of the right eye, direct stimulation may not occur, resulting in fixation disparity. In this figure, there is slight overconvergence of the right eye with stimulation of a point just nasal to the fovea. As this point falls within Panum's area, the stimuli to either eye are fused, resulting in a single image of the fixation target.

- **Distribution of highlights and shadows**.
- **Size of known objects**: when size is known the relative distance can be determined.
- **Aerial perspective**: knowledge of colours and hues.

FUSION

Central fusion occurs when the images of an object are perceived by each fovea and the area surrounding them, and are unified. This produces bifoveal binocular single vision with fusion. The highest levels of stereoacuity are associated with central fusion. Peripheral fusion results from unification of images outside the central region. Gross stereopsis is associated with peripheral fusion. Central and peripheral fusion usually function simultaneously. A patient's sensory status is considered crucial to the long-term stability of a successful surgical outcome. Fusion serves as the glue to maintain alignment (Burian 1941; Kushner & Morton 1992; Morris *et al.* 1993). It indicates the patient's ability to control his or her latent tendency for the eyes to drift. In order for fusion to occur, the images presented to each eye must be similar in size, brightness and sharpness. Peripheral fusion contributes significantly to the maintenance of binocular single vision (Bielchowsky 1935). If this is destroyed, even while maintaining good central vision, disruption of binocularity occurs.

The normal fusional range is 35/40 prism dioptres base out and 16 prism dioptres base in on near testing, and 16 prism dioptres base out and 8 prism dioptres base in on distance testing (Berens *et al.* 1927; Crone & Everhard-Halm 1975; Kertesz & Sullivan 1978; Guyton 1988; Sharma & Abdul-Rahim 1992).

Normal adults can fuse 8 degrees of cyclodisparity using sensory fusion (Guyton 1988). They can therefore use this ability to fuse torted images without diplopia. This ability derives from the receptive fields in the peripheral retina being large compared to those in the central retina. When measured with large field stimuli, 8 degrees of motor cyclovergence has been demonstrated in normals (Guyton 1988). This amount of motor cyclovergence combined with the 8 degrees of sensory cyclofusion allows normals to fuse up to 16 degrees of cyclodisparity.

RETINAL RIVALRY

When dissimilar images are presented to corresponding retinal areas, fusion becomes impossible and retinal rivalry occurs. When dissimilar targets are presented to each eye, the patient will see one target, then the other or a mosaic of contours, but not both simultaneously. Retinal rivalry is a physiological finding in binocular single vision and is distinct from suppression as it indicates a state of fluctuation between competing components. Retinal rivalry may be produced also by differences in colour and unequal illumination.

SUPPRESSION

Suppression is the mental inhibition of visual sensations of one eye in favour of those of the other eye when both eyes are open. This may occur in binocular single vision and commonly in manifest strabismus.

Physiological suppression is present in binocular single vision. Blurred images are suppressed when concentrating on one particular object. Pathological suppression is present in manifest strabismus and may alternate with alternating deviations (Fig. 2.6).

The area and density of suppression will vary according to the type of strabismus. A defined small central suppression scotoma exists in microtropia whereas larger angle strabismus shows an elliptical shaped scotoma extending horizontally, particularly in esotropia. Suppression can be more extensive involving the entire hemifield as has been reported in exotropia (Jampolsky 1955).

Suppression typically develops in childhood strabismus. There is debate as to whether adults can truly develop suppression. Inattention to diplopia and true suppression are different, but probably related, adaptive sensory strategies and additive factors other than the age of the patient may be involved (McIntyre & Fells 1996). Development of

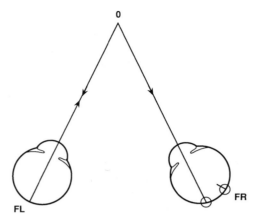

Figure 2.6   Projection in right esotropia with suppression. O is the fixation target which stimulates the fovea of the left eye and a nasal retinal point of the right eye. The nasal retinal point is suppressed which ensures a single perception of the fixation target.

'suppression' has been reported in adults with thyroid eye disease (Fells 1979), following retinal detachment surgery (Wright *et al*. 1999) and keratoconus (Sherafat *et al*. 2001). In adult onset strabismus, patients have a poor prognosis with regard to the ability to learn to suppress or ignore diplopia. Patients can have persistent troublesome diplopia that can be difficult or impossible to alleviate. An ability to develop suppression as an adult or an inattention to the diplopic image may reflect an element of plasticity in the mature binocular visual system.

Diplopia and confusion are not appreciated where suppression is present. Confusion is the simultaneous appreciation of two superimposed images due to the stimulation of corresponding retinal points by two different images. Binocular single vision is not present with pathological suppression and suppression obstructs attempts to obtain binocular single vision.

DIPLOPIA

Pathological binocular diplopia results from the presence of a manifest ocular deviation and is the simultaneous appreciation of two separate images caused by the stimulation of non-corresponding points by one object. It may be horizontal, vertical or torsional, or any combination.

Heteronymous diplopia is crossed binocular diplopia associated with exotropia in which the image of the fixation object is received on the temporal area of the retina of the deviating eye and is projected nasally. Homonymous diplopia is uncrossed binocular diplopia associated with esotropia in which the image of the fixation object is received on the

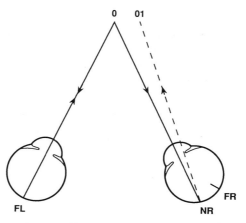

Figure 2.7   Projection in right esotropia with normal retinal correspondence and pathological diplopia. O is the fixation target which stimulates non-corresponding points of the left fovea and right nasal retina. The nasal retina projects temporally, resulting in uncrossed pathological diplopia.

nasal area of the retina of the deviating eye and is projected temporally (Fig. 2.7). Paradoxical diplopia is pathological binocular diplopia in which heteronymous diplopia occurs in esotropia or homonymous diplopia occurs in exotropia (Fig. 2.8).

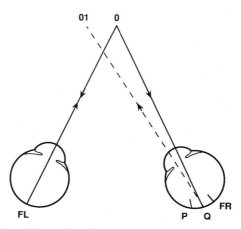

Figure 2.8   Projection in right esotropia with paradoxical diplopia. With abnormal retinal correspondence, there is sensory adaptation of the strabismic eye such that the pseudofovea and the fovea of the other eye become corresponding points. The retinal area between the fovea and pseudofovea of the strabismic eye which was originally nasal retina takes on the sensory function of temporal retina. With redirection of the strabismic eye, non-corresponding points are stimulated (FL and Q), resulting in crossed paradoxical diplopia.

REFERENCES

Berens C, Losey CC & Hardy LH. (1927) Routine examination of the ocular muscles and non-operative treatment. *American Journal of Ophthalmology*, 10: 910

Bielchowsky A. (1935) Congenital and acquired deficiencies of fusion. *American Journal of Ophthalmology*, 18: 925

Burian HM. (1941) Fusional movements in permanent strabismus. A study of the role of the central and peripheral retinal regions in the aetiology of binocular vision in squint. *Archives of Ophthalmology*, 26: 626

Crone RA & Everhard-Halm Y. (1975) Optically induced eye torsion. I Fusional cyclovergence. *Graefe's Archives of Clinical and Experimental Ophthalmology*, 195: 231

Erkelens CJ & Collewjin H. (1985) Eye movements and stereopsis during dichoptic viewing of moving random-dot stereograms. *Vision Research*, 25: 1689

Fells P. (1979) Confusion, diplopia and suppression. *Transactions of the Ophthalmic Society of the UK*, 99: 386

Flom MC & Kerr KE. (1967) Determination of retinal correspondence. Multiple testing results and the depth of anomaly concept. Archives of Ophthalmology, 77: 200

Flom MC & Weymouth F. (1961) Retinal correspondence and the horopter in anomalous correspondence. *Nature*, 89: 34

Guyton DL. (1988) Ocular torsion: sensorimotor principles. *Graefe's Archives of Clinical and Experimental Ophthalmology*, 226: 241

Hubel DH & Wiesel TN. (1968) Receptive fields and functional architecture of monkey striate cortex. *Journal of Physiology (London)*, 195: 215

Hyson MT, Julesz B & Fender DH. (1983) Eye movements and neural remapping during fusion of misaligned random-dot stereograms. *Journal of the Optical Society of America*, 73: 1665

Jampolsky A. (1955) Characteristics of suppression in strabismus. *Archives of Ophthalmology*, 54: 683

Kertesz AE & Sullivan MJ. (1978) The effect of stimulus size on human cyclofusional response. *Vision Research*, 18: 567

Kushner BJ & Morton GV. (1992) Postoperative binocularity in adults with longstanding strabismus. *Ophthalmology*, 99: 316

McIntyre A & Fells P. (1996) Bangerter foils: a new approach to the management of pathological intractable diplopia. *British Orthoptic Journal*, 53: 43

Morris RJ, Scott SE & Dickey CF. (1993) Fusion after surgical alignment of longstanding strabismus in adults. *Ophthalmology*, 100: 135

Piantanida TP. (1986) Stereo-hysterosis revisited. *Vision Research*, 26: 431

Rethy I. (1969) Development of simultaneous fixation from the divergent anatomic eye position of the neonate. *Journal of Pediatric Ophthalmology*, 6: 92

Sharma K & Abdul-Rahim AS. (1992) Vertical fusion amplitude in normal adults. *American Journal of Ophthalmology*, 114: 636

Sherafat H, White JEW, Pullum KW, Adams GGW & Sloper JJ. (2001) Anomalies of binocular function in patients with longstanding asymmetric keratoconus. *British Journal of Ophthalmology*, 85: 1057

Wright LA, Cleary M, Barrie T & Hammer HM. (1999) Motility and binocularity outcomes in vitrectomy versus scleral buckling in retinal detachment surgery. *Graefe's Archives of Clinical and Experimental Ophthalmology*, 237: 1028

FURTHER READING

Asher H. (1953) Suppression theory of binocular vision. *British Journal of Ophthalmology*, 37: 37

Awaya S, Nozaki H, Itoh T & Harada K. (1976) Studies of suppression in alternating constant exotropia and intermittent exotropia: with reference to the effects of fusional background. In: Moore S, Mein J & Stockbridge L (eds) *Orthoptics, Past, Present and Future*. Symposia Specialists, Miami, p. 531

Bagolini B & Capobianco NM. (1965) Subjective space in comitant squint. *American Journal of Ophthalmology*, 50: 430

Barlow HB, Blakemore C & Pettigrew JD. (1967) The normal mechanisms of binocular depth discrimination. *Journal of Physiology (London)*, 193: 327

Bishop PO & Pettigrew JD. (1986) Neural mechanisms of binocular vision. *Vision Research*, 26: 1587

Burian HM. (1945) Sensorial retinal relationship in concomitant strabismus. *Transactions of the American Ophthalmological Society*, 81: 373

Burian HM. (1951) Anomalous retinal correspondence: its essence and its significance in diagnosis and treatment. *American Journal of Ophthalmology*, 34: 237

Duane A. (1931) Binocular vision and projection. *Archives of Ophthalmology*, 5: 734

Jones RK & Lee DN. (1981) Why two eyes are better than one: the two views of binocular vision. *Journal of Experimental Psychology (Human Perception)*, 7: 30

Pratt-Johnson JA & Tillson G. (1984) Suppression in strabismus, an update. *British Journal of Ophthalmology*, 68: 174

Travers TAB. (1950) The practical importance of abnormal retinal correspondence. *Transactions of the American Academy of Ophthalmology and Otolaryngology*, 54: 561

Chapter 3
Ocular motility

A number of systems are responsible for producing eye movements and controlling fast (saccades), slow (smooth pursuit), disjugate (vergence) and involuntary (vestibular) movements. The eye movement system used depends on the nature of the visual input received and the response required for the visual stimulus. Visual information reaches the visual striate cortex (primary visual area 17, V1) via the visual pathway and attributes of this visual information such as fine features, colour, spatial localisation and motion are processed in separate secondary visual areas (Rowe 2003).

SACCADIC SYSTEM

Saccadic eye movements are rapid eye movements under both volitional and reflex control. Voluntary movements include willed refixations and those in response to command. Reflex movements include saccades in the direction of a new stimulus and usually are accompanied by head movement in the same direction. The visual stimulus for generation of saccadic eye movement is target displacement in space. Control decisions of movement size and velocity are made based on the continuous inflow of visual information from the retina (Rowe 2003).

The latency period is the interval from the appearance of a stimulus to the start of the eye movement in response. The ocular motor system for saccades responds after a latency or delay of 200–250 msec. Peak velocity and duration of saccade are dependent on size or amplitude of eye movement. Latencies are less when the fixation target is turned off before the peripheral target appears (gap stimulus) and greater when the fixation target remains illuminated after the peripheral target appears (overlap stimulus) (Kalesnykes & Hallett 1987).

The saccadic response consists of a period of acceleration to peak velocity followed by deceleration of the eyes as they approach the target position. Extraocular muscles use relative tension to hold the new eye position along with check ligaments and fatty tissue of the orbit.

A pulse-step mechanism is the process that generates a saccadic eye movement (Optican & Miles 1985). Burst and pause cells are the critical components of this mechanism (Sparks & Mays 1990; Enderle 2002). The saccadic pulse is a burst of activity that generates the forces necessary to overcome the drag from orbital tissue content and produce eye movement. Burst cells fire while pause cells are inhibited, thus constituting the pulse signal. Saccadic eye movement occurs and the neural integrator is activated for the new eye position which feeds back to tonic cells which activate to hold the eye in the new position which constitutes the step signal.

There are strong interconnections between the frontal and parietal lobes. The frontal eye field is involved with volitional, visually guided, purposive saccades and the parietal lobe is involved with a shift in attention to new targets appearing in the visual field. The inferior parietal lobe is involved with planning saccades and the frontal eye fields with intentional visual exploration. Other areas involved in the saccadic system include the dorsomedial supplementary motor area, which is important in learned ocular motor behaviour, and the dorsolateral frontal cortex which is involved in the programming of saccades and attention shifts to remembered target positions.

Fibres pass from cortical areas down through the internal capsule. Below this level there are different pathways including caudate nuclei, thalamic nuclei, superior colliculi and the pedunculopontine pathway to the cerebellum and to brainstem nuclei (Peirrot-Deseilligny *et al.* 1995; Deleu 1997; Enderle 2002). There is probable decussation at the level of the III nerve nuclei in the midbrain.

During a saccade the visual threshold is elevated about 0.5 log units (suppression) so that there is no awareness of the unstable visual environment during eye movement (Koerner & Schiller 1972).

The paramedian pontine reticular formation (PPRF) contains the nucleus pontis caudalis centralis which houses the pulse generator burst cells (Keller 1974). Inhibitory burst neurons for horizontal saccades can be found caudal to the VI nerve nuclei in the nucleus paragiganto-cellularis dorsalis (Scudder *et al.* 1988). Pause neurons lie in the nucleus raphe interpositus which is located in the midline between the rootlets of the VI nerve nucleus (Buttner-Ennerver *et al.* 1988; Horn *et al.* 1996). The horizontal integrator includes the nucleus prepositus hypoglossi (NPH), the medial vestibular nucleus and other cerebellar locations (Belknap & McCrea 1988).

The rostral interstitial nucleus of the medial longitudinal fasciculus (riMLF) contains burst neurons for vertical and cyclorotational movement (Vilis *et al.* 1989; Bhidayasiri *et al.* 2000; Buttner *et al.* 2002). Bilateral input is required for vertical gaze (Bender 1980). Each burst neuron in the riMLF projects to motoneurons supplying synergistic muscle pairs, e.g. superior rectus and inferior oblique (Bhidayasiri *et al.* 2000). Although each riMLF contains neurons for up- and downgaze, the nucleus contains neurons only in one direction for cyclorotational quick phases (e.g. right riMLF projects clockwise, left anticlockwise). Both riMLF nuclei are connected via the posterior commissure.

Upgaze commands pass from the riMLF dorsally through the posterior commissure to the III nerve nuclei. Downgaze commands pass dorsally and caudally to the III nerve and IV nerve nuclei. Inhibitory neurons for vertical saccades are probably also located in the riMLF (Robinson 1964; Boghen *et al*. 1974).

The riMLF projects to the interstitial nucleus of Cajal (INC) for vertical gaze holding (neural integrator) (Bhidayasiri *et al*. 2000; Buttner *et al*. 2002). The INC also receives input from vestibular nuclei, the

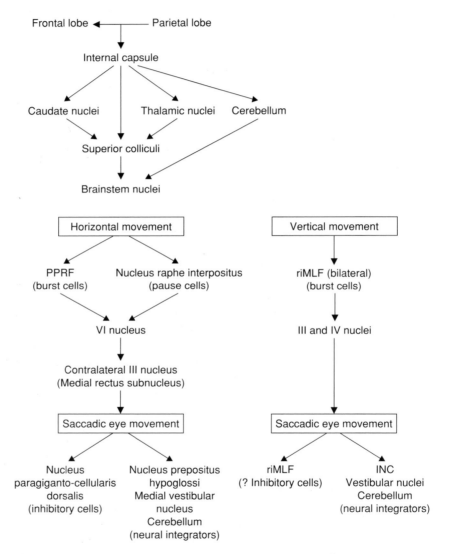

Figure 3.1 Saccadic eye movement control pathways. PPRF, paramedian pontine reticular formation; VI, VI nerve nucleus; III, III nerve nucleus; IV, IV nerve nucleus; riMLF, rostral interstitial nucleus of the medial longitudinal fasciculus; INC, interstitial nucleus of Cajal. (Reprinted with permission from: Rowe FJ. (2003) Supranuclear and internuclear control of eye movements. A review. *British Orthoptic Journal*, 60: 2.)

cerebellum (particularly the dorsal vermis) and the contralateral INC (King *et al.* 1981). Fibres pass from the vestibular nuclei for vertical eye movements to encode eye position signal and head velocity signal. These fibres are position-vestibular-pause cells (PVP). Medial vestibular nuclei and NPH contribute to vertical gaze holding but only to a small extent (Cannon & Robinson 1987). See Fig. 3.1 for a summary of the pathways involved in the generation of saccadic eye movements.

SMOOTH PURSUIT SYSTEM

Smooth pursuits are slow eye movements under a control system capable of continuous modification of motor output in response to visual input (Chen *et al.* 2002). For slow velocities the eye movement tracks the target accurately with velocity matching. For faster velocities the eye may not always match the target velocity, necessitating a catch-up saccade. The major stimulus for the generation of smooth pursuit movement is a fixated target that moves across the foveal and perifoveal retina. The input signal is therefore retinal error velocity (Yasui & Young 1975).

Movement is evoked after a latency of approximately 125 msec. Maximal sustained pursuit velocities are about 90 degrees per second. If a target is moving at a velocity greater than 50 degrees per second, the eyes, after lagging behind the target, may perform a saccade to catch up before continuing with the pursuit movement. A step-ramp of innervation is the result. The step is the jump in firing frequency and the ramp is the linear increase in frequency. Latency to ramp stimulus is approximately 100 msec (Carl & Gellman 1987) and step-ramp latency is approximately 150 msec (Tychsen & Lisberger 1986).

The detailed pathways for pursuit movements are not clearly understood. The brain requires information regarding target movement relative to the position of the head. Motion processing areas of the brain are therefore important in the production of a smooth pursuit eye movement. Visual information is received in the visual cortex and passed to areas 17–19 (occipital and parietal cortex), including the middle temporal visual area in the superior temporal sulcus, the medial superior temporal visual area and the posterior parietal area. There is a link with the frontal eye fields which contain neurons which discharge during smooth pursuit and aid programming of predictive pursuit movements, initiation and maintenance (Suzuki *et al.* 1999).

Efferent fibres from cortical areas pass through the internal capsule under the superior colliculi at the midbrain with a probable double decussation at the level of pons, medulla and cerebellum (Johnston *et al.* 1992), on to the dorsolateral pontine nuclei and the cerebellum (flocculus, paraflocculus and vermis) via the cerebral peduncles (Zeki *et al.* 1991). The visual information that is passed to the cerebellum is synthesised for pursuit signal and the cerebellum outputs to the vestibular nuclei which integrate the signal and pass this to the oculomotor nerves.

For horizontal smooth pursuit the signal is directed via the dorsolateral pontine nuclei, cerebellum, nucleus reticularis tegmenti pons and vestibular nuclei to the VI nerve nucleus (Suzuki *et al.* 1999). For vertical smooth pursuit the signal is directed to the III and IV nuclei. Medial vestibular nuclei and NPH link for velocity and position integration of horizontal smooth pursuit eye movements. The INC encodes neural integration predominantly for vertical and cyclorotatory smooth pursuit. See Fig. 3.2 for a summary of the pathways involved in the generation of smooth pursuit eye movements.

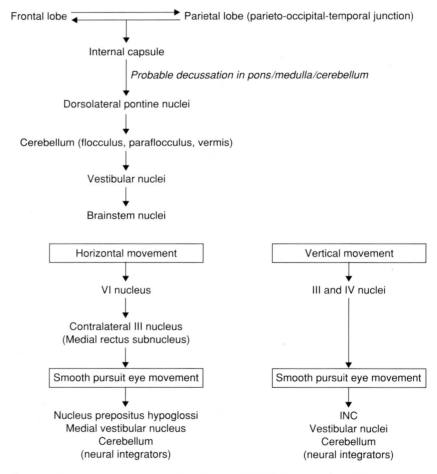

Figure 3.2   Smooth pursuit eye movement control pathways. VI, VI nerve nucleus; III, III nerve nucleus; IV, IV nerve nucleus; INC, interstitial nucleus of Cajal. (Reprinted with permission from: Rowe FJ. (2003) Supranuclear and internuclear control of eye movements. A review. *British Orthoptic Journal*, 60: 2.)

VERGENCE SYSTEM

Vergence movements are disjugate and smooth where one eye can move independently of the other. There is continuous control over the movement generated. Vergence movements occur as a synkinesis with accommodation of the lens and pupillary constriction. The medial and lateral recti motoneurons are reciprocally innervated during vergence movements.

The stimuli for this system include disparity between the location of images on the retina of each eye, which results in fusional vergence, and retinal blur caused by a loss of focus of images, which results in accommodative vergence. There is target displacement or motion along the y-axis (to or from the observer). There is generally a latency of 160 msec and maximum velocity of 20 degrees per second in the generation of vergence eye movements.

Higher control areas for the generation of vergence eye movements are poorly understood. Vergence eye movements may occur as saccadic or smooth pursuit movements and therefore cortical areas relating to the generation of these eye movement systems will be involved in the cortical processing of visual information necessitating a vergence eye movement response.

Neurons for control of vergence have been found in mesencephalic reticular formation (Judge & Cumming 1986) which is dorsolateral to the III nerve nuclei and contains different types of neurons: vergence tonic cells discharge in relation to vergence angle, vergence burst cells discharge in relation to vergence velocity, vergence burst tonic cells discharge in relation to both vergence angle and velocity. These cells may serve as a vergence integrator also (Mays *et al.* 1986). Lesions near the midbrain–diencephalic junction have been documented in pseudo abducens palsy which has been proposed as a manifestation of abnormal vergence activity (Pullicino *et al.* 2000). Pullicino *et al.* (2000) postulated that inhibitory descending pathways for convergence may pass through the thalamus and decussate in the subthalamic region.

Medial recti nuclei and VI nuclei discharge for vergence eye movements (Mays & Porter 1984). Medial rectus motoneurons are organised into different groups (A, B and C). Subgroup C may be specifically involved in vergence commands (Warwick 1953; Buttner-Ennerver & Akert 1981). There is also some cerebellar input to vergence control (Miles *et al.* 1980). The nucleus reticularis tegmenti pons (NRTP) houses neurons important for generating vergence position signal which may therefore serve as a vergence neural integrator (Gamlin & Clarke 1995). See Fig. 3.3 for a summary of the pathways involved in the generation of vergence eye movements.

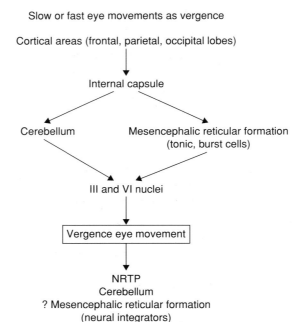

Slow or fast eye movements as vergence

Cortical areas (frontal, parietal, occipital lobes)

Internal capsule

Cerebellum

Mesencephalic reticular formation
(tonic, burst cells)

III and VI nuclei

Vergence eye movement

NRTP
Cerebellum
? Mesencephalic reticular formation
(neural integrators)

Figure 3.3 Vergence eye movement control pathways. III, III nerve nucleus; IV, IV nerve nucleus; NRTP, nucleus reticularis tegmenti pons. (Reprinted with permission from: Rowe FJ. (2003) Supranuclear and internuclear control of eye movements. A review. *British Orthoptic Journal*, 60: 2.)

VESTIBULO-OCULAR RESPONSE AND OPTOKINETIC RESPONSE

Head movement is the stimulus for vestibulo-ocular response (VOR). The VOR generates compensatory eye movements to stabilise visual images on the retina during head movements (Rambold *et al.* 2002). The latency between the onset of sudden head movements and the resultant eye movement can be as little as 15 msec (Gauthier & Vercher 1990).

This system integrates eye and body movements and is not dependent on ocular stimulation but is concerned with head position and balance. Input is received from:

- Semicircular canals. Each set of semicircular canals influences a particular pair of eye muscles. The horizontal canals produce lateral movement, posterior canals produce vertical movement and anterior canals produce rotary movements
- Neck proprioceptors.

The head movement is synthesised by semicircular canals to produce a neural signal proportional to head velocity. Stimulation of each set of

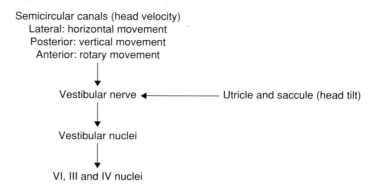

Semicircular canals (head velocity)
Lateral: horizontal movement
Posterior: vertical movement
Anterior: rotary movement

Vestibular nerve ◄——————— Utricle and saccule (head tilt)

Vestibular nuclei

VI, III and IV nuclei

Integration with slow and fast eye movement systems

Figure 3.4   Vestibulo-ocular and optokinetic response control pathways. VI, VI nerve nucleus; III, III nerve nucleus; IV, IV nerve nucleus. (Reprinted with permission from: Rowe FJ. (2003) Supranuclear and internuclear control of eye movements. A review. *British Orthoptic Journal*, 60: 2.)

semicircular canals influences a particular pair of eye muscles: horizontal/lateral canals produce lateral movement, posterior canals produce vertical movement and anterior canals produce rotary movement. The neural signal is transferred to the brainstem via the vestibular nerves and conversion of velocity data to position signal takes place in the vestibular nuclei and/or NPH. The utricle and saccule are the otolith organs. The otoliths are sensitive to tilts of the head and give rise to cyclorotational movement of the eyes to stabilise the visual image. This information is also transferred to the brainstem via the vestibular nerves.

If the head continues to rotate for more than a couple of seconds, the forces within the semicircular canals reduce to zero and no longer give a signal. The optokinetic response which is visually driven supplements the vestibulo-ocular response to continue the eye movements. The optokinetic response continues indefinitely in the presence of a moving visual field to generate compensatory eye movements. There is generally a latency of 100 msec and eye velocity slowly builds to a value equal to that of the surround. The vestibulo-ocular and opto-kinetic responses are most often combined as the visual vestibulo-ocular reflex. See Fig. 3.4 for a summary of the pathways involved in vestibulo-ocular and optokinetic eye movements.

BRAINSTEM CONTROL

Figs 3.5 and 3.6 depict the location of brainstem nuclei involved in the generation of eye movements. Fig. 3.7 depicts cortical areas involved in the generation of saccadic, smooth pursuit and vergence eye movements and which project to brainstem nuclei.

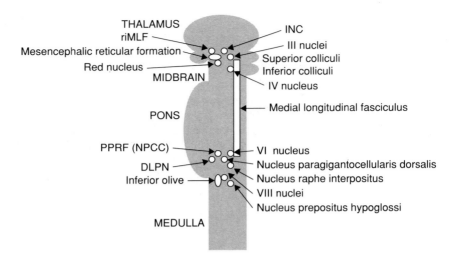

Figure 3.5 Sagittal cross-section of brainstem: schematic representation. riMLF, rostral interstitial nucleus of the medial longitudinal fasciculus; PPRF, paramedian pontine reticular formation; NPCC, nucleus pontis caudalis centralis; DLPN, dorsolateral pontine nuclei; INC, interstitial nucleus of Cajal; VI, VI nerve nucleus; III, III nerve nucleus; IV, IV nerve nucleus; VIII, vestibular nucleus. (Reprinted with permission from: Rowe FJ. (2003) Supranuclear and internuclear control of eye movements. A review. *British Orthoptic Journal*, 60: 2.)

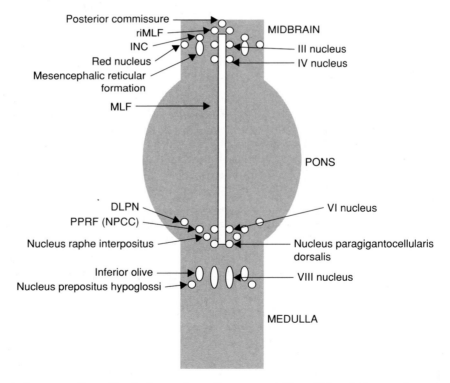

Figure 3.6 Coronal cross-section of brainstem: schematic representation. Abbreviations as for Figure 3.5. (Reprinted with permission from: Rowe, FJ. (2003) Supranuclear and internuclear control of eye movements. A review. *British Orthoptic Journal*, 60: 2.)

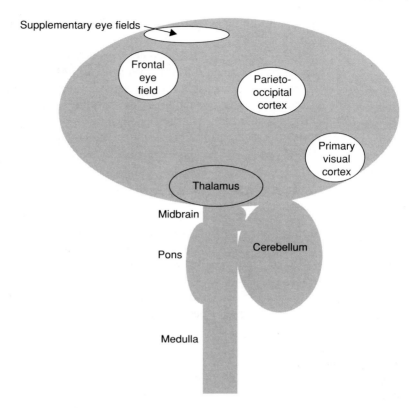

Figure 3.7   Sagittal view of cortical areas: schematic representation. (Reprinted with permission from: Rowe FJ. (2003) Supranuclear and internuclear control of eye movements. A review. *British Orthoptic Journal*, 60: 2.)

Horizontal gaze movements

The VI nuclei control horizontal conjugate gaze (Highstein & Baker 1978; Pola & Robinson 1978). They govern conjugate movement of both the ipsilateral lateral rectus and contralateral medial rectus. The nuclei house two neurons: abducens motoneurons to the lateral rectus and abducens internuclear neurons via the MLF to the contralateral medial

Figure 3.6   (*opposite*) Coronal cross-section of brainstem: schematic representation. riMLF, rostral interstitial nucleus of the medial longitudinal fasciculus; PPRF, paramedian pontine reticular formation; NPCC, nucleus pontis caudalis centralis; MLF, medial longitudinal fasciculus; DLPN, dorsolateral pontine nuclei; INC, interstitial nucleus of Cajal; VI, VI nerve nucleus; III, III nerve nucleus; IV, IV nerve nucleus; VIII, vestibular nucleus. (Reprinted with permission from: Rowe FJ. (2003) Supranuclear and internuclear control of eye movements. A review. *British Orthoptic Journal*, 60: 2.)

rectus motoneurons in the III nuclei (Highstein & Baker 1978; Strassman *et al*. 1986a, b).

For horizontal saccadic eye movement, saccadic commands originate from burst neurons of the paramedian pontine reticular formation which then project to the VI nerve nuclei. A descending smooth pursuit pathway probably projects to the VI nucleus via the flocculus and cerebellar fastigial nuclei (Leigh & Zee 1991). The VI nuclei receive vestibular and optokinetic inputs from the vestibular nuclei (McCrea *et al*. 1987).

Vertical and cyclorotatory gaze movements

Vertical gaze is under bilateral control from the cerebral cortex. Ocular motoneurons are in the III and IV nerve nuclei. For vertical saccadic eye movement, saccadic generation is from the riMLF (Moschovakis *et al*. 1991a, b). Neural signals for vertical vestibular and smooth pursuit eye movements ascend from the cerebellum, medulla and pons to midbrain oculomotor nuclei via the medial longitudinal fasciculus but also the superior cerebellar peduncle.

Vergence gaze movements

Premotor signals for vergence are found in neurons in the mesencephalic reticular formation near the III nerve nuclei. The NRTP is important for generating vergence position signal as the vergence integrator. VI and III neurons co-ordinate conjugate and vergence commands.

MUSCLE SEQUELAE

There are two relevant laws when assessing muscle sequelae:

- **Hering's law of equal innervation**: when a nervous impulse is sent to an ocular muscle to contract, an equal impulse is sent to its contralateral synergist to contract also.
- **Sherrington's law of reciprocal innervation**: when a muscle receives a nervous impulse to contract, an equal impulse is received by its antagonist to relax.

Every contraction of a muscle brings about a movement. The primary moving muscle is called an **agonist**. A movement in the opposite direction to that produced by an agonist is caused by its **antagonist**. Two muscles moving an eye in the same direction are **synergists**.

The **primary angle of deviation** is the deviation observed when fixing with the unaffected eye in paralytic incomitant strabismus. The **secondary angle of deviation** is the deviation observed when fixing with the affected eye in paralytic incomitant strabismus.

In the course of a paresis/paralysis, Hering and Sherrington's laws cause changes in the actions of other extraocular muscles. The extent to which this develops in different patients may vary markedly. The speed and amount of development can depend partly on which eye the patient prefers to use for fixation. Generally this is the normal eye but in some cases the paretic eye is preferred.

There are three stages in the development of muscle sequelae.

(1) **Overaction of the contralateral synergist.** According to Hering's law, both the paretic muscle and its yoke (synergist) muscle will receive an equal amount of innervation. Therefore, due to the paresis, the affected eye will require extra innervation to fixate and this innervation will also be received by the synergist, resulting in overaction of this muscle.

(2) **Overaction of the ipsilateral antagonist.** The antagonist of the affected muscle is acting more/less unopposed, depending on the extent of the paresis, and therefore it overacts.

(3) **Secondary underaction of the contralateral antagonist.** This occurs for two reasons. Since the direct antagonist of the affected muscle is acting more/less unopposed, this muscle requires less than normal innervation to move into its field of action. According to Hering's law, its yoke muscle will also receive the same little innervation and therefore underacts. The contralateral synergist of the affected muscle is overacting. According to Sherrington's law, its direct antagonist will receive an equal impulse to relax and since it is a normal muscle, this results in underaction of the muscle, for example, in right IV nerve palsy:

primary underaction = right superior oblique
overaction of contralateral synergist = left inferior rectus
overaction of ipsilateral antagonist = right inferior oblique
secondary underaction of contralateral antagonist = left superior rectus.

PAST-POINTING

This is the false localisation of objects in space, in patients with recent paresis, due to the sensory changes resulting from the altered alignment of the eyes. If the patient is asked to point at an object in the field of action of the paretic muscle while the sound eye is covered, he will point beyond the object (Ambrose & von Noorden 1976).

BELL'S PHENOMENON

In most individuals, the eyes normally rotate up and out when both lids are closed. This is demonstrated by asking the patient to try to close the lids while the examiner holds the lids open or by asking the patient to keep the lids closed while the examiner tries to open them. Presence of Bell's phenomenon indicates an intact infranuclear pathway and indicates the elevating muscles are receiving innervation.

REFERENCES

Ambrose PS & von Noorden GK. (1976) Past-pointing in comitant strabismus. *Archives of Ophthalmology*, 94: 1896

Belknap DB & McCrea RA. (1988) Anatomical connections of the prepositus and abducens nuclei in the squirrel monkey. *Journal of Comparative Neurology*, 268: 13

Bender MB. (1980) Brain control of conjugate horizontal and vertical eye movements: a survey of the structural and functional correlates. *Brain*, 103: 23

Bhidayasiri R, Plant GT & Leigh RJ. (2000) A hypothetical scheme for the brainstem control of vertical gaze. *Neurology*, 23: 1985

Boghen D, Troost BT, Daroff RB, Dell'Osso LF & Birkett JE. (1974) Velocity characteristics of normal human saccades. *Investigative Ophthalmology*, 13: 619

Buttner U, Buttner-Ennever JA, Rambold H & Helmchen C. (2002) The contribution of midbrain circuits in the control of gaze. *Annals of the New York Academy of Science*, 956: 99

Buttner-Ennever J & Akert K. (1981) Medial rectus subgroups of the oculomotor nucleus and their abducens internuclear input in the monkey. *Journal of Comparative Neurology*, 197: 17

Buttner-Ennever JA, Cohen B, Pause M & Fries W. (1988) Raphe nucleus of the pons containing omnipause neurons of the oculomotor system in the monkey and its homologue in man. *Journal of Comparative Neurology*, 267: 307

Cannon SC & Robinson DA. (1987) Loss of the neural integrator of the oculomotor system from brainstem lesions in monkeys. *Journal of Neurophysiology*, 57: 1383

Carl JR & Gellman RS. (1987) Human smooth pursuit: stimulus-dependent responses. *Journal of Neurophysiology*, 57: 1446

Chen Y, Holzman PS & Nakayama K. (2002) Visual and cognitive control of attention in smooth pursuit. *Progress in Brain Research*, 140: 255

Deleu D. (1997) Selective vertical saccadic palsy from unilateral medial thalamic infarction: clinical, neurophysiologic and MRI correlates. *Acta Neurologica Scandinavica*, 96: 332

Enderle JD. (2002) Neural control of saccades. *Progress in Brain Research*, 140: 21

Gamlin PD & Clarke RJ. (1995) Single-unit activity in the primate nucleus reticular tegmenti pontis related to vergence and ocular accommodation. *Journal of Neurophysiology*, 73: 2115

Gauthier GM & Vercher JL. (1990) Visual vestibular interaction; vestibulo-ocular reflex suppression with head-fixed target fixation. *Experimental Brain Research*, 81: 150

Highstein SM & Baker R. (1978) Excitatory termination of abducens internuclear neurons on medial rectus motoneurons; relationship to syndrome of internuclear ophthalmoplegia. *Journal of Neurophysiology*, 41: 1647

Horn AKE, Buttner-Ennever JA & Buttner U. (1996) Saccadic premotor neurons in the brainstem; functional neuroanatomy and clinical implications. *Neuro-Ophthalmology*, 16: 229

Johnston JL, Sharpe JA & Morrow MJ. (1992) Paresis of contralateral smooth pursuit and normal vestibular smooth eye movements after unilateral brainstem lesions. *Annals of Neurology*, 31: 495

Judge SJ & Cumming BG. (1986) Neurons in the monkey midbrain with activity related to vergence eye movement and accommodation. *Journal of Neurophysiology*, 55: 915

Kalesnykes RP & Hallett PE. (1987) The differentiation of visually guided and anticipatory saccades in gap and overlap paradigms. *Experimental Brain Research*, 68: 115

Keller EL. (1974) Participation of medial pontine reticular formation in eye movement generation in monkey. *Journal of Neurophysiology*, 37: 316

King WM, Fuchs AF & Magnin M. (1981) Vertical eye movement-related responses of neurons in midbrain near interstitial nucleus of Cajal. *Journal of Neurophysiology*, 46: 549

Koerner F & Schiller PH. (1972) The optokinetic response under open and closed loop conditions in the monkey. *Experimental Brain Research*, 14: 318

Leigh RJ & Zee DS. (1991) *The Neurology of Eye Movements*. Davis, Philadelphia

Mays LE & Porter JD. (1984) Neural control of vergence eye movements; activity of abducens and oculomotor neurons. *Journal of Neurophysiology*, 52: 743

Mays LE, Porter JD, Gamlin PDR & Tello CA. (1986) Neural control of vergence eye movements; neurons encoding vergence velocity. *Journal of Neurophysiology*, 56: 1007

McCrea RA, Strassman A, May E & Highstein SM. (1987) Anatomical and physiological characteristics of vestibular neurons mediating the horizontal vestibulo-ocular reflex of the squirrel monkey. *Journal of Comparative Neurology*, 264: 547

Miles FA, Fuller JH, Braitman DJ & Dow BA. (1980) Long-term adaptive changes in primate vestibuloocular reflex. III Electrophysiological investigations in flocculus of normal monkeys. *Journal of Neurophysiology*, 43: 1437

Moschovakis AK, Scudder CA & Highstein SM. (1991a) Structure of the primate oculomotor burst generator. I Median-lead burst neurons with upward on-directions. *Journal of Neurophysiology*, 65: 203

Moschovakis AK, Scudder CA, Highstein SM & Warren JD. (1991b) Structure of the primate oculomotor burst generator. II Median-lead burst neurons with downward on-directions. *Journal of Neurophysiology*, 65: 218

Optican LM & Miles FA. (1985) Visually induced adaptive changes in primate saccadic oculomotor control signals. *Journal of Neurophysiology*, 54: 940

Pierrot-Deseilligny C, Rivand S, Gaymard B, Muri R & Vermersch AI. (1995) Cortical control of saccades. *Annals of Neurology*, 37: 557

Pola J & Robinson DA. (1978) Oculomotor signals in medial longitudinal fasciculus of the monkey. *Journal of Neurophysiology*, 41: 245

Pullicino P, Lincoff N & Truax BT. (2000) Abnormal vergence with upper brainstem infarcts: pseudoabducens palsy. *Neurology*, 8: 352

Rambold H, Churchland A, Selig Y, Jasmin L & Lisberger SG. (2002) Partial ablations of the flocculus and ventral paraflocculus in monkeys cause linked deficits in smooth pursuit eye movements and adaptive modification of the VOR. *Journal of Neurophysiology*, 87: 912

Robinson DA. (1964) The mechanics of human saccadic eye movements. *Journal of Physiology (London)*, 174: 245

Rowe FJ. (2003) Supranuclear and internuclear control of eye movements. A review. *British Orthoptic Journal*, 60: 2

Scudder CA, Fuchs AF & Langer TP. (1988) Characteristics and functional identification of saccadic inhibitory burst neurons in the alert monkey. *Journal of Neurophysiology*, 59: 1430

Sparks DL & Mays LE. (1990) Signal transformations required for the generation of saccadic eye movements. *Annual Review of Neuroscience*, 13: 309

Strassman A, Highstein SM & McCrea RA. (1986a) Anatomy and physiology of saccadic burst neurons in the alert squirrel monkey; I Excitatory burst neurons. *Journal of Comparative Neurology*, 249: 337

Strassman A, Highstein SM & McCrea RA. (1986b) Anatomy and physiology of saccadic burst neurons in the alert squirrel monkey; II Inhibitory burst neurons. *Journal of Comparative Neurology*, 249: 358

Suzuki DA, Yamada T, Hoedema R & Yee RD. (1999) Smooth-pursuit eye-movement deficits with chemical lesions in macaque nucleus reticularis tegmenti pontis. *Journal of Neurophysiology*, 82: 1178

Tychsen L & Lisberger SG. (1986) Visual motion processing for the initiation of smooth pursuit eye movements in humans. *Journal of Neurophysiology*, 56: 953

Vilis T, Hepp K, Schwarz U & Henn V. (1989) On the generation of vertical and torsional rapid eye movements in the monkey. *Experimental Brain Research*, 77: 1

Warwick R. (1953) Representation of the extraocular muscles in the oculomotor nuclei of the monkey. *Journal of Comparative Neurology*, 98: 449

Yasui S & Young LR. (1975) Perceived visual motion as effective stimuli to pursuit eye movement system. *Science*, 190: 906

Zeki S, Watson JDG, Lueck CJ, Friston KJ, Kennard C & Frackowiak RS. (1991) A direct demonstration of functional specialisation in human visual cortex. *Journal of Neuroscience*, 11: 641

FURTHER READING

Boeder P. (1961) The co-operation of the extraocular muscles. *American Journal of Ophthalmology*, 51: 469

Boeder P. (1962) Co-operative action of the extraocular muscles. *British Journal of Ophthalmology*, 46: 397

Clement RA. (1982) Computer simulation of extraocular muscle co-operation: an evaluation. *Ophthalmic and Physiological Optics*, 2: 107

Gordon OE. (1954) A study of primary and auxillary ocular rotations. *Transactions of the American Academy of Ophthalmology and Otolaryngology*, 58: 553

Guyton D. (1988) Ocular torsion; sensorimotor principles. *Graefe's Archives of Clinical and Experimental Ophthalmology*, 226: 241

Harbridge H & Thomson C. (1948) Methods of investigating eye movements. *British Journal of Ophthalmology*, 32: 581

Rashbass C & Westheimer G. (1961) Independence of conjugate and disjunctive eye movements. *Journal of Physiology (London)*, 159: 361

Robinson DA. (1965) The mechanics of human smooth pursuit eye movement. *Journal of Physiology (London)*, 180: 569

Robinson DA. (1966) The mechanics of human vergence movement. *Journal of Pediatric Ophthalmology*, 3: 31

Westheimer G. (1954) Mechanism of saccadic movements. *Archives of Ophthalmology*, 52: 710

Chapter 4
Orthoptic investigative procedures

This chapter deals with the methods used to detect the presence of strabismus or abnormal ocular movements, to measure any deviation and to assess binocular function. Methods of assessing and measuring visual acuity and additional tests for investigation of incomitant strabismus are also discussed.

VISUAL ACUITY

The visual perception of an object is resolved according to light sense, form sense and colour sense. Form sense may be divided into central (the ability to discriminate fine high contrast detail) and peripheral (the field of vision) vision.

Central visual acuity is dependent on:

- the minimal visible angle. This is based on the target subtending the smallest angle which elicits a positive visual response
- the minimal separable angle. This requires the identification of two sharp, black edges separated by a white interval of known dimension.

Visual acuity is a function of the dioptric apparatus of the eye and also of the retina, the nervous pathways and central nervous mechanisms. It is determined by the smallest retinal image whose form can be appreciated. This is the minimal separable angle and is measured by the smallest object which can be clearly seen at a certain distance. The minimal visible angle is produced at the nodal point and represents the diameter of a cone which is approximately 0.004 mm.

For two separate points to be distinguished, it is necessary for their images to be formed upon cones which are not adjacent to one another, but are separated by at least one cone which is unstimulated. In order to produce this, the object of fixation must subtend a visual angle of 1 minute of arc at the nodal point of the eye. This is taken as the minimum visual angle of the normal eye (Fig. 4.1).

Variables affecting visual acuity include:

- retinal stimulation (central stimulation involves the fovea with higher acuity function)

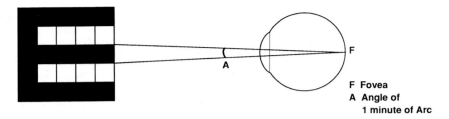

Figure 4.1   Optics of visual acuity.

- luminance (brightness of target)
- contrast (sensitivity to background lighting)
- eye movements (even when looking steadily at targets there are constant refixation movements to maintain central fixation)
- contour interaction (it is easier to identify a target presented singly than one with other surrounding stimuli).

Clinical vision tests

Qualitative (observation of visual response)

Fixation: observe pursuit movement and fixation preference (Calcutt 1995). Fixation preference testing reliability detects amblyopia only if the deviation exceeds 10 prism dioptres (Zipf 1976).

Cover test: uniocular fixation and objection to occlusion.

Visually directed reaching: reaction to visual stimulus by reaching towards the object of interest.

100s and 1000s: response to small sweets and indicates acuity of approximately 6/24.

Catford drum (Atkinson *et al.* 1981): moving dots or gratings.

Stycar rolling/mounted balls: graded balls in various sizes either mounted or rolled along the floor.

Stycar matching toys.

10 dioptre prism (Wright *et al.* 1981): the 10 prism dioptre test is specifically designed to assess fixation preference in preverbal children who are not strabismic or who have small deviations. It may be performed base down or base up. It is recommended that the prism is held base up in cases of ptosis to aid accuracy in detecting eye movement response (Whittaker *et al.* 2000). A 25 dioptre base-in prism may also be used (Cassin 1992).

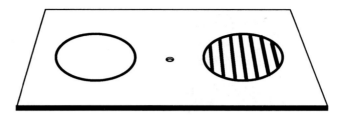

Figure 4.2   Forced choice preferential looking.

Quantitative (measurement of visual response)

Forced choice preferential looking cards (FCPL) (Katz & Sireteanu 1990) (Fig. 4.2): the principle of this test is that a child prefers to look at a patterned background than at a plain background (Fantz 1958; Dobson *et al.* 1978; Quinn *et al.* 1993). The test cards consist of a black and white grating placed on the left or right of the card. The child's response to look towards the pattern is noted. The gratings are graded in size. FCPL may be used with a screen to exclude observer bias. The observer sits behind the screen and the baby in front. The observer records the direction of head movements in response to the appearance of the striped stimulus.

Visual acuities determined with FCPL range from approximately 6/240 in the newborn to 6/60 at three months and 6/6 at 36 months (Mayer *et al.* 1995). Grating acuity is better than recognition acuity (Mayer *et al.* 1984) and this difference is exaggerated in children with amblyopia (Mayer 1986; Ellis *et al.* 1988; Katz & Sireteanu 1990; Sireteanu *et al.* 1990).

Teller acuity cards: Teller (1997) introduced a set of 16 cards which consist of a grey background with a square wave grating on one side. An FCPL process is undertaken.

Keeler cards: Moseley *et al.* (1988) introduced a circular pattern of square wave gratings to prevent identification of the pattern by its edge. An FCPL process is undertaken.

LogMAR (Bailey-Lovie) chart; LOGarithm of the Minimal Angle of Resolution (Sloan 1959; Frank 1986) (Fig. 4.3): this letter chart consists of letters of almost equal legibility with the same number of letters on each row. The between letter spacing is equal to one letter width and the between row spacing is equal to the height of the letters in the smaller row. The chart is designed for a standard testing distance of 6 m, giving a visual acuity range of 6/60 to 6/3, the log unit for 6/60 acuity being 1.0 and for 6/6, 0. This test is considered one of the more accurate forms of visual acuity assessment.

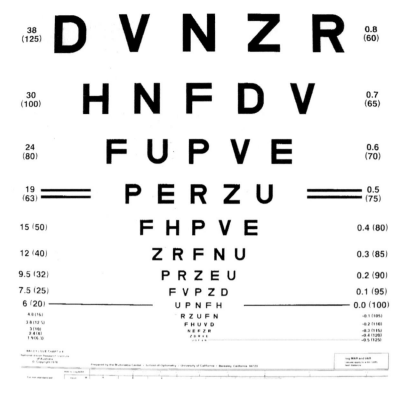

Figure 4.3   LogMAR test.

Snellen test type (Fig. 4.4): this test is the most widely used assessment of visual acuity. It consists of a chart of letters, starting with one letter at 6/60 level and with additional letters on each line progressing to 6/4 level. There is no related letter spacing or row spacing according to the size of letters on each line, which renders the test less accurate than logMAR.

Sheridan Gardiner singles/linear test type (Fig. 4.5): this test uses seven letters (X, U, T, O, H, A, V). The letters are presented singly on a card or as a linear chart in rows and the patient is required to match the letters with those on a key card. The letters are graded from 6/60 to 6/3.

Kay's pictures (Fig. 4.6): a variety of pictures which are graded in size are presented singly on a card. The patient is required to identify the picture by naming it or matching it with a key card. These pictures range from 6/60 to 6/3. Kay pictures are also available in logMAR format.

Cardiff acuity cards (Woodhouse *et al.* 1992; Horwood 1994) (Fig. 4.7): this test is based on the principle of vanishing optotypes. It consists of a series of cards displaying a picture on each. The defining outer lines which form the pictures decrease in size until the picture appears to fade into the grey background. The patient's ability to recognise each picture is noted.

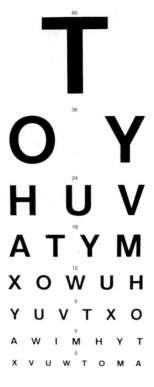

Figure 4.4   Snellen test.

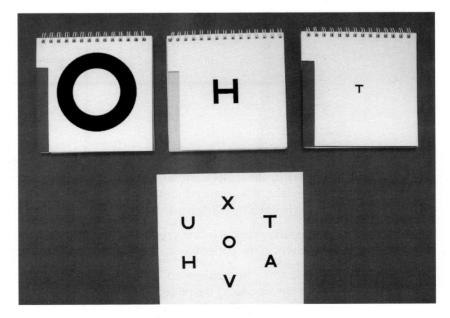

Figure 4.5   Sheridan Gardiner test.

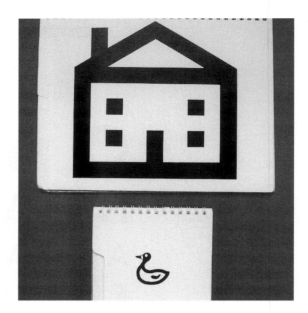

Figure 4.6   Kay's pictures.

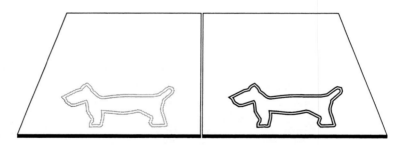

Figure 4.7   Cardiff acuity cards.

Cambridge crowding cards (Atkinson *et al*. 1988): five letters (H, O, T, V, X) are used in this test. Each letter to be matched is surrounded by the other letters, which introduces a crowding effect. The patient identifies the centre letter on a key card.

Sonksten-Silver test: this test presents six letters (X, O, U, H, V, T) in linear format which the patient matches with letters on a key card.

Stycar letters: three groups of letters may be presented, depending on the patient's age, and the patient is required to match the letters on a key card. The first group contains five letters (V, T, O, H, X), the second group contains seven letters (the first five plus A and U) and the third group has nine letters (the existing seven plus L and C). The letters are graded from 6/60 to 6/4.

Ffookes symbols: this test presents the shapes of a circle, square and triangle which the patient matches with a hand-held corresponding shape.

Illiterate E test: capital letter Es are presented with the letter directed up, down, right or left. The patient identifies the relevant orientation of the letter.

Landolt C test: this test is similar to the illiterate E test in that the capital letter C is presented with the letter directed up, down, right or left. The patient is required to indicate the position of the gap in the letter.

Sjogren hand test: a black hand with the fingers pointing up, down, right or left is presented and the patient identifies the orientation of the position of the fingers.

Near tests

(1)   Reduced Snellen test
(2)   Reduced Sheridan Gardiner
(3)   Reduced E test
(4)   Maclure book
(5)   Moorfields bar reading book
(6)   N series test

Pinhole test

This can be used to assess whether or not reduced vision is caused by an uncorrected refractive error. One eye is occluded, a pinhole is placed before the other eye and the visual acuity is tested. When vision improves, this is strongly indicative of a refractive error. If no improvement occurs, there is amblyopia or some organic cause for the reduced vision.

Crowding phenomenon

It is easier to see a single optotype than a letter on a linear chart. The reduced visual acuity is due to the additional stimuli from surrounding letters and results in confusion. Crowding is specifically caused by contour interaction and attentional factors (Leat *et al.* 1999). This is noted in particular with reduced visual acuity in amblyopes (see Chapter 8).

Delayed visual maturation

With delayed visual maturation there is apparent blindness in a normal child until approximately 12 weeks of age. This is thought to be due to a delay in the myelination of the visual fibres. Children usually demon-strate normal visual development thereafter.

Age indications for use of visual acuity tests

Age	Test
0–6/12	Forced choice preferential looking, visual evoked response, optokinetic nystagmus, observation, fixation, pursuit, visually directed reaching, objection to occlusion, cover test, Catford drum.
6/12–2 years	100s and 1000s, visually directed reaching, Stycar balls, forced choice preferential looking, Cardiff acuity cards.
2–3 years	Kay's pictures, Stycar toys, illiterate E test, ffookes symbols, Sjogren hand test, logMAR.
3+ years	Sheridan Gardiner test, Cambridge crowding cards, Sonksten-Silver test, Landolt C test, Stycar letters, Snellen test, logMAR.

Refractive errors

Assessment of the presence of refractive errors is important to the investigation and management of strabismus and amblyopia.

A cycloplegic refraction is required for infants and young children to ensure non-accommodation in order to obtain an accurate result. Usually 1% cyclopentolate is used. However, since this may cause a transient increase in blood pressure in infants, 0.5% is used and a drop of 2.5% phenylephrine hydrochloride may be added if mydriasis is unsatisfactory.

Hypermetropia

This occurs where parallel rays of light come to a focus behind the retina when the eye is at rest.

Myopia

This occurs where parallel rays of light come to a focus in front of the retina when the eye is at rest.

Astigmatism

This refractive error occurs where a point of focus cannot be formed on the retina owing to unequal refraction in different meridians.

Against the rule astigmatism occurs when the vertical meridian is relatively hypermetropic and the horizontal meridian is relatively myopic. With the rule astigmatism occurs where the refractive power of the vertical meridian is the greatest.

Regular astigmatism is a refractive anomaly where the two maximally differing meridians of the eye are at right angles. Oblique astigmatism has the maximally differing meridians at oblique angles.

Anisometropia

This is a difference in refractive error between the two eyes.

COVER TEST

The cover test is one of the most important diagnostic tests used in orthoptic practice. It is an objective dissociative test to elicit the presence of a manifest or latent deviation. It relies on the observation of the behaviour of the eyes whilst fixation is maintained and each eye is covered and uncovered in turn.

Equipment

- **Occluder** (Fig. 4.8): a card/paddle which is opaque and large enough to cover one eye should be used so that the patient cannot see through or around it. A Spielmann occluder is a translucent occluder through which the patient can only see diffuse light without contours but with which the observer can see the patient's eyes (Spielmann 1986).
- **Fixation target** (Fig. 4.9): a small object which will maintain the patient's interest, such as a picture for a child and a letter for an adult, should be used at 1/3 m. This will make the patient

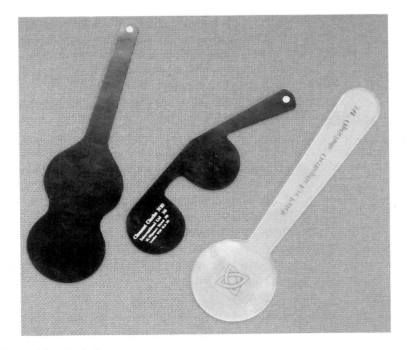

Figure 4.8   Occluders.

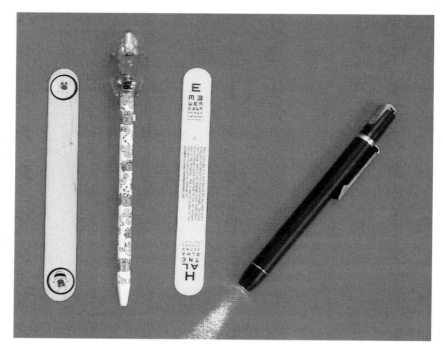

Figure 4.9   Fixation targets.

accommodate and is therefore also called an accommodative target. A Snellen letter or picture at 6 m from the eyes is also required. Visual acuity must be good enough to see the fixation target with a minimum of 6/60 for Snellen's fixation. Otherwise, corneal reflections must be monitored.

● **Pen torch**: this should project a single spot of light.

Cover/uncover test

Manifest deviation

The test is performed both with and without spectacles and also with and without any abnormal head posture. The patient looks at a spot-light held at eye level 1/3 m away. The examiner should also be at the patient's eye level. Corneal reflections are noted to see if there is an obvious deviation.

One eye is covered with an opaque occluder and the other eye is observed. If the uncovered eye moves to take up fixation, a manifest deviation of that eye is present (Fig. 4.10). The deviation is present in the opposite direction to the take-up of fixation, as in the following examples:

● temporal movement indicates a convergent (eso) deviation
● nasal movement indicates a divergent (exo) deviation

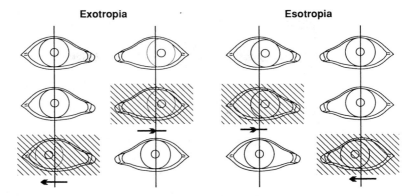

Figure 4.10   Cover/uncover test in manifest strabismus. The left exotropic eye does not move when an occluder is placed before the left eye. On occlusion of the right eye, the left eye moves inwards to take up fixation. The right esotropic eye does not move under cover of the occluder. It moves outwards to take up fixation on occlusion of the left eye.

- downward movement indicates an upward (hyper) deviation
- upward movement indicates a downward (hypo) deviation.

If no movement of the uncovered eye is seen, there is usually no manifest deviation present. The exception is if eccentric fixation is present where a manifest deviation may be noted whilst observing the corneal reflections.

The test is then repeated with the other eye covered, using a fixation target placed first at 1/3 m and then at 6 m. A target may need to be placed at a distance of greater than 6 m if a significant increase or decrease in the angle of deviation is noted between near and distance fixation. This may occur particularly in exodeviations. The deviation will alternate in cases of alternating heterotropia.

Latent deviation

The patient fixates a spotlight at 1/3 m. One eye is completely covered. The cover is removed and any movement of the covered eye is noted (Fig. 4.11). The test is then repeated for the other eye with fixation targets for 1/3 m and 6 m and also for greater than 6 m where there is a significant increase or decrease in the angle of deviation between near and distance fixation, particularly in exodeviations.

Alternate cover test

The patient fixates a spotlight at 1/3 m. One or other eye is covered alternately throughout the test to ensure the complete dissociation which is necessary to detect latent deviations. Movement of the

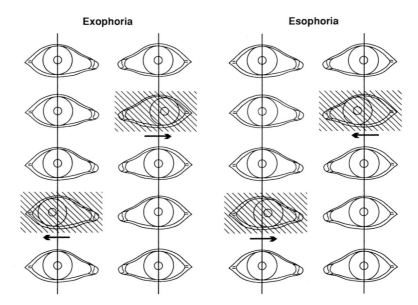

Figure 4.11   Cover/uncover test in latent strabismus. With latent deviations, the eye deviates under cover of the occluder. With exophoria, the eye moves outwards under cover and on removal of the occluder it moves inwards to refixate and binocular single vision is regained. With esophoria, the eye moves inwards under cover and on removal of the occluder it moves outwards to refixate and binocular single vision is regained.

uncovered eye is noted as the cover is changed from one eye to the other (Fig. 4.12). The test is then repeated with a fixation target at both 1/3 m and 6 m. Finally the cover/uncover test is repeated to ensure that full recovery and not partial recovery to a manifest deviation has occurred.

Information gained from cover testing

Manifest deviation

(1)   Type of deviation: eso-, exo-, hyper-, hypo-, cyclo-.
(2)   Size of deviation: slight, small, moderate, marked.
(3)   Speed to take up fixation. This gives a good indication of the level of vision in the eye. Rapid uptake indicates the presence of reasonable vision in the deviating eye; slow uptake indicates poor vision; a wandering eye indicates non-central fixation with very poor vision. Eyes which show alternating fixation are often favoured equally and as a result have equal vision.
(4)   The effect of accommodation on the deviation can be determined by comparing the deviation on cover test to a light and detailed fixation target.

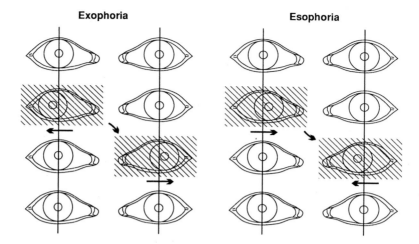

Figure 4.12 Alternate cover test. The eyes move outwards under cover with exophoria and move inwards to refixate. The eyes move inwards under cover with esophoria and move outwards to refixate.

(5) Nystagmus. Manifest nystagmus is seen before the cover test is performed but latent nystagmus is only elicited when one eye is covered (see Chapter 17).
(6) Dissociated vertical deviation (DVD) (see Chapter 6).
(7) Incomitance. The angle of deviation will vary depending on which eye is covered.

Latent deviation
(1) Type of deviation.
(2) Size of deviation.
(3) Rate of recovery to achieve binocular single vision, e.g. rapid, moderate, slow, delayed; deviation decompensates further to produce a manifest deviation. The rate of recovery indicates the strength of control over the deviation.
(4) Partial recovery. There is recovery to a small manifest deviation, usually microtropia (see Chapter 7).

OCULAR MOTILITY

Versions are rotary movements of both eyes from the primary position in the same direction. Ductions are rotary movements of one eye from the primary position. Since the eye has an essentially fixed centre of rotation, it can rotate around one of three axes, all going through the centre of rotation (Boeder 1957) (Fig. 4.13):

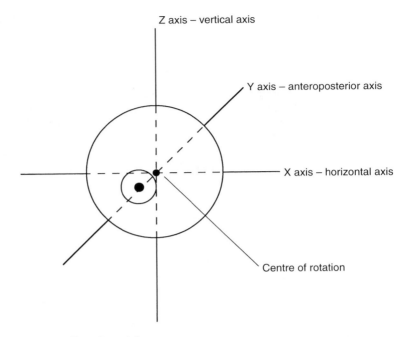

Figure 4.13   Rotation of the eye.

- X-axis: horizontal axis around which vertical movements occur, perpendicular to the line of sight
- Y-axis: anterior/posterior axis for torsional movements, coincident with the line of sight
- Z-axis: vertical axis for horizontal movements, perpendicular to the line of sight.

Saccadic movement

The patient is asked to look from one target to another, one held in the primary position and the other:

- to each side of the head for horizontal movement
- above and below the head for vertical movement.

The movement, speed and accuracy of both eyes are compared and any asymmetry between the eyes is noted.
   Testing of saccadic eye movements is useful in:

- comparing movement of the two eyes as this may show slight limitations
- suspected myasthenia gravis as fatigue may become evident
- suspected internuclear ophthalmoplegia as dysmetria may be evident.

Smooth pursuit movement

Versions are tested binocularly using a spotlight to observe the movement from the primary position into the eight cardinal positions of gaze with the head erect and immobile. The corneal reflections are observed and a cover test is performed in each position.

Ductions are tested monocularly to compare with versions and the following noted:

- excursion
- behaviour of both eyes
- whether the movement is smooth or jerky
- nystagmus
- change in position of the lids or globe
- effect of fatigue
- torsional movement
- any discomfort on movement
- abnormal head movements.

Ocular movements may be recorded in written or graphic form.

Optokinetic movement

This assesses the integrity of both saccadic and smooth pursuit pathways by movement of high contrast repetitive targets (black and white) across the field of vision.

Optokinetic nystagmus may be tested with an OKN/Barany drum (Fig. 4.14) or OKN scarf. It is tested horizontally with movement

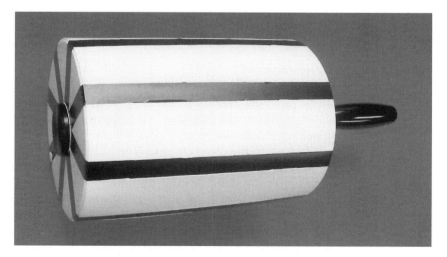

Figure 4.14   Optokinetic nystagmus drum.

right and left and vertically with movement up and down. The patient is asked to watch the stripes in turn and the following are noted:

- movement present or absent
- difference between eyes
- difference in movement to either side or up and down
- smooth pursuit movement (slow phase)
- saccadic movement (fast phase).

Vestibular movement

Doll's head testing

This is a rapid, passive head rotation used to elicit an initial con-traversion deviation of the eyes followed by a prompt recentering. The head is moved quickly by the examiner to the right and left for horizontal movement and up and down for vertical movement. A normal response is of the eyes moving in the opposite direction to the head movement.

Swinging baby test

A similar response to the doll's head test is seen. It is based on the observation of a conjugate deviation of the eyes in response to head movement induced by rotation and is useful with babies who will not respond to conventional testing.

The infant is held upright facing the examiner. The examiner rotates him/herself and the infant through 360 degrees while observing the infant's eyes. An indication of the extent of ocular movement is gained and also an indication of the level of visual acuity. Post-rotational nystagmus in sighted babies will only persist for a few seconds before being suppressed.

Induced vestibular nystagmus

This results from altered input from the VIII nerve. Caloric testing alters input by instilling warm or cold water into one ear. Warm water produces a slow phase to the opposite side and fast phase to the same side. Cold water produces a slow phase to the same side and a fast phase to the opposite side. Vertical caloric nystagmus is induced by stimulating both ears. Rotational testing produces nystagmus which is induced by seating the patient in a Barany chair with the head forward 30 degrees and rotating the chair. By rotating the chair to the right, there is a fast phase to the right and slow phase to the left. Post-rotational nystagmus in the opposite direction follows on ceasing the rotation. The patient is aware of this movement and may feel nauseated.

ACCOMMODATION AND CONVERGENCE

Accommodation

Accommodation is the ability to increase the convexity of the crystalline lens in order to obtain a clear image of a near object. It is closely associated with convergence and pupil constriction.

The **far point of accommodation** is the furthest distance at which an object can be seen clearly, while the **near point** is the nearest point at which an object can be seen clearly. The **range of accommodation** is the distance over which accommodation is effective, the distance between the near and far points. The **amplitude of accommodation** is the difference in the focus power of the eye whilst fixating for near distance and fixating for far distance. Relative accommodation is the amount by which accommodation can be increased or relaxed whilst convergence remains constant.

Measurement of accommodation

Accommodation is measured in dioptres. One dioptre has a focal distance of 1 m and therefore accommodation is calculated in terms of the reciprocal of the fixation distance.

The **near point of accommodation** is assessed using the RAF rule (Fig. 4.15). The rule cheek pads are placed on the patient's cheeks and held in a slightly depressed reading position. The patient wears distance spectacles (if any) but may need to repeat the test using reading spectacles. Using the N series target, the patient observes the smallest line seen with either eye.

With both eyes open, the carrier is moved towards the patient from the end of the rule and the patient asked to state when the print becomes blurred. The monocular near point of accommodation is also assessed to determine any difference between the monocular and binocular accommodative states. The results are recorded in centimetres and

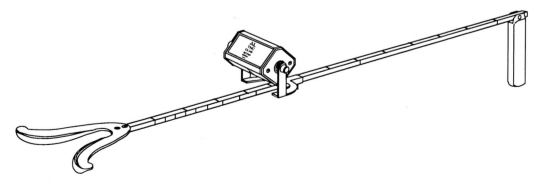

Figure 4.15   RAF rule.

repeated three times, both binocularly and uniocularly, to assess the effect of fatigue.

The examiner is able to identify whether the level of accommodation is adequate for the patient's age from the age scale and the amount of accommodation exerted at a given distance can be determined from the dioptre scale. The patient's blur point is an indication of the amplitude of accommodation.

The amplitude of accommodation can also be assessed using trial lenses. The patient is seated 6 m from a Snellen test type wearing the appropriate prescription and with one eye occluded. Whilst viewing the smallest print which can be seen clearly, minus lenses are introduced in steps of 0.5–1 dioptre until the print blurs. The sum of the strength of lens through which the patient can no longer see clearly is equivalent to the amplitude of accommodation.

The **accommodative facility** is a measure of how fast a patient can report that clarity has been restored following a rapid change of focus. Assessment involves stimulation followed by relaxation of accommodation using −2.00 and +2.00 DS lenses (Henshall & Rowe 2002).

Convergence

Convergence is a disjugate movement in which both eyes rotate inwards. There are four types of convergence.

(1)   Tonic, which is due to the tone of the extraocular muscles initiating movement from the anatomical position of rest.
(2)   Accommodative, which is initiated by the stimulus of accommodation.
(3)   Fusional, which is initiated by a fusional stimulus. This is an involuntary vergence movement to maintain binocular single vision.
(4)   Proximal, which is induced by the awareness of a near object.

Relative convergence is the degree of convergence produced relative to the amount of accommodation exerted and may be positive (increased) or negative (decreased) in order to maintain binocular single vision. The 'metre angle' is one unit measurement for the amount of convergence present. One metre angle equals the amount of convergence required for each eye to fixate an object, located at a distance of 1 m, in the median plane having moved from fixating a distant object.

Measurement of convergence

The near point of convergence is assessed objectively using either a fixation target or the fixation target on the RAF rule. Normal convergence is to 6 cm. The fixation target or the RAF rule is held in the primary position. The target is gradually moved, from at least 1/3 m away from the patient, slowly and steadily towards the patient's eyes. The patient is instructed to maintain fixation on the target and states when the target blurs, jumps or becomes double. The examiner notes the point at which this occurs by observing the break of convergence in the patient's eyes. Pupil dilation may be observed at this stage which is an additional indicator of convergence failure. Convergence gives an indication of the strength of binocular single vision (Capobianca 1952).

AC/A ratio

This is the amount of accommodative convergence which is induced by each dioptre of accommodation exerted and is measured in prism dioptres. It is a fixed relationship, so that an equal amount of convergence occurs for each dioptre of accommodation. This is inborn and remains virtually unchanged from childhood to at least presbyopic age, provided that the stimulus to accommodate is kept within narrow limits. The normal range is 2–4:1.

The AC/A ratio can be modified permanently by surgery of the extraocular muscles and temporarily by drugs and lenses which reduce the accommodation requirement and hence the resulting accommodative convergence.

Methods of measurement of AC/A ratio

Gradient method

(1) Near measurement, using convex lenses. A prism cover test (PCT) is performed for near fixation with and without convex lenses (usually +3.0 DS).
(2) Distance measurement using concave lenses. A prism cover test is performed for distance with and without concave lenses (usually −3.0 DS).

$$AC/A \text{ ratio} = \frac{\text{PCT with accom. exerted} - \text{PCT without accom. exerted}}{\text{Amount of accom. exerted}}$$

Heterophoric method

A prism cover test is performed for near and distance fixation and the interpupillary distance (IPD) is measured. A positive sign is used for esodeviations and a negative sign for exodeviations.

$$AC/A \text{ ratio} = IPD \text{ (in cm)} + \frac{\text{Near PCT} - \text{distance PCT}}{\text{Amount of accom. exerted}}$$

Graphic method

The angle of deviation is measured for distance fixation on the synoptophore or using the prism cover test. This is repeated using concave lenses, starting with −1.0 DS and increasing in 1 D steps to −4.0 DS if possible. A Snellen test type chart is used and the patient is instructed to fixate the same line of letters at each measurement. A graph is plotted showing change in convergence in prism dioptres against the change in accommodation in dioptres.

Uses of AC/A ratio

- Diagnosis of convergence excess type intermittent esotropia (see Chapter 6).
- Differential diagnosis of true and simulated intermittent distance exotropia (see Chapter 6).

RETINAL CORRESPONDENCE

Tests which are used to investigate retinal correspondence are often dissociative and usually subjective and include:

- **diplopia based**: e.g. Bagolini glasses and Worth's four light test. These tests rely on the subjective localisation of a single object whose image is formed on the retinal elements stimulated.
- **haploscope–synoptophore**: two dissimilar objects are presented in the binocular field of view and the patient is required to super-impose the two images.

Bagolini glasses test

This is a minimally dissociative diplopia based test which investigates the presence of retinal correspondence. The test may be used in lorgnette form or separately in a trial frame. Each glass is made of plain glass incorporating fine parallel striations placed before both eyes with the striations at 45 and 135 degrees (Fig. 4.16). A spotlight viewed through the glass produces a line image seen perpendicular to the striations.

The patient is asked how many line images and spotlights are seen and what form the lines make. Possible results include:

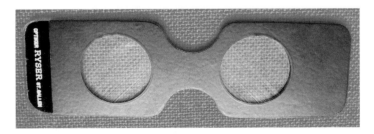

Figure 4.16   Bagolini glasses.

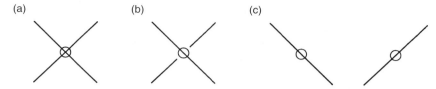

Figure 4.17   Results with Bagolini glasses.

- one spotlight with two line images forming a cross through the middle of the light, which indicates normal or abnormal retinal correspondence (Fig. 4.17a). A gap in one of the lines around the light indicates a suppression scotoma (Fig. 4.17b)
- two lights with the two lines displaced, which indicates a manifest deviation with diplopia. Normal retinal correspondence is present if a cross response is achieved when the angle of deviation is corrected (Fig. 4.17c)
- one light with one line image, which indicates suppression.

Worth's four light test

This test is used to investigate the presence of retinal correspondence. The subject may be tested at 1/3 m and 6 m. It consists of four circular lights on a black/grey background – one red, one white, two green – which are set in a diamond pattern and illuminated from within. The patient views these lights using red and green glasses, with the red filter before the right eye.

This is a dissociative diplopia based test and uses complementary colours. The white light is common to both eyes and therefore provides a fusional stimulus. The patient views the lights and is asked to state how many are seen. Possible results include:

- four lights – one red, two green and one light which is a mixture of red and green; this indicates normal or abnormal retinal correspondence (Fig. 4.18a)
- five lights, which indicates a manifest deviation with diplopia. The lights are displaced according to the type of deviation present. Two red lights on the left and three green lights on the right are seen with exodeviations, while with esodeviations the green lights will be on the left and the red on the right. Normal retinal correspondence is present if four lights are seen when the deviation is corrected (Fig. 4.18b)
- three or two lights, which indicates suppression. Three green lights indicate right suppression and two red lights indicate left suppression (Fig. 4.18c).

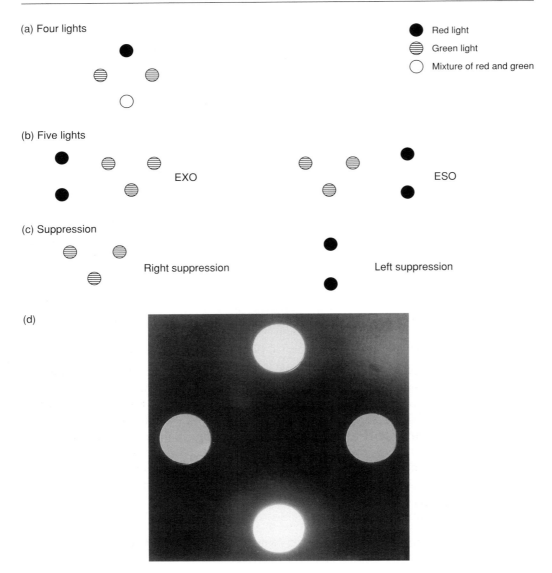

Figure 4.18   Worth's four light test.

After-image test

When the eye is exposed to a bright flash of light, the subjective sensations last longer than the stimulus itself. This sensation is the after-image. The after-image test uses fovea/foveal projection to demonstrate the relationship between the foveal projection of both eyes. There is bifoveal stimulation but not simultaneous stimulation. It is a test of retinal correspondence because it compares the retinal areas which have the same visual direction during binocular single vision (Bielchowsky 1937).

An after-image is presented to each eye in turn in the form of a linear bright light, either horizontal or vertical, with a central fixation target on each linear light. The horizontal line image is presented to the fixing eye first, followed by a vertical image to the deviating eye (this minimises suppression).

An after-image may be produced by an electronic flash gun or by using the synoptophore. The flash stimulus produced by an electronic flash gun is presented to each eye in turn and the subjective responses are recorded.

The synoptophore may be used to produce an after-image when an autoflash device has been incorporated into the instrument. After-image slides of the line images are required. Controls are set at zero and the opal filters are removed. The slides are inserted with the horizontal image before the fixating eye and the vertical image before the deviating eye. The autoflash is adjusted to rapid and simultaneous settings and the light intensity is increased to maximum strength.

The tube is switched on before the fixing eye for 10 seconds and then switched off. This is followed by the same procedure before the deviating eye. The opal filters are then replaced, the slides removed and the autoflash is switched on. The patient looks into the synoptophore or at a blank wall and describes the subjective after-image. Possible results include:

- foveae which project to the same point in space, indicating normal retinal correspondence
- a displaced after-image is produced by the deviating eye in cases of manifest strabismus because the foveae project to different points in space. This includes cases with abnormal retinal correspondence as the stimulus is to the fovea and not the pseudofovea in the deviating eye.

Prism adaptation test

This test assesses the state of binocular function. The angle of deviation is overcorrected by 5–10 prism dioptres with fresnel prisms. The patient's motor response is observed after a period of at least 24 hours. Possible results include:

- the visual axes may assume a straight position or a microtropia, demonstrating binocular single vision
- the visual axes may resume their original position which indicates abnormal retinal correspondence
- the visual axes remain in the overcorrected position, indicating absence of any binocular function.

Vertical prism test

In cases of manifest horizontal strabismus with suppression, a 10 or 15 prism dioptre vertical prism may be used to displace an image onto the superior or inferior retina and produce diplopia. A second horizontal prism is used to place the images in vertical alignment.

Normal retinal correspondence is present if the strength of the second prism is equivalent to the objective measurement of the angle of deviation. If the second prism strength is equivalent to the patient's subjective angle of deviation, then abnormal retinal correspondence is present. If the patient is unable to appreciate the images in vertical alignment, then suppression is present and retinal correspondence cannot be determined.

Synoptophore

Simultaneous perception slides are used. The method is described further later in the chapter (see page 80).

Botulinum toxin A

Botulinum toxin A can be used to decrease the angle of deviation in order to assess the potential for post-operative binocular single vision. In esotropia, the medial rectus is injected and in exotropia the lateral rectus is injected with botulinum toxin to paralyse the muscle's function. The eye takes up a straighter or overcorrected angle post injection. When the eye is in a 'straight' position, the state of retinal correspondence and potential for binocular single vision can be assessed.

FUSION

Sensory fusion is the ability to perceive simultaneously two images, one formed on each retina, and interpret them as one. It has been advocated that sensory fusion may be assessed using Bagolini glasses and Worth's lights. However, these tests are only an assessment of retinal correspondence indicating the ability or inability of the patient to superimpose images. Sensory fusion may be assessed on the synoptophore or the Sbiza bar can be used (Hocking & Gage 2002).

Motor fusion is the ability to maintain sensory fusion through a range of vergence movements. The strength of binocular single vision is indicated by measuring the range of motor fusion.

Motor fusion may be measured qualitatively by:

- cover test recovery

and quantitatively by:

- prism fusion range
- prism reflex test
- binocular visual acuity
- synoptophore.

Cover test recovery

The recovery movement is assessed on removal of the cover from either eye as this movement denotes the presence of binocular single vision and therefore fusion. Full recovery, in which the eyes move back to a straight position, indicates normal binocular single vision.

Prism fusion range

If a base-out prism is placed before one eye, the target image is displaced in the direction of the prism apex (Figs 4.19, 4.20). In order to maintain binocular single vision, the eye turns inwards by a corrective amount. The strongest base-out prism through which binocular single vision can be maintained marks the limit of the patient's convergent fusion range.

When assessing the divergent fusion range with base-in prisms, the target image is displaced towards the prism apex and the eye turns outwards by a corrective amount. The strongest base-in prism through which binocular single vision can be maintained marks the limit of the patient's divergent fusion range.

Horizontal fusion range

Latent deviation

The patient fixates a target at 1/3 m or 6 m held in the primary position. A horizontal prism bar is placed before one eye and, starting with the weakest prism strength, is moved through the range until the patient is no longer able to maintain binocular single vision. This can be determined by observing the patient's eyes to ensure that the prism is overcome. The strength of prism at which the patient no longer makes a fusional movement to overcome it marks the limit of the fusional range.

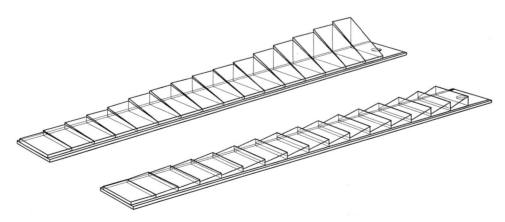

Figure 4.19   Prism bars.

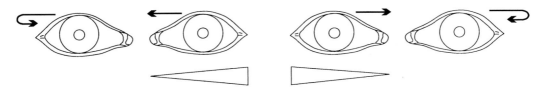

Figure 4.20   Response to overcome a base-out prism. A base-out prism is placed before the left eye. Both eyes make a conjugate movement to the right and the right eye makes a refixation movement to the left. When the prism is placed before the right eye, a similar response is obtained, with a conjugate movement of both eyes to the left followed by a refixation disjugate movement of the left eye to the right.

The eyes are seen to diverge and the patient may appreciate diplopia. If unsure of the break point, Bagolini glasses may be used as a control. The cross response will split into two separate lines on break of fusion. When fusion breaks, allow time to re-fuse the images if the patient is able. Once fusion is lost, decrease the prisms until the patient is able to regain fusion; this is usually at a level 4–6 prism dioptres lower than the break point. If the level is more than this, there may be an underlying problem with compensation. The blur point measures the limits within which accommodation can clear the image of the fixation target in spite of increased convergence. The amount of fusional convergence that can be elicited between the blur point and break point represents the absolute convergence.

The test is performed with the prisms held base out and base in. On increasing the base-out prisms (convergence range), the patient may appreciate a decrease in size of the image (micropsia). On increasing the base-in prisms (divergence range), the patient may appreciate an increase in the size of the image (macropsia). Quite often, the patient will be aware of blurring of the image before the image actually splits on break of fusion. This is termed the blur point of fusion (Narbheram & Firth 1997).

Manifest deviation

The angle of deviation is first corrected with prisms which are then gradually altered (increased and decreased) in strength to assess the motor fusion range. Bagolini glasses may be used as a control to ensure that the patient does not suppress one image.

Vertical and cyclovertical fusion range

This is an important test for the differential diagnosis of long-standing decompensating IV nerve palsy and acquired IV nerve palsy. Base-down prisms are used to assess supravergence and base-up prisms for infravergence. The normal range is 3 prism dioptres base down and 3 prism dioptres base up (Sharma & Abdul-Rahim 1992).

Prism reflex test

Babies and young children who are unable to co-operate with a prism fusion range test may be assessed using single base-out prisms. Using a 20 dioptre prism base out, the prism is placed before either eye in turn with the examiner looking for a movement of the eyes to overcome the effect of the prism and looking at the rate of recovery and extent of recovery. If the patient does not overcome the 20 dioptre prism, the test should be repeated with lower strength prisms down to a 10 dioptre prism before recording absence of fusional movements.

Binocular visual acuity

This test is used to assess the strength of binocular single vision. The test is important as patients can exert accommodation to control their deviation. Therefore, during testing intermittent occlusion acts as dissociation and control can break at a level of visual acuity less than each monocular visual acuity.

The patient is required to read decreasing sizes of print whilst maintaining binocular single vision at both 1/3 m and 6 m. The examiner must record the level of monocular visual acuity first. The patient is then instructed to read slowly down the letter chart. The examiner observes the eyes for a manifest strabismus. A cover/uncover test is performed for each size of letter to determine if binocular single vision is still present.

If a latent deviation becomes manifest, the binocular visual acuity is recorded for the previous line of letters. The maximum level of binocular visual acuity is equivalent to the weakest monocular visual acuity.

Synoptophore

This can be used to assess the presence of sensory fusion. Motor fusion is assessed by converging and diverging the tubes. This will be further discussed later in the chapter.

STEREOPSIS

Depth may be perceived in two forms: binocular disparity (stereopsis) and monocular depth clues in the absence of binocular single vision.

Stereopsis is the perception of the relative depth of objects on the basis of binocular disparity which reflects the slight difference in images presented to each eye.

Stereoacuity is the angular measurement of the minimal resolvable binocular disparity which is necessary for the appreciation of stereopsis. The ability to demonstrate stereopsis indicates the presence of retinal correspondence, the normal level of stereopsis being 40 seconds of arc with normal equal visual acuity in each eye. The level of stereoacuity decreases with reduction in visual acuity (Oguz & Oguz 2000).

Lang two pencil test

This is a test for gross stereopsis. The patient attempts to place a pencil on top of one held by the examiner (Fig. 4.21). Patients who possess stereopsis will find it easier to perform the test with both eyes open than monocularly. The two pencil test gives stereopsis estimates of 3000–5000 seconds of arc (LaRoche & von Noorden 1982).

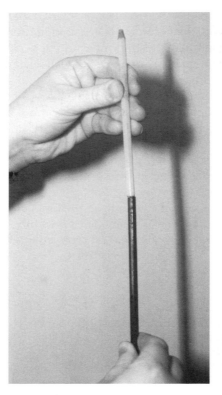 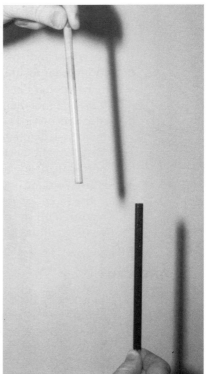

Figure 4.21   Lang two pencil test.

Frisby stereotest

This uses random shapes with displacement and consists of three plastic plates of different thickness: 6 mm, 3 mm and 1 mm. On each plate, there are four squares produced by random shapes printed on one side and on the other, corresponding to one of the squares, and a disparity is

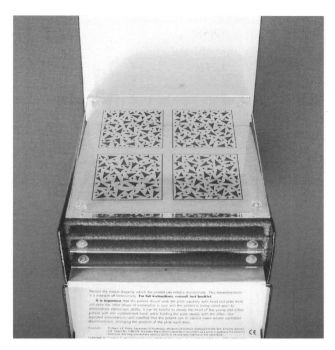

Figure 4.22   Frisby stereotest.

created by printing a circle with random shapes (Fig. 4.22). This gives a real-time 3D appearance. The disparity is affected by the thickness of the plate and the distance at which the plate is held from the patient. When held at 40 cm, stereopsis of 340, 170 and 55 seconds of arc can be achieved with the 6, 3 and 1 mm plates respectively. The Frisby stereotest is very useful for assessing stereopsis in very young children and patients with easily dissociative strabismus.

Principle of random dot stereograms

Random dot stereograms are images formed of dots which are displaced in relation to each other. The space created by this is filled randomly by dots, those seen by one eye having no relation to those seen by the other eye. This produces disparity of viewing as both eyes will see different dots. With stereopsis, these disparate images are fused and depth is appreciated.

Random dot tests lack monocular clues but are more difficult (Simons 1981). The inability to perform on random dot may be due to a crowding effect from closely placed random dots.

Random dot stereogram tests include:

- Lang stereotest
- TNO stereotest
- Synoptophore.

Lang stereotest

This is based on the use of random dot stereograms and cylindrical grating placement (panography) spaced at 24 cylinders per centimetre. Beneath each cylinder, there are two strips of an image, one seen by the right eye and the other seen by the left eye. The two images are fused and the disparity produces stereopsis (Lang 1983). The first Lang stereotest consists of three images – cat, car and star. The second consists of four images – the star is a control image and can be seen in the absence of stereopsis while the car, elephant and moon are seen in the presence of stereopsis up to 200 seconds of arc (Fig. 4.23).

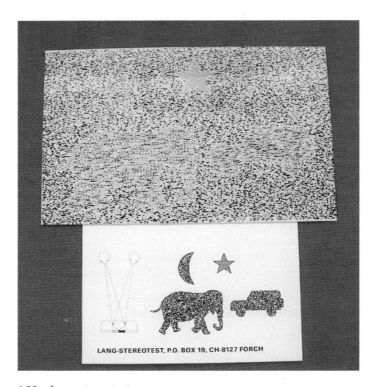

Figure 4.23   Lang stereotest.

TNO stereotest

This is based on the use of random dot stereograms. Computer generated random dots are printed as red and green analyphs. Red and green glasses are worn which are complementary colours to the red and green

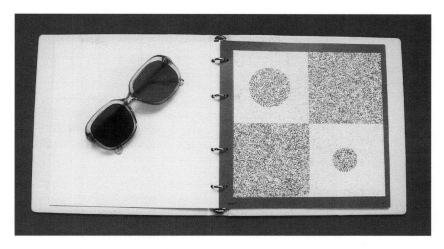

Figure 4.24   TNO stereotest.

random dots used. Three gross stereoplates are used, a suppression plate and three graded plates with segmented circle shapes which give a result of 480 to 15 seconds of arc (Okuda *et al.* 1977) (Fig. 4.24). This is considered the most accurate test for stereopsis as there are no monocular clues.

Synoptophore

There are two different groups of slides in use.

(1)   Graded stereoscopic slides which contain two dissimilar images. Each has a control but there is an inbuilt disparity between the images which when fused will produce gross stereoscopic vision.
(2)   Braddick slides consist of pairs of random dots, each slide stimulating slightly disparate retinal points, resulting in depth disparity.

Principle of linear polarisation

Polaroid filter glasses are worn and a vertical image of a light source is seen through one filter and a horizontal image of the light is seen through the other. The targets are presented as vectographs and consist of two polarised surfaces with a slight crossed disparity between them. The disparity produced by either eye results in stereopsis.

Linear polarisation stereotests include:

•   Titmus/Wirt stereotest
•   Randot stereotest.

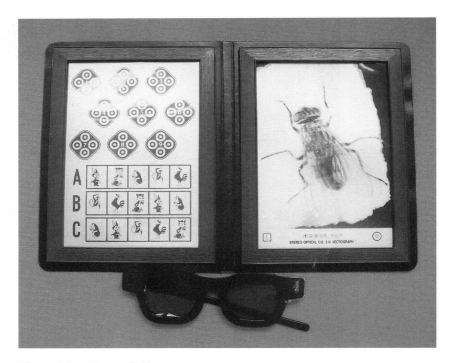

Figure 4.25   Titmus/Wirt stereotest.

Titmus/Wirt stereotest

This is based on linear polarisation and consists of two plates (Fig. 4.25). One plate contains the image of a fly and three rows of animals. Gross stereopsis is demonstrated if the wings of the fly are perceived as standing out from the body of the fly. The image of one animal in each row also appears to stand out and stereopsis of up to 100 seconds of arc may be achieved. The second plate consists of nine boxes, each containing four circles. One circle is displaced to produce disparity and stereopsis of up to 40 seconds of arc may be achieved.

The Titmus stereotest has limitations due to monocular clues. False positive responses with Titmus are reported (Simons & Reinecke 1974), the most obvious of which is lateral displacement of targets (Cooper & Warshowsky 1977). True stereoacuity may be confirmed by rotating the test target 180 degrees. The previously elevated target should sink below the plane of the book.

Randot stereotest

This is based on linear polarisation and consists of two plates containing random forms (Fig. 4.26). The perception of random dot shapes gives a result of 500 to 250 seconds of arc. Appreciation of depth with the animals and circles gives a result of 400 to 20 seconds of arc.

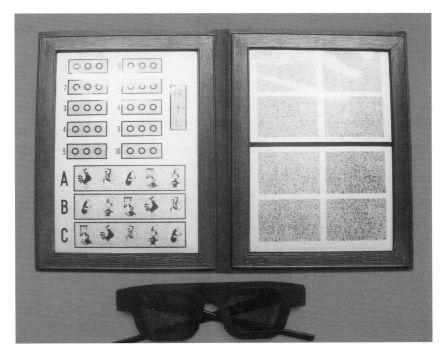

Figure 4.26   Randot stereotest.

SUPPRESSION

The presence of suppression can be detected by using Bagolini glasses, Worth's lights, the synoptophore and the 4 dioptre prism test. Various stereopsis tests also incorporate a suppression test plate, e.g. TNO.

The area and density of suppression may also be measured.

Area of suppression

The area of suppression may be plotted using the synoptophore with simultaneous perception slides. The tube is locked at zero before the fixating eye. It is then rotated horizontally and then vertically before the suppressing eye and the angles at which the image of the deviating eye disappears and then reappears are recorded. This forms an area of suppression.

Different sizes of graded simultaneous perception slides may also be used to assess a suppression scotoma. The patient will only be aware of both slides if the picture in front of the suppressing eye is large enough to lie outside the suppression scotoma. It follows that the larger the slide required in front of the deviating eye to enable it to be seen, the larger the size of the suppression scotoma.

The area of suppression may also be assessed with prisms in the same way that post-operative diplopia is assessed. Prisms are placed before the suppressing eye and gradually increased in strength until diplopia is noticed. Prisms are introduced base out, base in, base up and base down to assess the complete area of suppression.

Depth/density of suppression

A Sbiza (Bagolini filter) bar is used to investigate the depth of suppression in patients with amblyopia approaching the age of seven years who require treatment. If suppression is very dense, the decision may be taken to occlude carefully. The Sbiza bar consists of a series of red filters of increasing density from very pale to very dark. This decreases the illumination in front of the fixating eye to induce fixation with the deviating eye and therefore diplopia. The patient fixates a spotlight held at 1/3 m in the primary position. The Sbiza bar is introduced before the fixating eye, commencing with the palest filter. The filter strength is increased until the patient sees one white and one red light as a result of diplopia. The strength of filter at which this occurs represents the density of suppression.

Post-operative diplopia test

This test is used to investigate the likelihood of a patient experiencing diplopia post-operatively. It may be performed on any patient over the age of seven years who is being considered for cosmetic strabismus surgery. It investigates the area of suppression and therefore the possible occurrence of post-operative diplopia if surgery were to result in ocular alignment in which images fall outside the suppression area. At this stage, the patient would be unable to resuppress and would appreciate intractable diplopia.

The patient fixates a spotlight at 1/3 m and prisms are introduced initially at the lowest strength and then gradually increased in order to first undercorrect, then correct the angle of deviation and eventually overcorrect it. For each strength of prism, the patient is asked to state what is seen, i.e. single image or diplopia, and the test is then repeated at 6 m. Red and green glasses may be used to facilitate the appreciation of diplopia, but in clinical practice the test is often performed without these glasses as this is more representative of the patient's everyday viewing conditions (Gray *et al.* 1996).

Possible results include the following:

- Should the patient continue to see one light, it is unlikely that intractable diplopia would pose a problem post-operatively.
- Diplopia may be appreciated when the deviation is overcorrected and this would alert the surgeon not to overcorrect the deviation.

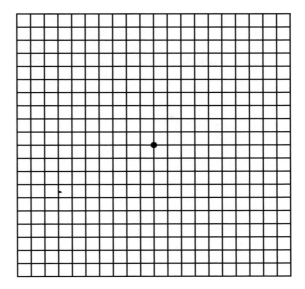

Figure 4.27   Amsler chart.

- Diplopia may be appreciated intermittently when undercorrected and this may be a contraindication to surgery.

Should the patient appreciate diplopia, it is important to assess whether this may be ignored, particularly if vision in one eye is poor. When diplopia is appreciated, the patient is asked whether they are capable of ignoring or resuppressing the second image and how easy this is to achieve. Where it is relatively easy to ignore the second image, the patient may feel that the cosmetic appearance warrants the risk of diplopia post-operatively.

Where further information regarding post-operative diplopia is required, use of botulinum toxin may be considered to align the eyes temporarily.

Amsler charts

These may be used to plot central and paracentral scotomas. The chart usually consists of a square grid of black lines on a white background (Fig. 4.27). The patient describes or draws how the grid appears, thus demonstrating the scotoma.

SYNOPTOPHORE

This is a haploscopic device in which each eye looks through a separate tube, viewing a picture on a slide on a plane mirror (Figs 4.28, 4.29). The

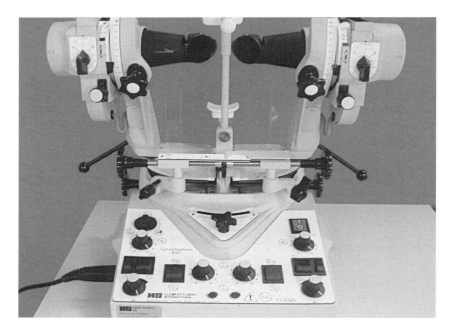

Figure 4.28   Synoptophore.

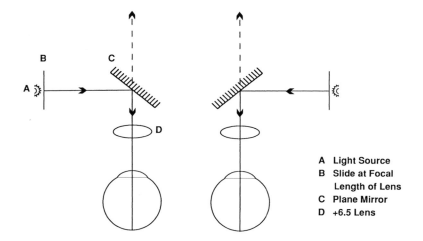

A Light Source
B Slide at Focal
   Length of Lens
C Plane Mirror
D +6.5 Lens

Figure 4.29   Optics of the synoptophore.

strength of the lenses within the eye pieces are +6.5 DS and, as a result, it is considered to be a distance test.

Slides

There are a range of slides. The sizes of the pictures on the slides subtend visual angles of differing degrees at the nodal point. Foveal simultaneous perception (SP) is the ability to perceive simultaneously and to superimpose two dissimilar images subtending angles not greater than 1 degree at the nodal point. Macular SP is the ability to perceive simultaneously and to superimpose two dissimilar images subtending angles greater than 1 degree but not greater than 3 degrees at the nodal point. Paramacular SP is the ability to perceive simultaneously and to superimpose two dissimilar images subtending angles greater than 3 degrees but not greater than 5 degrees at the nodal point. Peripheral SP is the ability to perceive simultaneously and to superimpose two dissimilar images subtending angles greater than 5 degrees at the nodal point.

- SP slides are red in colour and are used to measure IPD and angle of deviation and for assessing SP.
- Fusion slides are green in colour and are used to measure sensory and motor fusion.
- Stereopsis slides are yellow in colour. Sizes include gross, detailed or Braddick.

Uses of the synoptophore

Measurement of interpupillary distance

The interpupillary distance is the distance between the two pupil centres. This procedure is performed on all patients so that they are aligned properly such that each eye is looking centrally down each tube. The average for an adult is 65 mm when the eyes are fixing in the distance, the average for a child is 50 mm. The set-up and measurement of IPD must be correct before any other measurements may be made.

Measurement of the angle of deviation

The test may be performed either objectively or subjectively, both with and without spectacles, fixing either eye, in nine cardinal positions. The tubes are rotated horizontally and/or vertically by up to 25 degrees (elevation, adduction and abduction) and 35 degrees (depression) for this purpose and horizontal, vertical and torsional angles of deviation are obtained.

Simultaneous perception slides appropriate to the visual acuity are used. However, Maddox slides are used for measurement of incomitant deviations (Fig. 4.30). The tube is locked before the fixing eye and an alternate cover test performed by extinguishing the light in each tube to act as an occluder. With esodeviations, the tubes are converged before the deviating eye and for exodeviations, the tubes are diverged. The cover test is repeated and the procedure continued until no further movement to take up fixation is seen. The angle of deviation, in degrees, is obtained from the scale. If there is poor vision and the patient is

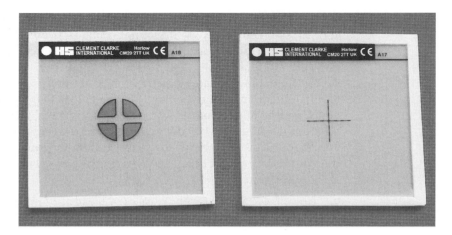

Figure 4.30   Maddox slides.

unable to fixate with one eye, the deviation may be measured by assessing the position of corneal reflections. The tube is moved before the deviating eye until the corneal reflections are symmetrical.

When assessing the subjective angle of deviation, the patient is asked to move the tube before the deviating eye so that the images overlap. Vertical deviations are measured by moving one of the slides vertically until the patient states that there is no vertical movement of the images.

Assessment of retinal correspondence

Simultaneous perception

Simultaneous perception slides are dissimilar (Fig. 4.31). Subjectively, the patient moves the tube before the non-fixating eye and attempts to overlap the images. Simultaneous perception is absent if the patient is unable to see the two images at the same time or if one image repeatedly disappears or the images jump. It is easier to superimpose with larger slides, and if simultaneous perception is not achieved with smaller slides, it is useful to reassess with peripheral slides before assuming lack of SP.

Fusion

Sensory fusion is present if, at the subjective angle, the patient is able to superimpose both fusion slide images (Fig. 4.32) and is able to see both control images (one from each slide). The motor fusion range is assessed by converging and diverging the tubes whilst asking the patient to state when fusion breaks. The patient will appreciate diplopia or will suppress one of the controls. If the patient has difficulty viewing the targets or loses one of the controls, larger slides may be used. Foveal fusion is more difficult to maintain than peripheral.

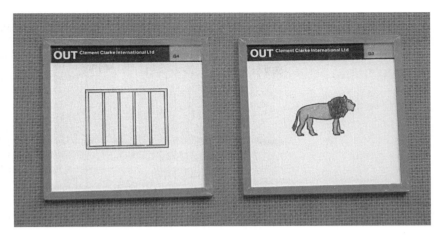

Figure 4.31   Simultaneous perception slides.

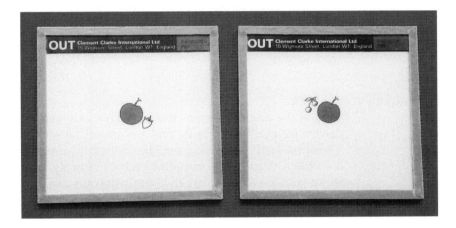

Figure 4.32   Fusion slides.

Stereoacuity

Both tubes are locked at the fusion angle. Gross stereopsis slides (Fig. 4.33) are inserted and the patient asked whether or not there is a stereoscopic effect. Detailed stereopsis (Fig. 4.33) is assessed using Braddick slides.

Assessment of aniseikonia

Ruben's slides are used to establish the difference in image size between either eye (see Chapter 9).

Assessment of after-images to investigate retinal correspondence

Please see pages 64–65 for a full description.

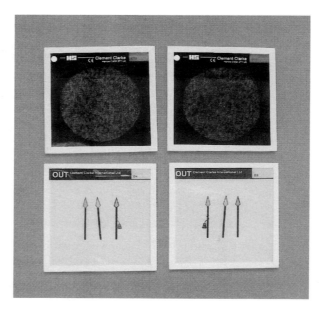

Figure 4.33   Stereopsis slides. *Above*: detailed stereopsis. *Below*: gross stereopsis.

Measurement of angle kappa

This is the angle between the pupillary axis and visual axis and is caused by a failure of the optical and visual axes of the eye to coincide. The optical axis is a line connecting the optical centres of the cornea and lens when aligned. The visual axis is the line of sight which connects the fovea with the fixation target. Usually the optical axis touches the retina slightly nasal and inferior to the fovea. As a result, the corneal reflection is slightly nasal to the centre of the pupil (normal positive angle kappa). If there is a large positive angle kappa, this may give the appearance of a divergent deviation. If the fovea is nasal to the optical axis, the corneal reflection will appear on the temporal side of the pupil centre and this may give the appearance of a convergent deviation.

Fig. 4.34 illustrates angle kappa and Fig. 4.35 illustrates the slide used for measurement of the angle.

Angle kappa is measured monocularly on the synoptophore. The slides have a horizontal series of letters and numbers separated by intervals of 1–2 degrees. A row of animals is placed below the horizontal line of letters and numbers on some slides for use with children. The patient looks at the central fixation point and then on to each subsequent number until the corneal reflections appear symmetrical. This gives a measurement of a positive angle kappa. With a negative angle kappa, the patient looks at each subsequent letter progressively outwards until the corneal reflections appear symmetrical.

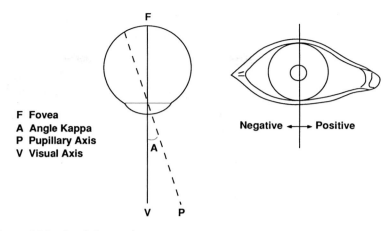

F Fovea
A Angle Kappa
P Pupillary Axis
V Visual Axis

Negative ◄─┼─► Positive

Figure 4.34   Angle kappa.

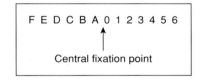

F E D C B A 0 1 2 3 4 5 6

Central fixation point

Figure 4.35   Angle kappa slide assessment.

Haidinger's brushes

These are rarely used in current orthoptic practice but have been used in pleoptic treatment for eccentric fixation to stimulate the fovea and re-educate foveal fixation (see Chapter 8). This is an entoptic phenomenon caused by the effect of polarised light at the fovea and consists of polarised and blue filters. The background of blue light enhances this effect which may be prolonged by rotating the axis of polarisation so that the brushes also rotate.

FIXATION

Visuscope (fixation ophthalmoscope)

This test is used to assess fixation in cases of amblyopia and manifest strabismus. The visuscope incorporates a four-pointed star with a clear central area as the fixation target. A green filter is occasionally used to produce a red free image of the retina. The normal eye is assessed initially, to ensure patient understanding and co-operation, followed by the amblyopic eye. The position of fixation is recorded in relation to the foveola (central, parafoveal, macular, peripheral) and according to the state of fixation (steady, unsteady, wandering or eccentric) (Fig. 4.36).

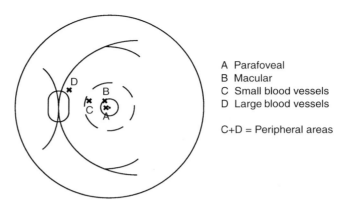

Figure 4.36   Fixation.

A Parafoveal
B Macular
C Small blood vessels
D Large blood vessels

C+D = Peripheral areas

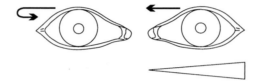

Figure 4.37   Fusion response with four dioptre prism test. When a base-out prism is placed before the left eye, both eyes move conjugately to the right. The right eye then makes a disjugate refixation movement to the left.

Four dioptre prism test

This test assesses the presence of bifoveal fixation. The following response is expected in the presence of normal bifoveal fixation. On placing a 4 dioptre prism base out before the right eye, the eyes make a conjugate movement to the left. A subsequent disjugate fusional movement of the left eye is seen. A prism placed before the left eye produces a similar fusional movement (Fig. 4.37).

In the presence of a central suppression scotoma, with the prism placed before the normal eye, a conjugate movement is seen to the opposite side. However, a disjugate fusional movement is not seen in the affected eye because the image has been displaced into the suppression scotoma. When the prism is placed before the affected eye, no movement is seen in either eye because the image is already within the suppression scotoma (Fig. 4.38) (Bagolini *et al.* 1985).

The test may also be performed with the prism base in, particularly in cases of micro-exotropia (Romano & von Noorden 1969; Epstein & Tredici 1972).

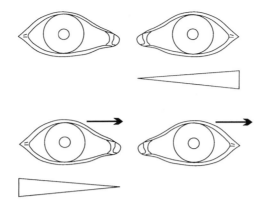

Figure 4.38 Suppression scotoma response with four dioptre prism test. When a base-out prism is placed before the left eye, no movement of the eyes is seen as the image of the fixation target falls within the left suppression scotoma. When the base-out prism is placed before the right eye, a conjugate movement of both eyes is seen to the left but there is no refixation movement of the left eye, as the image has fallen within the suppression scotoma of the left eye.

MEASUREMENT OF DEVIATIONS

Neutralisation

On cover test a movement of the eyes will be observed indicating the presence of either a manifest or latent deviation. By using prisms to displace light across the retina the deviation may be reduced and eventually neutralised when no movement of the eyes occurs. There will be no movement of the eyes when the selected prism causes the image to fall on the fovea. The prism cover test uses this principle.

Estimation

When an accurate measurement of a deviation cannot be obtained due to age, lack of co-operation or poor visual acuity, an estimation of a manifest deviation may be made by observation of the corneal reflections and additionally by using a prism to displace the image until the corneal reflections appear symmetrical. The prism reflection and Krimsky tests use this method.

Objective tests

- Prism cover test (see page 87)
- Simultaneous prism cover test (see page 87)
- Prism reflection test (see page 88)

- Krimsky test (see page 88)
- Hirschberg's test (see page 88)
- Synoptophore (see page 79–80)

Subjective tests

- Maddox rod (see page 88–90)
- Maddox wing (see page 90)
- Synoptophore (see page 79–80)

Difficulties with prisms

Test accuracy is limited by the optical properties of prisms. The stronger the prism, the greater the error. When using prisms, significant errors are produced when a low power prism is added to a high power prism, i.e. stacking prisms.

Errors in quantitative measurements of strabismus can also be induced by not placing prisms accurately while measuring the deviation (Thompson & Guyton 1983). Glass prisms are calibrated for use in the Prentice position (posterior face of prism held perpendicular to the line of sight of the deviating eye). Plastic prisms are calibrated for use in the frontal place with the position parallel to the infraorbital rim (Fig. 4.39).

The measurement error introduced by using the Prentice position increases as prisms greater than 20 prism dioptres are used. When deviations exceed the amount of the largest available prism, the examiner should not stack prisms. The error can be minimised by holding one prism before each eye. Prisms may be stacked, however, if they are used to simultaneously measure vertical and horizontal misalignment which are independent of each other. Prisms should be held close to the eyes as the power needed to neutralise the deviation with near fixation will

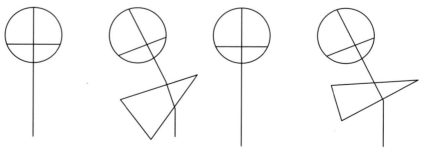

Prentice position   Frontal plane

Figure 4.39   Prism position.

increase as prisms are held further from the cornea (Thompson & Guyton 1985).

High refractive corrections may also affect measurement. Plus lenses reduce and minus lenses increase the deviation due to the prismatic effect of the spectacle correction.

Prism cover test

This is an objective dissociative test used to measure the angle of deviation. The test may be performed at 1/3 m, 6 m and greater than 6 m and indicates the maximum angle of deviation. Both horizontal and vertical angles can be measured in manifest and latent deviations. The prism cover test is generally the test of choice in the majority of cases.

The patient must fixate the target accurately and have adequate visual acuity to be able to fix with either eye. The test is performed both with and without spectacles with the patient holding and fixating a target at 1/3 m, at eye level. A prism bar is held in front of the deviating eye usually in manifest deviations and before either eye in latent deviations. The other eye is occluded. An alternate cover test is performed by moving the occluder from one eye to the other whilst watching the movement of the eye behind the prism as it takes up fixation. The prism strength is then increased gradually until the movement decreases and eventually there is no movement to take up fixation. By continuing to increase the prism strength until a reverse movement is seen and then decreasing again until there is no movement, the 'null' point can be verified from both directions. The prism strength is noted and is equivalent to the maximum measurement of the angle of deviation. The test may be repeated for 6 m and greater than 6 m if required.

Advantages are that the test provides accurate measurements, is performed under natural conditions and provides the maximum angle of deviation. Disadvantages are that the patient must have central fixation in either eye with at least 6/60 visual acuity to see the fixation target. It is difficult with young or unco-operative patients and prism bars have a range of only 45 prism dioptres.

Simultaneous prism cover test

The aim of this test is to neutralise the deviation without complete dissociation. It is used in cases of microtropia with an associated heterophoria, in order to isolate and measure the angle of the manifest deviation. A prism is placed before the deviating eye and, simultaneously, an occluder is placed before the other eye. The aim is to neutralise the movement of the deviating eye when it moves to take up fixation, thereby giving the angle of manifest deviation.

Prism reflection test

This test is used with small children unable to co-operate with the prism cover test or with patients with poor vision who do not have foveal fixation. The prism bar is placed before the deviating eye and the patient fixates a spotlight at 1/3 m. The examiner observes the position of the corneal reflections and the prism strength is gradually increased until the corneal reflections appear symmetrical. This prism strength is noted. The test may also be performed using loose prisms.

Krimsky test

This test is similar to the prism reflection test but the prism is placed before the fixing eye (Krimsky 1943). The patient fixates a spotlight at 1/3 m and the prism strength is increased until the corneal reflections are symmetrical. The optical principle is different from the prism reflection test as the prism is placed before the fixing eye and the fixing eye moves to overcome the prism and maintain fixation in the primary position. Because of Hering's law (each eye will make a conjugate movement of the same amount), if an increasing prism strength is placed before the fixing eye, this will centralise the corneal reflections of the deviating eye.

Hirschberg's test

This test is based on the presence of comparable corneal reflections by assessing the position of the corneal reflection in the squinting eye compared with that of the fixing eye.

An indication of the angle of manifest deviations can be obtained. A spotlight is shone into the patient's eyes and an estimated measurement is taken as to the angle of deviation, by observing the position of the corneal reflection of the deviating eye; 1 mm displacement is equivalent to 7 degrees or 15 prism dioptres in adults (Brodie 1987) or 20–22 prism dioptres in children (Hasebe *et al.* 1998) (Fig. 4.40).

Corneal reflections viewed at the pupil margin are roughly equivalent to a displacement of 10–15 degrees (20–30 prism dioptres), those situated half way between the pupil and the limbus to 25 degrees (50 prism dioptres) and those at the limbus to 45 degrees (90 prism dioptres). Reflections displaced temporally indicate the presence of an esodeviation whilst nasal displacement indicates an exodeviation.

Maddox rod

This is a subjective, diplopia based test used to measure the angle of deviation in heterophorias and small heterotropias provided normal

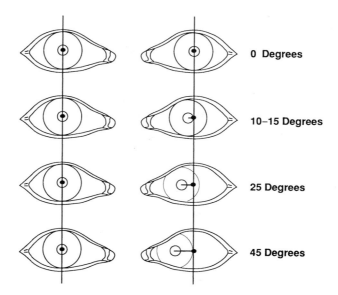

Figure 4.40   Hirschberg's corneal reflections.

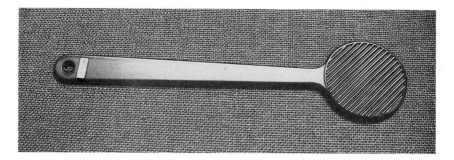

Figure 4.41   Maddox rod.

retinal correspondence is present. It is a series of parallel high power plano-convex cylinders which convert a point source of light into a line seen perpendicular to the axis of the cylinders which are traditionally coloured red or blue. The Maddox lenses may also be in the form of a Maddox hand frame or Franceshetti frame (Fig. 4.41).

The test is performed with and without spectacles at 1/3 m and 6 m and fixating with either eye.

Horizontal deviation

The patient fixates a spotlight held at eye level. The rod is placed before the non-fixing eye and is rotated in order to produce a vertical line. The patient is asked to state where the line is in relation to the light. If the line passes through the light, there is no horizontal deviation.

The eyes are dissociated as the stimulus to fuse has been removed because dissimilar images are presented to the eyes. If the line is seen to one side of the light, a horizontal deviation is present and the line is displaced according to the deviation present.

Uncrossed displacement occurs with esodeviations and crossed displacement with exodeviations. In order to correct the displacement, corrective prisms of increasing strengths are placed before the rod until the patient states that the line passes through the light. This prism strength is noted.

Vertical deviation

The rod is rotated to produce a horizontal line image and the patient is asked to state the position of the line in relation to the light. If the line passes through the light, there is no vertical deviation. If the line is above the light, there is a hypodeviation and if below the light, there is a hyperdeviation. Corrective prisms of increasing strengths are used until the patient states that the line passes through the light. This prism strength is noted.

Maddox wing

This is a subjective test used to measure the angle of deviation in heterophorias and small heterotropias provided normal retinal correspondence is present. The instrument consists of a metal plate bearing a horizontal row of white numbers graded from right to left (22…01…15) and a white arrow (Fig. 4.42). It also contains a vertical row of numbers graded from top to bottom (22…01…13) and a red arrow.

The wing is situated at 1/3 m from the eyes and is supported by a septum and handle which connects it to the eye pieces containing trial lens holders. The septum is arranged so that the patient sees the arrows with the right eye and numbers with the left eye. The test is performed with and without spectacles and the patient asked to state which white number the white arrow is pointing to. If it points to an even number, there is a divergent deviation while an odd number is indicative of an esodeviation. The size of deviation corresponds in prism dioptres to the number stated.

For vertical deviations, the patient observes the red arrow and states which red number it points to. Between the numbers 22…01, there is a left/right deviation and between 01…13, there is a right/left deviation.

Torsion may also be assessed by asking the patient whether the red arrow is parallel to the white line of numbers. If not, the arrow can be moved until it is parallel and the amount of torsion recorded in degrees from the scale situated at the right side of the metal plate.

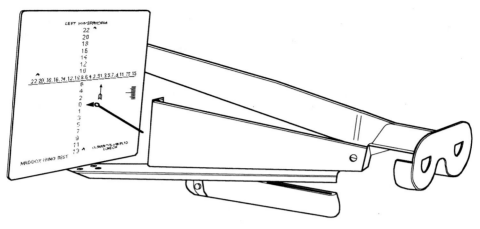

Figure 4.42 Maddox wing.

Synoptophore

The uses of this instrument are described in detail earlier in the chapter (pages 79–80).

HESS CHARTS

Hess charts are used in the investigation of incomitant strabismus in order to assess the paretic element (see Chapters 14–16). By means of dissociation, it is possible to indicate the position of the non-fixing eye when the other eye is fixing, in specified positions of gaze. A field is plotted in this way for each eye. Each point on the inner field represents fixation at 15 degrees from the primary position and on the outer field, represents fixation at 30 degrees from the primary position at 30 degrees. Defects which are present on more extreme gaze than this will not necessarily be evident on the Hess chart. It is essential to interpret these results together with the assessment of ocular movements. Information is gained from the chart by comparing the fields with each other and with the normal field printed on the chart.

Hess screen

This consists of a screen incorporating a tangent pattern on a black/grey background (Fig. 4.43). It may be manually or electrically operated. Red and green glasses are worn by the patient, with the red filter before the fixing eye. The patient is seated at 50 cm from the screen.

Dissociation is achieved by means of complementary colours. The fixing eye sees only a tangent pattern with red points or lights while

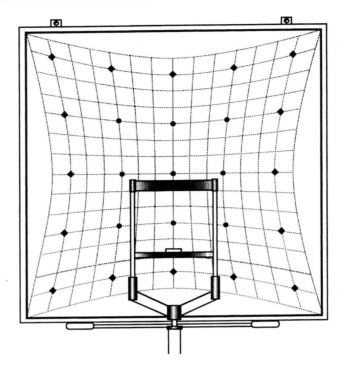

Figure 4.43   Hess screen.

the deviating eye sees only a green spot projected into the screen by a torch held by the patient. There must be macular/macular projection to ensure that either eye can maintain fixation. The position of the field will therefore reflect the true extent of the deviation.

Lees screen

This consists of two opalescent screens placed at 90 degrees to each other and a two-sided mirror septum at 45 degrees to the screens which dissociates the visual fields (Fig. 4.44). The mirror must be a true plane mirror and bisect the screens exactly. Each screen incorporates a tangent grid with an inner and outer field. There must be macular/macular projection.

The Lees screen possesses a number of advantages over the Hess screen:

- accurate dissociation
- greater contrast between tangent scale and background
- increased ease and speed of performance
- illumination is constant.

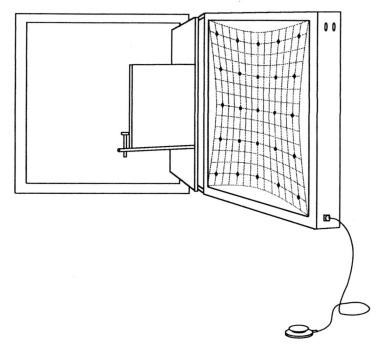

Figure 4.44   Lees screen.

Interpretation of results

The patient must possess normal retinal correspondence and central fixation. The test may be performed in the presence of abnormal retinal correspondence if a record of motility is required for comparison from visit to visit.

Comparing fields with each other

(1) Size of fields. The smaller field represents the affected eye. Any difference in size indicates incomitance, which is usually indicative of recent onset paresis. Similar size indicates concomitance.

(2) Sloping sides to fields indicates an A/V pattern.

Comparing each field with the normal field

(1) Smaller field: the deviation in the primary position is the primary deviation. The greatest negative (inward) displacement represents the primary underaction and is seen in the direction of the main action of the affected muscle. Positive (outward) displacement indicates an overaction.

(2)   Larger field: the deviation in primary position is the secondary deviation. The greatest positive displacement is the main overaction and the maximum displacement often occurs in the direction of the main action of the overacting contralateral synergist in the larger field. It is important to note any difference in the deviation in other positions of gaze.

Outer fields

These may show a defect when the central fields appear normal, particularly with mechanical defects or very slight paresis.

Information obtained

(1)   Underactions and overactions.
(2)   Affected eye.
(3)   A or V pattern.
(4)   Type of deviation in the primary position and other positions of gaze.
(5)   Size of deviation. Each box on the chart represents 5 degrees.
(6)   Primary and secondary deviations.
(7)   Muscle sequelae. There are limited sequelae with mechanical defects. The presence of full or part developed muscle sequelae aids in the differential diagnosis of concomitance and incomitance and recent and long-standing deviations.
(8)   Comparison between clinic visits.
(9)   Comparison between pre- and post-operative visits.
(10) It is possible to measure torsion using the Lees screen. This is described on page 97.

Characteristics of mechanical defects

(1)   Compressed fields.
(2)   Limited muscle sequelae.
(3)   The deviation in the primary position does not reflect the extent of the defect. Binocular single vision is often present in the primary position.

Characteristics of neurogenic defects

(1)   Sloping fields. These are indicative of an A or V pattern, not torsion.
(2)   Muscle sequelae are not limited and will eventually attain relative concomitance.
(3)   The deviation in the primary position reflects the extent of the palsy and therefore binocular single vision may or may not be present in the primary position.

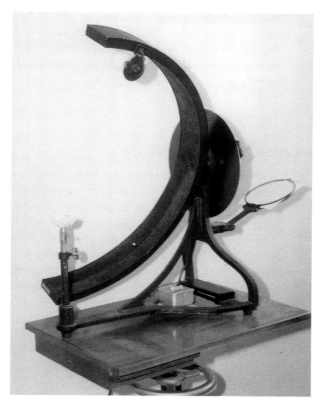

Figure 4.45   Arc perimeter.

FIELD OF BINOCULAR SINGLE VISION

The binocular field is plotted using an arc perimeter (Fig. 4.45) with a single chin rest; the rest is used to place the head in a central position with both eyes level and aligned with the fixation target. It is plotted for patients with incomitant deviations who appreciate diplopia but have an area of single vision and is used to monitor the progress of the condition, the effects of any treatment and for pre- and post-operative comparison. The patient is seated level with the fixation target and with the eyes in the primary position.

With both eyes open, the patient observes the target as it is moved slowly away from the primary position and is asked to state when it appears double. At this point, the examiner stops and marks the chart. The target is returned to the primary position and the arc is rotated (usually through 30 degree intervals) and the test repeated through 360 degrees. On completion, the marked dots on the chart are joined and the area of single vision is shaded.

At certain points, the facial contours (e.g. the nose) may obscure one eye. A cover test should be performed to ensure single vision is present because the patient will not appreciate diplopia in this situation. The test is performed without spectacles because the frame obscures vision.

If diplopia is present in the primary position, the target is moved into the area of single vision, recorded and moved again until diplopia is again perceived.

UNIOCULAR FIELD OF VISION

This may be plotted using an arc perimeter with a double chin rest which places the head in an off-centred position and each eye is aligned with the fixation target in turn. One eye is occluded during the test and the patient must maintain foveal fixation which is monitored by ensuring that the patient perceives clear vision. The test is indicated in patients who have very limited ocular movements and where responses obtained from the Hess chart are confused and overlapping.

The test can also be plotted using a Goldmann perimeter. The fixation target is typically a small letter which blurs when not fixated foveally. A red target may be used as an alternative and the foveal threshold value can be determined using Goldmann perimetry. Adaptations have considerably improved test/retest and intraobserver reliability by measuring the field using only six positions corresponding to the main action of each extraocular muscle.

MEASUREMENT OF TORSION

Torsion may be measured objectively or subjectively. An objective measure is obtained by observing the fovea–optic disc relationship ophthalmoscopically in congenital cases. If torsion is present, the disc will appear displaced and either intorted or extorted in relation to the fovea (Fig. 4.46) (Bixenman & von Noorden 1982). Subjective measurement methods include:

- Synoptophore
- Adapted Lees screen
- Maddox wing
- Awaya cyclo test
- Bagolini glasses
- Maddox double rod.

Synoptophore

Maddox slides are used and the degree of torsion is measured subjectively. The cross is placed before the fixing eye and the segmented circle is placed before the non-fixing eye. The patient superimposes the cross within the segmented circle, so that all lines are parallel at 90 and

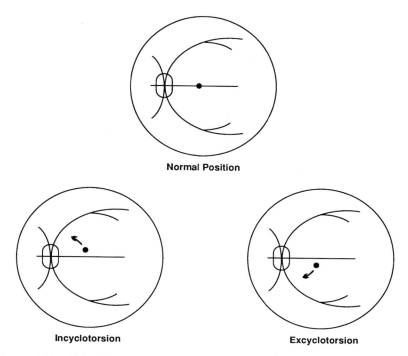

Normal Position

Incyclotorsion

Excyclotorsion

Figure 4.46   Objective assessment of torsion.

180 degrees. Torsion is adjusted by rotating the slide with the tilted image and the amount recorded in degrees. Torsion may be assessed fixing either eye and in the nine cardinal positions of gaze.

Adapted Lees screen

Linear targets are used (Dulley & Harden 1974). The patient places a short bar, mounted on a pointer, on sequential dots with the bar lying along the horizontal grid line. In the presence of torsion, the bar will slope and the position of its ends should be marked on the screen using a non-permanent marker. The amount of torsion is measured on completion of the test, using a protractor mounted on a Perspex block, which is pivoted around a fixed centre of rotation. The block is placed parallel to the horizontal grid line and the protractor is rotated until its base is in line with the marked position of the bar. Measurement of torsion is given in degrees.

Maddox wing

Torsion is present if the horizontal red arrow is not parallel to the white line composed of numbers. The arrow may be moved until it is parallel and the amount of torsion is indicated on a separate measurement scale. Each division on the scale is equivalent to 2 degrees of arc. The arrow is usually moved by the patient, giving a subjective measurement.

Awaya cyclo test

The test is presented in book form presenting 13 pairs of half moons. One half of each pair is red and the other green and each pair is spaced 10 mm apart. The green half moons are tilted in gradations of 1 degree. Initially the plate of parallel half moons is shown to the patient. Should the green half moon appear tilted clockwise there is extorsion and if it appears tilted anticlockwise there is intorsion. The patient wears red and green glasses with the red filter before the right eye if there is extorsion and the red filter before the left eye if there is intorsion. The patient decides which pair of half moons are parallel and this measurement is noted.

Bagolini glasses

Two Bagolini glasses are placed in a trial frame, one before either eye. The striations are placed vertically so that two horizontal line images are seen. In the presence of a vertical deviation, the lines will be seen one above the other. If there is no vertical deviation, a small vertical prism is introduced in order to separate the images. The patient is asked to state whether or not the lines are parallel. If tilted, the image can be straightened by rotating one of the Bagolini glasses and the degree of intorsion or extorsion measured from the trial frame. The test may be performed with either eye fixating (Ruttum & von Noorden 1984).

Maddox double rod

The test is conducted in the same manner as that described above for Bagolini glasses. Two Maddox rods are placed in a trial frame with the cylinder axes vertical.

PARKS-HELVESTON THREE STEP TEST

This triple procedure may assist in the diagnosis of vertical muscle palsies.

(1)   A cover test is performed in the primary position and the hypertropic eye is recorded.

(2)   An alternate cover test is then performed on dextroversion and laevoversion and the direction of the greater vertical deviation is recorded.

(3) The Bielchowsky head tilt test is performed. This differentiates between a superior oblique and a contralateral superior rectus palsy.

The patient fixates a target at 3 m and a cover test is performed in the primary position and with the patient's head tilted maximally to the left and then to the right. The difference in the degree of vertical deviation is recorded. An increase in the vertical angle when the head is tilted to the affected side is indicative of a superior oblique palsy. Results can, however, be misleading with regard to differential diagnosis. A positive test result has been observed with superior rectus palsy, inferior oblique overaction and cases of DVD.

DIPLOPIA CHARTS

These are used to evaluate and document the type of diplopia present. Red and green glasses are worn with the red filter usually placed before the right eye. A linear light source is used so that torsion may also be assessed. The patient's head should be still and erect. The patient is asked to describe diplopia in the nine cardinal positions of gaze, starting with the primary position, and also to describe the relative position of the lines of light in each position of gaze. The results are recorded in chart form as if one is looking through the patient's eyes. The position at which diplopia occurs, the type of diplopia, the maximum separation of images and the distal image are all recorded (Figs 4.47, 4.48).

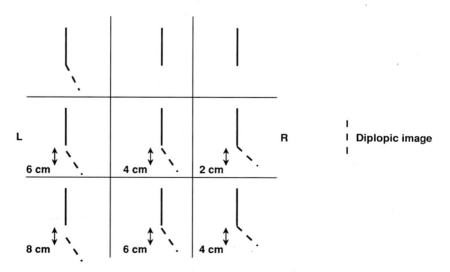

Figure 4.47 Diplopia chart of right IV nerve palsy.

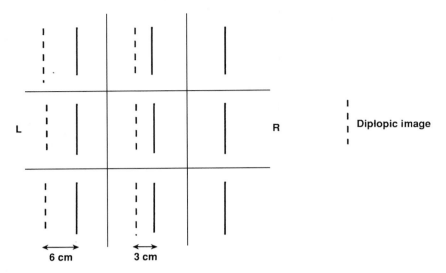

Figure 4.48   Diplopia chart of left VI nerve palsy.

BIELCHOWSKY PHENOMENON (DARK WEDGE TEST)

This is a clinical test used to differentiate between DVD and alternating hyperphoria. One eye is occluded (a Spielmann occluder is preferable) and is seen to elevate under cover. With a spotlight at 6 m, a Sbiza bar (Fig. 4.49) is placed before the fixating eye and the filter density is gradually increased. The examiner observes the occluded eye, which will make a downward movement and may often pass below the midline if DVD is present. The occluded eye will start to elevate when the filter density is again decreased. By contrast, the elevated position of the occluded eye will remain unchanged when increasingly dense filters are placed before the fixing eye in cases of alternating hyperphoria.

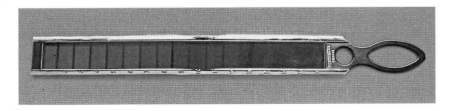

Figure 4.49   Sbiza bar.

FORCED DUCTION TEST

This test is used to assess the passive movement of the globe when active movement is restricted. It is used to determine the tone of the muscle by attempting to move the eye with forceps in different directions. The eye is anaesthetised and then gripped at opposite limbal points with two pairs of fine-toothed forceps. The eye is rotated into each position of gaze to assess the extent and ease of eye movement. A limitation of passive movement indicates a mechanical restriction (Stephens & Reinecke 1967).

FORCED GENERATION TEST

This test assesses the active muscle force in eye movement. By evaluating the amount of contraction force present in an apparently paresed muscle, an indication of muscle potential is gained. The anaesthetised eye is gripped at opposite limbal points with two pairs of fine-toothed forceps and held firmly. The patient is asked to move the eyes in the direction of gaze of the limited movement. The extent of muscle action can be felt by the examiner during the attempt to rotate the eye.

ORTHOPTIC EXERCISES

Orthoptic exercises are indicated in certain conditions:

- to increase control in latent deviations
- to increase control in intermittent deviations
- pre- or post-operatively to consolidate the result
- to achieve good binocular convergence.

Patients must be well motivated before receiving exercises.

Bar reading

Bar reading is based on the principle of crossed physiological diplopia. The patient's binocular visual acuity is assessed and the test commenced with print which is one size larger than the level of binocular visual acuity. The patient holds the book with the bar held against the bottom of the page. The bar will thus be at 8 cm from the page. The bar must be held steadily with the book at 1/3 m in a slightly depressed reading position. The patient is then instructed to read along the lines of the book (Fig. 4.50).

The head must be kept still and erect so that the patient does not look around the bar. Where binocular single vision is present, when the bar obstructs the vision of one eye looking at a word, the word is still seen by the other unobstructed eye and reading is therefore not impaired by the presence of the bar.

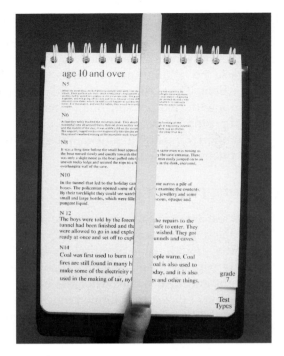

Figure 4.50   Bar reading.

Indications for use

- Treatment of intermittent fully accommodative esotropia.
- To improve binocular single vision.
- Treatment of decompensating heterophoria.
- Differential diagnosis between intermittent fully accommodative esotropia and convergence excess esotropia. Bar reading is not achieved with cases of convergence excess esotropia.

Stereograms

Stereograms are based on the principle of physiological diplopia, the ability to fuse dissimilar images giving rise to stereoscopic vision, and relative convergence.

Types of stereogram (Fig. 4.51)

- Non-stereoscopic – cats.
- Stereoscopic – buckets (clear and filled), RAF (ABC or 123).

The patient must have some form of binocular single vision to be able to appreciate stereograms.

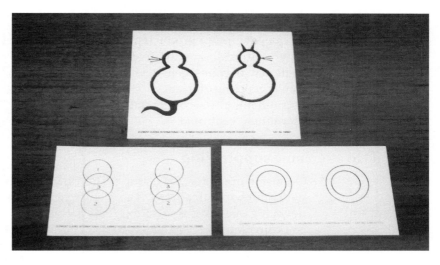

Figure 4.51   Stereograms.

Stereograms may be used in two positions using either near or distance fixation.

Near position

This position induces positive relative accommodative convergence. When the stereoscopic effect is perceived, the patient's eyes are converged on the fixation target but accommodation is exerted to a lesser extent to perceive a clear image of the images on the stereogram card.

The card should be held at arm's length in the primary position and the patient fixates a target between the card and the eyes. Three images should be appreciated on the card. If four images are seen, the position of the target should be adjusted until the middle two images are fused. The middle image should have all control features. When using a stereoscopic stereogram, ensure that depth is perceived. The patient should aim to see the three images clearly.

Distance position

This position induces negative relative convergence. When the stereoscopic effect is perceived, the patient's eyes are aligned on the distant fixation target but accommodation is exerted to a greater extent to perceive a clear image of the images on the stereogram card.

The patient fixates a target in the distance in the primary position and the card is held at about 1/3 m from the nose. The upper border of the card should appear to be just underneath the distance target. Three images should be appreciated and the middle image should have all control features present. The patient should aim to see all three images clearly.

Indications for use

- Cases of symptom-producing heterophoria. Stereograms are used in the near position with divergent deviations and in the distance position with convergent deviations.
- Convergence insufficiency.
- Intermittent fully accommodative esotropia.
- Intermittent exotropia.

Methods to overcome suppression

(1) Occlusion or monocular reading. This may be used in conjunction with amblyopia treatment. The fixing eye is occluded so that the deviating eye takes up fixation. This is combined with hand/eye co-ordination exercises.

(2) Red filter drawing. The patient wears a red filter over the deviating eye and an occluder over the other eye. A complementary coloured pen is used. This exercise may be used for 10–15 minutes daily. Diplopia is appreciated when the filter and occlusion are removed.

(3) Recognition of diplopia with red and green glasses and a spotlight.

(4) Sbiza bar. This is placed before the fixing eye in increasing density until the deviating eye fixates and diplopia is appreciated. The filter density is gradually reduced so that the deviating eye is still used and diplopia is present continually.

(5) Synoptophore. Suppression exercises include chasing (examiner moves one tube and patient chases with the other tube), flashing the light in the tube before the deviating eye, kinetic stimulation, tapping (moving the slide image before the deviating eye), and altering the rheostat intensity. Mayou slides may be used where the patient places a target into large boxes and the box size is gradually decreased.

(6) Septum. This dissociates the eyes in free space using an opaque card between the eyes.

(7) Vertical prism. This overcomes vertical suppression. The prism strength is gradually decreased while diplopia is appreciated.

(8) Cheiroscope. The patient looks through two eye pieces which are separated by an oblique mirror septum which is placed at an angle of 45 degrees. One eye sees a pad of paper and the other eye sees a pen which the patient is holding. The patient is instructed to draw pictures/shapes.

REFERENCES

Atkinson H, Braddick O, Pimm-Smith E, Ayling L & Sawyer R. (1981) Does the Catford drum give an accurate estimate of visual acuity? *British Journal of Ophthalmology*, 65: 652

Atkinson J, Anker S, Evans C, Hall R & Pimm-Smith E. (1988) Visual acuity testing of young children with the Cambridge crowding cards at 3 and 6 years. *Acta Ophthalmologica*, 66: 505

Bagolini B, Campos EC & Chiese C. (1985) The Irvine 4 dioptre prism test for the diagnosis of suppression: a reappraisal. *Binocular Vision*, 1: 77

Bielchowsky A. (1937) Application of the after image test in the investigation of squint. *American Journal of Ophthalmology*, 20: 408

Bixenman WW & von Noorden GK. (1982) Apparent foveal displacement in normal subjects and in cyclotropia. *Ophthalmologica*, 89: 58

Boeder P. (1957) An analysis of the general type of ocular rotations. *Archives of Ophthalmology*, 57: 200

Brodie SE. (1987) Photographic calibration of the Hirschberg test. *Investigative Ophthalmology and Visual Science*, 28: 736

Calcutt C. (1995) Is fixation preference assessment an effective method of detecting strabismus amblyopia? *British Orthoptic Journal*, 52: 29

Capobianca NM. (1952) The subjective measurement of the near point of convergence and its significance in the diagnosis of convergence insufficiency. *American Orthoptic Journal*, 2: 40

Cassin B. (1992) Alternate fixation in the non-strabismic child. *American Orthoptic Journal*, 32: 111

Cooper J & Warshowsky J. (1977) Lateral displacement as a response cue in the Titmus stereotest. *American Journal of Ophthalmic and Physiological Optics*, 54: 537

Dobson V, Teller D, Lee CP & Wade B. (1978) A behavioural method for efficient screening of visual acuity in young infants. I Preliminary laboratory development. *Investigative Ophthalmology and Visual Science*, 17: 1142

Dulley B & Harden A. (1974) Cyclo-torsion: a new method of measurement. *British Orthoptic Journal*, 31: 70

Ellis GS, Hartmann EE, Love A, May JG & Morgan KS. (1988) Teller acuity cards versus clinical judgement in the diagnosis of amblyopia with strabismus. *Ophthalmology*, 96: 788

Epstein DL & Tredici TJ. (1972) Use of the 4 dioptre base-in prism test in microexotropia. *American Journal of Ophthalmology*, 73: 340

Fantz RL. (1958) Pattern vision in young infants. *Psychological Research*, 8: 43

Frank JW. (1986) Scaling of visual acuity; applying a logarithmic scale. *American Orthoptic Journal*, 36: 11

Gray C, Anson A & Spencer A. (1996) The method of testing and recording of the postoperative diplopia test. *British Orthoptic Journal*, 53: 51

Hasebe S, Ohtsuki H, Kono R & Nakahira Y. (1998) Biometric confirmation of the Hirschberg ratio in strabismic children. *Investigative Ophthalmology and Visual Science*, 39: 2782

Henshall VS & Rowe FJ. (2002) Diagnostic, aetiological and management considerations in accommodative insufficiency. *British Orthoptic Journal*, 59: 19

Hocking GE & Gage JE. (2002) The relationship between the strength of sensory fusion and motor fusion amplitude. *British Orthoptic Journal*, 59: 45

Horwood AM. (1994) The Cardiff acuity test in amblyopic children. *British Orthoptic Journal*, 51: 19

Katz B, Sireteanu R. (1990) The Teller acuity card test: a useful method for the clinical routine? *Clinical Visual Science*, 5: 307

Krimsky E. (1943) The binocular examination of the young child. *American Journal of Ophthalmology*, 26: 624

Lang J. (1983) A new stereotest. *Journal of Pediatric Ophthalmology and Strabismus*, 20: 72

LaRoche R & von Noorden GK. (1982) Theoretical and practical evaluation of a simple stereotest. *Investigative Ophthalmology and Visual Science*, 22 (suppl): 266

Leat SJ, Li W & Epp K. (1999) Crowding in central and eccentric vision; the effects of contour interaction and attention. *Investigative Ophthalmology and Visual Science*, 40: 504

Mayer DL. (1986) Acuity of amblyopic children for small field gratings and recognition stimuli. *Investigative Ophthalmology and Visual Science*, 27: 1148

Mayer DL, Beiser AS, Warner AF, Pratt EM, Raye KN & Lang JM. (1995) Monocular acuity norms for the Teller acuity cards between ages one month and four years. *Investigative Ophthalmology and Visual Science*, 36: 671

Mayer L, Fulton A & Rodier D. (1984) Grating and recognition acuities of pediatric patients. *Ophthalmology*, 91: 947

Moseley MJ, Fielder AR, Thompson JR, Minshull C & Price D. (1988) Grating and recognition acuity of young amblyopes. *British Journal of Ophthalmology*, 72: 50

Narbheram J & Firth AY. (1997) Prism fusion range; blur point, break point and recovery point. *British Orthoptic Journal*, 54: 2

Oguz H & Oguz V. (2000) The effects of experimentally induced anisometropia on stereopsis. *Journal of Pediatric Ophthalmology and Strabismus*, 37: 214

Okuda F, Apt L & Wanter B. (1977) Evaluation of the TNO random-dot stereogram test. *American Orthoptic Journal*, 27: 124

Quinn GE, Berlin JA & James M. (1993) The Teller acuity card procedure: three testers in a clinical setting. *Ophthalmology*, 100: 488

Romano PE & von Noorden GK. (1969) Atypical responses to the 4 dioptre prism test. *American Journal of Ophthalmology*, 67: 935

Ruttum M & von Noorden GK. (1984) The Bagolini striated lens test for cyclotropia. *Documenta Ophthalmologica*, 58: 131

Sharma K & Abdul-Rahim AS. (1992) Vertical fusion amplitude in normal adults. *American Journal of Ophthalmology*, 114: 636

Simons K. (1981) A comparison of the Frisby, random-dot E, TNO and Randot circles stereotests in screening and office use. *Archives of Ophthalmology*, 99: 446

Simons K & Reinecke RD. (1974) A reconsideration of amblyopia screening and stereopsis. *American Journal of Ophthalmology*, 78: 707

Sireteanu R, Franius M & Katz B. (1990) A perspective on psychophysical testing in children. *Eye*, 4: 794

Sloan LC. (1959) New test charts for the measurement of visual acuity at far and near. *American Journal of Ophthalmology*, 48: 807

Spielmann A. (1986) A translucent occluder for studying eye positions under unilateral and bilateral cover test. *American Orthoptic Journal*, 36: 65

Stephens KF & Reinecke RD. (1967) Quantitative forced duction. *Transactions of the American Academy of Ophthalmology and Otolaryngology*, 71: 324

Teller DY. (1997) First glances: the vision of infants (Friedenwald lecture). *Investigative Ophthalmology and Visual Science*, 38: 2183

Thompson JT & Guyton DL. (1983) Ophthalmic prisms: measurement errors and how to minimise them. *Ophthalmology*, 90: 204

Thompson JT & Guyton DL. (1985) Prisms: deviant behaviour at near. *Ophthalmology*, 92: 684

Whittaker KW, O'Flynn E & Manners FM. (2000) Diagnosis of amblyopia using the 10 dioptre fixation test; a proposed modification for patients with unilateral ptosis. *Journal of Pediatric Ophthalmology and Strabismus*, 37: 21

Woodhouse JM, Adoh TO, Oduwaiye KA *et al.* (1992) New acuity test for toddlers. *Ophthalmology Physiology and Optics*, 12: 249

Wright KW, Kalonker F & Edelman P. (1981) 10-dioptre fixation test for amblyopia. *Archives of Ophthalmology*, 99: 1242

Zipf RF. (1976) Binocular fixation pattern. *Archives of Ophthalmology*, 94: 401

FURTHER READING

Abrams D. (1993) *Duke Elder's Practice of Refraction*, 10th edn. Churchill Livingstone, Edinburgh

Adler FH & Jackson FE. (1947) Correlations between sensory and motor disturbances in convergent squint. *Archives of Ophthalmology*, 38: 289

Ambrose PS & von Noorden GK. (1976) Past-pointing in comitant strabismus. *Archives of Ophthalmology*, 94: 1896

Archer SM. (1988) Stereotest artefacts and the strabismic patient. *Graefe's Archives of Clinical and Experimental Ophthalmology*, 226: 313

Archer SM, Miller KK & Helveston EM. (1987) Stereoscopic contours and optokinetic nystagmus in normal and stereoblind subjects. *Vision Research*, 27: 841

Avilla C & von Noorden GK. (1981) Limitation of the TNO random dot stereo test for visual screening. *American Orthoptic Journal*, 31: 87

Bagolini B. (1967) Anomalous correspondence: definition and diagnostic methods. *Documenta Ophthalmologica*, 23: 346

Bagolini B. (1976) I Sensorial anomalies in strabismus (suppression, anomalous correspondence amblyopia). *Documenta Ophthalmologica*, 41: 1

Bagolini B. (1976) II Sensori-motorial anomalies in strabismus (anomalous movements). *Documenta Ophthalmologica*, 41: 23

Bagolini B. (1982) Anomalous fusion. In: van Balen AThM & Houtman WA (eds) *Documenta Ophthalmologica Proceedings Series, No. 32*. Junk, The Hague, p. 41

Bailey IL & Lovie JE. (1976) New design principles for visual acuity letter charts. *American Journal of Optometry and Physiological Optics*, 53: 740

Birch E, Shimojo S & Held R. (1985) Preferential looking assessment of fusion and stereopsis in infants aged 1–6 months. *Investigative Ophthalmology and Visual Science*, 26: 366

Boothe RG, Dobson V & Teller DY. (1985) Postnatal development of vision in human and non-human primates. *Annual Review of Neurosciences*, 8: 495

Brown EVL. (1938) Net average yearly change in refraction of atropinized eyes from birth to beyond middle age. *Archives of Ophthalmology*, 19: 719

Burian HM. (1941) Fusional movements in permanent strabismus. A study of the role of the central and peripheral retinal regions in the aetiology of binocular vision in squint. *Archives of Ophthalmology*, 26: 626

Burian HM. (1945) Sensorial retinal relationship in concomitant strabismus. *Transactions of the American Ophthalmological Society*, 81: 373

Burian HM. (1951) Anomalous retinal correspondence: its essence and its significance in diagnosis and treatment. *American Journal of Ophthalmology*, 34: 237

Cashell GTW & Durran IM. (1980) *Handbook of Orthoptic Principles*, 4th edn. Churchill Livingstone, Edinburgh

Dobson V & Teller D. (1978) Visual acuity in human infants: a review and comparison of behavioural and electrophysiological studies. *Vision Research*, 18: 1469

Fincham EF. (1955) The proportion of muscle force required for accommodation. *Journal of Physiology*, 128: 99

Fincham EF & Walton J. (1957) The reciprocal actions of accommodation and convergence. *Journal of Physiology (London)*, 135: 488

Firth AY & Whittle JP. (1994) Clarification of the correct and the incorrect use of ophthalmic prisms in the measurement of strabismus. *British Orthoptic Journal*, 51: 15

Friendly DS, Jaafer MS & Morillo DL. (1990) A comparative study of grating and recognition visual acuity testing in children with anisometropic amblyopia without strabismus. *American Journal of Ophthalmology*, 110: 293

Frisby JP, Mein J, Saye A & Stanworth A. (1975) Use of random dot stereograms in the clinical assessment of strabismic patients. *British Journal of Ophthalmology*, 59: 545

Georgievski Z. (1994) The effects of central and peripheral binocular visual field masking on fusional-disparity vergence. *Australian Orthoptic Journal*, 30: 41

Goodier HM. (1981) The evaluation of the Bielchowsky head tilt test. In: Mein J, Moore S (eds) *Orthoptics, Research and Practice*. Kimpton, London, p. 189

Gorman TJ, Cogan DG & Gellis SS. (1957) Apparatus for grading visual acuity of infants on basis of optokinetic nystagmus. *Pediatrics*, 19: 1088

Guyton DL. (1988) Ocular torsion: sensorimotor principles. *Graefe's Archives of Clinical and Experimental Ophthalmology*, 226: 241

Harrad R, Sengpiel F & Blakemore C. (1996) Physiology of suppression in strabismic amblyopia. *British Journal of Ophthalmology*, 80: 373

Held R. (1988) Normal visual development and its deviations. In: Lennerstrand D, von Noorden GK, Campos EC (eds) *Strabismus and Amblyopia*. Wenner Gren International Symposium Series No. 49. Macmillan Press, London, p. 247

Held R, Birch E & Gwiazda J. (1980) Stereoacuity in human infants. *Proceedings of the National Academy of Science (USA)*, 77: 5572

Hendrickson AE. (1994) Primate foveal development: a microcosmos of current questions in neurobiology. *Investigative Ophthalmology and Visual Science*, 35: 3129

Hinchliffe HA. (1978) Clinical evaluation of stereopsis. *British Orthoptic Journal*, 35: 46

Hugonnier R & Hugonnier S. (1969) *Strabismus, Heterophoria, Ocular Motor Paralysis. Clinical Ocular Muscle Imbalance*. Mosby, St Louis

Irvine SR. (1944) A simple test for binocular fixation: clinical application useful in the appraisal of ocular dominance, amblyopia ex anopsia, minimal strabismus and malingering. *American Journal of Ophthalmology*, 27: 740

Jampolsky A. (1955) Characteristics of suppression in strabismus. *Archives of Ophthalmology*, 54: 683

Jampolsky A. (1971) A simplified approach to strabismus diagnosis. In: *Symposium on Strabismus. Transactions of the New Orleans Academy of Ophthalmology*. Mosby, St Louis, p. 66

Jampolsky A. (1986) Management of vertical strabismus. In: Allen JH (ed) *Pediatric Ophthalmology and Strabismus. Transactions of the New Orleans Academy of Ophthalmology*. Raven Press, New York, p. 141

Johnson F, Harcourt B & Fox A. (1987) The clinical assessment of cyclodeviation. In: Lenk-Schafer M, Calcutt C, Doyle M & Moore S (eds) *Transactions of the Sixth International Orthoptic Congress*. British Orthoptic Society, London, p. 179

Kay H. (1984) A new picture visual acuity test. *British Orthoptic Journal*, 41: 77

Ketley MJ, Powell CM, Lee JP & Elston J. (1987) Botulinum toxin adaptation test: the use of botulinum toxin in the investigation of the sensory state in strabismus. In: Lenk-Schafer M, Calcutt C, Doyle M & Moore S (eds) *Transactions of the Sixth International Orthoptic Congress*. British Orthoptic Society, London, p. 289

Kertesz AE & Sullivan MJ. (1978) The effect of stimulus size on human cyclofusional response. *Vision Research*, 18: 567

Kohler L & Stigmar G. (1973) Vision screening in 4 year old children. *Acta Paediatrica Scandinavica*, 62: 17

Kushner BJ, Kraft SE & Vrabec DP. (1984) Ocular torsional movements in humans with normal and abnormal ocular motility. Part 1: objective measurements. *Journal of Pediatric Ophthalmology and Strabismus*, 21: 172

Kushner GJ, Lucchese NJ & Morton GV. (1995) Grating acuity with Teller cards compared to Snellen acuity in literate patients. *Archives of Ophthalmology*, 113: 485

Lancaster WB. (1939) *Detecting, measuring, plotting and interpreting ocular deviations*. AMA, New York

Lang J. (1991) Nine years experience with the Lang stereotest. In: Tillson G, Doyle M, Louly M & Verlohr D (eds) *Transactions of the Seventh International Orthoptic Congress*. Nurnberg, Germany, p. 163

Levine MH. (1969) Evaluation of Bielchowsky's head tilt test. *Archives of Ophthalmology*, 82: 433

Luke NE. (1970) Antisuppression exercises in exodeviations. *American Orthoptic Journal*, 20: 100

Lyle TK & Wybar KC. (1967) *Lyle and Jackson's Practical Orthoptics in the Treatment of Squint*, 5th edn. Lewis, London

Marsh WR, Rawlings SC & Mumma JV. (1980) Evaluation of clinical stereoacuity tests. *Ophthalmology*, 87: 1265

Martens TG & Ogle KN. (1959) Observations on accommodative convergence, especially on its non-linear relationships. *American Journal of Ophthalmology*, 47: 455

McDonald M, Dobson V, Sebris SL, Baitch L, Verner D & Teller DY. (1985) The acuity card procedure: a rapid test of infant visual acuity. *Investigative Ophthalmology and Visual Science*, 26: 1158

McKenzie L. (1991) The ocular motor development of infants. *Australian Orthoptic Journal*, 27: 19

Moore S. (1963) Orthoptic treatment for intermittent exotropia. *American Orthoptic Journal*, 13: 14

Ogle KN. (1951) Distortion of the image by prisms. *Journal of the Optical Society of America*, 41: 1023

Plenty J. (1988) A new classification for intermittent exotropia. *British Orthoptic Journal*, 45: 19

Pratt-Johnson J & Tillson G. (1994) *Management of Strabismus and Amblyopia. A Practical Guide*. Thieme, New York

Price D, Minshull C, Moseley M & Fielder A. (1987) The acuity card procedure: its use in orthoptics. *British Orthoptic Journal*, 44: 34

Reinecke R & Simons K. (1974) A new stereoscopic test for amblyopia screening. *American Journal of Ophthalmology*, 78: 714

Rowe FJ. (1994) Measurement of manifest deviations using corneal reflections. *Optometry Today*, 21: 36

Ruttum M & von Noorden GK. (1983) Adaptation to tilting of the visual environments in cyclotropia. *American Journal of Ophthalmology*, 96: 229

Scattergood KD, Brown M & Guyton D. (1983) Artefacts introduced by spectacle lens in the measurement of strabismic deviations. *American Journal of Ophthalmology*, 96: 439

Sheridan MD. (1969) Visual screening procedures for very young or handicapped children. In: Gardiner P, MacKeith R & Smith V (eds) *Aspects of Developmental and Pediatric Ophthalmology*. Heinemann Medical, London, p. 39

Slataper FJ. (1950) Age norms of refraction and vision. *Archives of Ophthalmology*, 43: 466

Sloan L, Sears ML & Jablonski MD. (1960) Convergence–accommodation relationships. *Archives of Ophthalmology*, 63: 283

Stuart J & Burian H. (1962) A study of separation difficulty. Its relationship to visual acuity in normal and amblyopic eyes. *American Journal of Ophthalmology*, 53: 471

Veronneau-Troutman S. (1994) *Prisms in the Medical and Surgical Management of Strabismus*. Mosby, St Louis

von Noorden GK. (1986) Superior oblique paralysis. *Archives of Ophthalmology*, 104: 1771

von Noorden GK & Crawford MLJ. (1980) The sensitive period. *Transactions of the Ophthalmological Society of the United Kingdom*, 99: 442

Wisnicki HJ & Guyton DL. (1986) A modified corneal light reflex test with distance fixation. *American Journal of Ophthalmology*, 102: 661

Yuodelis C & Hendrickson A. (1986) A qualitative and quantitative analysis of the human fovea during development. *Vision Research*, 26: 847

SECTION II

Chapter 5
Heterophoria

Where heterophoria is present, both visual axes are directed towards the fixation point but deviate on dissociation. Orthophoria occurs where both visual axes are directed towards the fixation point and do not deviate on dissociation.

Classification

- Esophoria
  - convergence excess
  - divergence weakness
  - non-specific
- Exophoria
  - convergence weakness
  - divergence excess
  - non-specific
- Hyperphoria/hypophoria
- Alternating hyperphoria/hypophoria
- Cyclophoria

Aetiology

Esophoria
- anatomical – enophthalmos, narrow IPD, extraocular muscle anomalies
- refractive – suprable hypermetropia, anisohypermetropia
- high AC/A ratio
- weak negative fusional reserves

Exophoria
- anatomical – exophthalmos, wide IPD, extraocular muscle anomalies
- refractive – acquired myopia, presbyopia, anisomyopia
- weak positive fusional reserves
- passage of time

Hyperphoria/hypophoria
- refractive – high myopia (heavy eye syndrome)
- weak vertical fusional reserves
- anatomical – displaced globes, abnormal extraocular muscles, ptosis

Cyclophoria
- oblique astigmatism

A compensated or controlled heterophoria is asymptomatic and accounts for the majority of the population. Decompensation occurs with the inability to control the angle of deviation which produces symptoms in older age groups.

Causes of decompensation

- **Optical**. Under-, over- or uncorrected refractive errors. Wrongly prescribed or badly fitting spectacles. Aniseikonia.
- **Medical**. Poor general health. Fatigue. Head injury affecting fusional abilities. Drugs affecting accommodation. Alcohol. Dissociative, e.g. an eye pad for an ocular infection may decompensate an existing large angle heterophoria. Visual field loss.

Esophoria

The eyes become convergent on dissociation.

- **Convergence excess**: esophoria is greater on near fixation than distant fixation.
- **Divergence weakness**: esophoria is greater on distant fixation than near fixation.
- **Non-specific**: esophoria which does not vary significantly in degree for any distance.

Exophoria

The eyes become divergent on dissociation.

- **Convergence weakness**: exophoria is greater on near fixation than distant fixation.
- **Divergence excess**: exophoria is greater on distant fixation than near fixation.
- **Non-specific**: exophoria which does not vary significantly in degree for any distance.

Hyperphoria/hypophoria

A vertical deviation occurring on dissociation in which one eye rotates upwards and the other downwards, depending on the fixation.

Alternating hyperphoria

Either eye rotates upwards on dissociation as a result of extraocular muscle imbalance.

Alternating hypophoria

Either eye rotates downwards on dissociation as a result of extraocular muscle imbalance.

Cyclophoria

Either eye wheel rotates on dissociation, so that the upper end of the vertical axis is nasal (incyclophoria) or temporal (excyclophoria).

Incomitant heterophoria

The angle of deviation differs fixing either eye and in different positions of gaze. This is often due to an extraocular muscle underaction and treatment usually involves use of prisms or surgery.

Hemifield slide

Significant visual field loss in either eye that includes the macula may result in loss of fusion and dissociation of heterophoria to esotropia or exotropia. Complete bitemporal deficit in particular interferes with fusion. The loss of temporal visual field in both eyes disrupts stimulation of corresponding retinal points and results in failure to generate corrective fusional vergences, leading to decompensation of heterophoria (Fisher *et al.* 1968; Roper-Hall 1976; Fritz & Brodsky 1992).

Hemifield slide occurs where the visual fields of the two eyes are separated from each other as in bitemporal hemianopia and cannot be joined by the normal fusional vergence reflex, creating reading problems (Shainberg *et al.* 1995; Rowe 1996). Patients have a blind area distal to the fixation point which is termed post-fixational blindness (Fig. 5.1). When they fixate bifoveally they are unable to locate targets beyond the fixation target and cannot respond to uncrossed physiological diplopia or base-in prisms because of the loss of divergence disparity (Shainberg *et al.* 1995; Rowe 1996).

Investigation of heterophoria

Case history   Symptoms of decompensation are those of headaches, asthenopia, blurring of print, intermittent diplopia and confusion if the deviation has become manifest. Predisposing factors include a change in occupation, poor general health, general fatigue and change in refractive error.

Visual acuity   Ensure acuities are appropriately corrected with any required refractive error.

Cover test   The rate of recovery and the size of heterophoria should be noted as these factors will denote the state of control of the deviation.

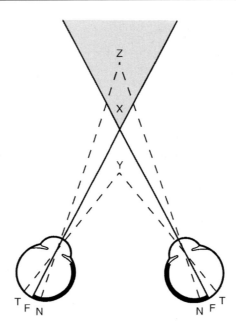

Figure 5.1   Post-fixational blindness. X is the object of fixation and Z is a point behind the point of fixation. The image falls on impaired nasal retina and is not seen. Y is a point in front of the point of fixation. The image falls on temporal retina and is seen as physiological crossed diplopia

Convergence   This is important with exodeviations as a reduced or remote near point indicates decompensation, in part, of the exophoria.

Binocular function   Fusional reserves may be reduced and it is necessary to assess the range of fusional convergence and divergence which are used to compensate for exo- and esodeviations respectively. Binocular visual acuity will show decompensation when accommodation is interrupted.

Measurements   The near point of accommodation, stereopsis and angle of deviation are assessed.

Monocular occlusion   Ocular and non-ocular symptoms may be differentiated by using monocular occlusion during reading for a period of at least 1 hour. Symptoms will improve if ocular.

Management

Indications for treatment include:

- symptom-producing deviations
- children where there is a possibility of decompensation in later life
- where necessary to achieve specific standards required for certain careers.

Correct any existing refractive error as an uncorrected refractive error may result in decompensation of a heterophoria.

Orthoptic exercises. For esophoria, it is important to improve negative relative convergence with stereograms, bar reading and fusional exercises with base-in prisms and the divergent range on the synoptophore. For exophoria, it is important to improve positive relative convergence, binocular convergence, fusional exercises with base-out prisms and the convergent range on the synoptophore.

Prisms may be used with moderate or large angle deviations. The deviation should be only partially corrected (often half the prism cover test measurement) so that fusional vergences continue to be exercised.

Surgery. With moderate or large angles it may be necessary to reduce the angle surgically as fusional vergences may not be sufficient to maintain comfortable control at all times.

Botulinum toxin can be used both diagnostically and therapeutically and a single administration may be sufficient to allow a return to asymptomatic binocular single vision.

REFERENCES

Fisher NF, Jampolsky A & Flom MC. (1968) Traumatic bitemporal hemianopia: II Binocular co-operation. *American Journal of Ophthalmology*, 65: 574

Fritz KJ & Brodsky MC. (1992) Elusive neuro-ophthalmic reading impairment. *American Orthoptic Journal*, 42: 125

Roper-Hall G. (1976) Effect of visual field defects on binocular single vision. *American Orthoptic Journal*, 26: 74

Rowe FJ. (1996) Visual disturbances in chiasmal lesions. *British Orthoptic Journal*, 53: 1

Shainberg MJ, Roper-Hall G & Chung SM. (1995) Binocular problems in bitemporal hemianopia. *American Orthoptic Journal*, 45: 132

FURTHER READING

Abrahamson M, Fabian G & Sjostrand J. (1992) Refraction changes in children developing convergent or divergent strabismus. *British Journal of Ophthalmology*, 76: 723

Albert DG & Hiles DA. (1969) Myopia, bifocals and accommodation. *American Orthoptic Journal*, 19: 59

Hugonnier R & Clayette-Hugonnier S. (1969) *Strabismus, Heterophoria, Ocular Motor Paralysis: Clinical Muscle Imbalance* (trans. Veronneua-Troutman S). Mosby, St Louis

Knapp P. (1975) The use of membrane prisms. *Transactions of the American Academy of Ophthalmology and Otolaryngology*, 79: 718

Lynburn EG & MacEwen CJ. (1994) Botulinum toxin in the management of heterophoria. *British Orthoptic Journal*, 51: 38

Neikter B. (1994) Effects of diagnostic occlusion on ocular alignment in normal subjects. *Strabismus*, 2: 67

Paris V & Weiss JB. (1995) Treatment of symptomatic heterophoria by small prisms. In: Louly M, Doyle M, Hirai T & Tomlinson E (eds) *Transactions of the Eighth International Orthoptic Congress.* Japan, p. 113

Veronneau-Troutman S. (1971) Fresnel prism membrane in the treatment of strabismus. *Canadian Journal of Ophthalmology,* 6: 249

Chapter 6
Heterotropia

Heterotropia is a condition in which one or other visual axis is not directed towards the fixation point. The incidence of strabismus is 5–8% in the general population. Concomitant strabismus is strabismus in which the angle of deviation remains the same in all directions of gaze, whichever eye is fixing.

There are a number of different forms of heterotropia:

- esotropia
- exotropia
- hypertropia
- hypotropia
- cyclotropia
- dissociated vertical deviation (DVD)
- dissociated horizontal deviation (DHD).

Esotropia

Esotropia is a condition in which one or other eye deviates nasally.

Classification

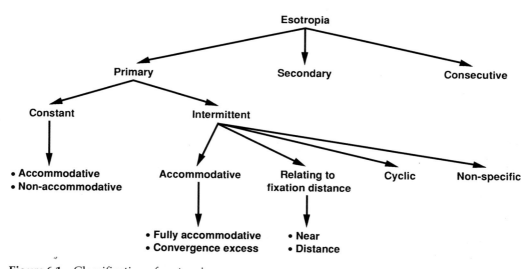

Figure 6.1　Classification of esotropia.

Aetiology

Primary esotropia

Constant
- Accommodative: anatomical, proprioceptive, hereditary, always with hypermetropia or high AC/A ratio
- Non-accommodative: anatomical (narrow IPD, enophthalmos, muscle anomalies), proprioceptive, hereditary, congenital nystagmus, high congenital myopia, unknown

Intermittent
- Fully accommodative: suprable hypermetropia, < +6.0 DS
- Convergence excess: high AC/A ratio
- Near: proximal convergence, muscle anomalies
- Distance: muscle anomalies
- Cyclic: biorhythms, general hyperactivity of the central nervous system
- Non-specific: any of above, weak fusion

Secondary esotropia
- Loss/impairment of vision: 6 months to 7 years as accommodative convergence is most active

Consecutive esotropia
- Surgical overcorrection of divergent deviation

Factors necessary for development of binocular single vision

(1) Normal anatomy of the eye and orbit.
(2) Normal refractive systems.
(3) Normal sensory, psychomotor and motor pathways.
(4) Normal mental development.

Interruption of any of these factors can result in development of a manifest deviation.

Primary esotropia

The convergent deviation constitutes the initial defect.

CONSTANT ESOTROPIA WITH AN ACCOMMODATIVE ELEMENT

The esotropia is present under all conditions and increases when accommodation is exerted.

Investigation

Case history   An early, insidious onset, generally between 1 and 3 years, is documented. Check for precipitating causes and family history.

Refraction	A hypermetropic error, often associated with astigmatism and aniso-metropia, is detected.
Visual acuity	Amblyopia may be present, particularly in cases of constant unilateral strabismus.
Cover test	The angle of deviation decreases when hypermetropia is corrected and may be less marked for distance fixation, although the deviation remains manifest. There may be an associated DVD (see page 144–6) and/or vertical deviation which is most often due to inferior oblique overaction.
Convergence	Convergence to 6 cm with the same angle of deviation indicates abnormal retinal correspondence (Moore 1990). Convergence with reducing angle of deviation to intersection of the visual axes followed by symmetrical convergence of either eye indicates normal retinal correspondence. Divergence following intersection of the visual axes indicates absence of retinal correspondence. Retinal correspondence cannot be estimated where there is convergence to 6 cm with reducing angle of deviation as intersection of the visual axes does not occur.
Binocular function	Free space tests may be used to assess the presence of abnormal retinal correspondence with the strabismic angle of deviation and normal retinal correspondence at the corrected angle. A binocular response is indicative of abnormal retinal correspondence but will generally be seen in small angle deviations. Free space fusion and stereopsis may be further tested to examine the quality of abnormal retinal correspondence. Suppression responses on free space tests do not give an indication of retinal correspondence.
	Retinal correspondence may be evaluated in full using the synoptophore. Normal retinal correspondence is present where superimposition is achieved at the full corrected angle of deviation. Abnormal retinal correspondence is present where superimposition is achieved at the angle of deviation. Quality of retinal correspondence, whether normal or abnormal, may be determined by assessing the fusion and stereopsis responses at these angles.
	Where suppression responses are obtained it is not possible to determine retinal correspondence. Further assessments may therefore be undertaken, including after-images and using vertical prisms to move the image out of the suppression area and align the vertically displaced images using horizontal prisms. Where there is suppression and the patient is aged seven years or greater, the depth and area of suppression should be measured in order to assess the risk of postoperative diplopia.
Angle of deviation	This should be measured with and without the hypermetropic correction and for near and distance fixation.
AC/A ratio	This is assessed preferably by the gradient method and may be high.

Management

Correct the refractive error and treat amblyopia if present. Surgery may be for a cosmetic or functional result.

- Cosmetic: the aim is to undercorrect the deviation to guard against a later onset of consecutive exotropia.
- Functional: the aim is to obtain parallel visual axes to restore binocular single vision when wearing the corrective prescription, thereby resulting in a fully accommodative esotropia which may then be treated if indicated.

Surgery may be in the form of a unilateral medial rectus recession and lateral rectus resection or bilateral medial recti recessions. DVD and associated muscle overactions may be corrected when performing the horizontal muscle surgery.

CONSTANT ESOTROPIA WITHOUT AN ACCOMMODATIVE ELEMENT

The esotropia is present under all conditions and is unaffected by the state of accommodation. Presence of latent nystagmus, DVD, horizontal monocular asymmetry of smooth pursuit and monocular asymmetry of OKN aid the diagnosis of early versus late onset strabismus (Schor *et al.* 1997).

Infantile esotropia (Fig. 6.2)

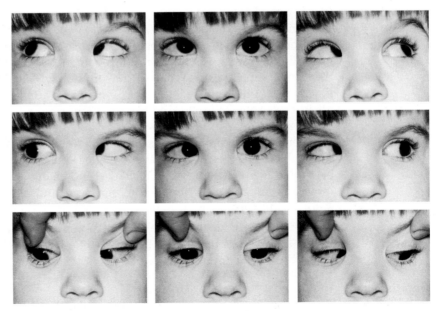

Figure 6.2   Infantile esotropia.

Infantile esotropia occurs in 0.1–1% of the population (Graham 1974; Nixon *et al.* 1985). It can be called the essential infantile esotropia syndrome because of its specific association with DVD and manifest latent nystagmus.

Investigation

Case history   Infantile esotropia is associated with an early onset within the first six months of life (Nixon *et al.* 1985; Friedrick & de Decker 1987).

Refraction   There may be an associated degree of hypermetropia.

Abnormal head posture   There may be a face turn to adduct the fixing eye.

Visual acuity   There is a low incidence of amblyopia due to alternation of the deviation. Amblyopia is more common in infantile esotropia after treatment (Costenbader 1961; von Noorden 1988a; Shauly *et al.* 1994) but not before (Friedman *et al.* 1980; Calcutt & Murray 1998).

Cover test   A large angle alternating esotropia is demonstrated and there may be associated DVD and latent nystagmus which is usually detected after the age of 2 years (Lang 1968).

Ocular motility   Cross-fixation is characteristic and limited abduction may be noted.

Stimulation of the vestibulo-ocular reflex by swinging is useful in assessing the degree of abduction in a young infant. Cross-fixation occurs where the patient uses the right eye to fix in the left field of gaze and the left eye to fix in the right field of gaze.

Optokinetic nystagmus   This response is often asymmetrical with an absent or defective nasal to temporal response (Mein 1983; Demer & von Noorden 1988).

Binocular function   Patients are usually too young for assessment of retinal correspondence but in older patients this may be assessed by correcting the angle of deviation either in free space or using the synoptophore.

Angle of deviation   Measurement of the deviation is most often assessed by corneal reflections in this younger age group. The measurement often exceeds 30 prism dioptres.

Associated syndromes   Congenital strabismus syndrome (Lang 1968) includes esotropia, latent nystagmus and DVD.

Ciancia syndrome includes infantile esotropia, latent nystagmus, abnormal head posture to adduct the eye and apparently limited abduction in either eye (Helveston 1993).

Nystagmus block esotropia

This is a condition in which manifest nystagmus is 'blocked' either totally or partially by placing one or both eyes in an adducted position. The presence of nystagmus in the primary position is often not detectable.

Investigation

Case history   An early onset within the first six months of life is typical. Esotropia develops as the patient constantly adducts the fixing eye to compensate for congenital nystagmus, leading to constant esotropia. There is often an abnormal head posture to maintain one eye in adduction (Dell'Osso *et al.* 1983).

Visual acuity   Amblyopia is common.

Abnormal head posture   Face turn to adduct fixating eye.

Cover test   A variable large angle esotropia is present and is usually unilateral although both eyes often appear to be convergent.

Ocular motility   An increase in the amplitude of nystagmus on lateroversions is seen. On attempted abduction, the nystagmus often becomes apparent.

Angle of deviation   It is difficult to measure the angle with a prism bar as the eye continues to adduct on using base-out prisms. The position of corneal reflections is assessed using Hirschberg's method to estimate the angle of deviation.

Normosensorial esotropia

This later onset esotropia occurs after a period of normal development of binocular single vision.

Investigation

Case history   Onset is from the age of 2–4 years. The deviation may be intermittent for a short period of time but soon becomes constant and diplopia is appreciated by the older age group (Lang 1981, 1986). It may occur after temporary occlusion of one eye, resulting in disruption of fusion, or may be spontaneous and possibly precipitated by illness.

Cover test   A large angle of deviation is demonstrated.

Binocular function   Normal retinal correspondence and fusion are demonstrable on correction of the deviation.

Differential diagnosis   It is important to ensure that the deviation is not due to an acquired VI nerve palsy. The optic discs should be examined to exclude the presence of papilloedema.

Esotropia with myopia

This occurs in a small percentage of patients with non-accommodative esotropia. Binocular convergence develops so that the patient may use the far point but is not relaxed on distance viewing, resulting in esotropia. The deviation then becomes constant and progressively increases in angle.

Investigation

Case history   This esotropic deviation may present in childhood but is more common in adults and diplopia may be appreciated (Hugonnier & Clayette Hugonnier 1969).

Refraction	A high degree of myopia is detected.
Visual acuity	The level of acuity is often affected by degenerative myopic fundus changes.
Cover test	The deviation progressively increases on dissociation.
Ocular motility	An associated limitation of abduction may be noted.
Binocular function	Normal retinal correspondence and fusion should be demonstrable on correction of the deviation but are often difficult to assess due to the reduced levels of visual acuity and the marked angle of deviation.
Differential diagnosis	It is necessary to ensure that the deviation is not due to thyroid eye disease as both have prominent eyes and may show limited abduction.

Management of constant non-accommodative esotropia

Correct the refractive error and treat amblyopia if present. Surgery may be for a cosmetic or functional result.

Congenital/infantile. Aim for parallel visual axes. It is often advocated that if surgery is performed before two years of age, there is a greater potential for achieving binocular vision (normal retinal correspondence or more commonly abnormal retinal correspondence) (Ing 1983; Parks 1984). The procedure may involve bilateral medial rectus recessions or bilateral medial rectus recessions combined with unilateral lateral rectus resection if there is a large angle deviation. Surgery may also include use of Faden sutures (Rizk 1999). Treatment, however, is usually with bilateral medial recti recessions (Ing *et al.* 1966; von Noorden *et al.* 1972; Prieto-Diaz 1980, 1985; Helveston *et al.* 1983; Kushner & Morton 1984; Weakley *et al.* 1991). Botulinum toxin has been used as a sole therapeutic intervention with some success in achieving long-term alignment of the visual axes (Campos *et al.* 2000; McNeer *et al.* 2000).

Nystagmus block syndrome. Surgery is unpredictable. A similar procedure to that in infantile esotropia is employed (von Noorden & Wong 1986).

Normo-sensorial. Aim for parallel visual axes or overcorrect slightly as a functional result is indicated.

Esotropia with myopia. Disappointing results are common as the deviation tends to recur.

INTERMITTENT ESOTROPIA

The esotropia is only present under certain conditions.

ACCOMMODATIVE ESOTROPIA

The convergent deviation is affected by the state of accommodation and this is the primary factor in the aetiology of the squint.

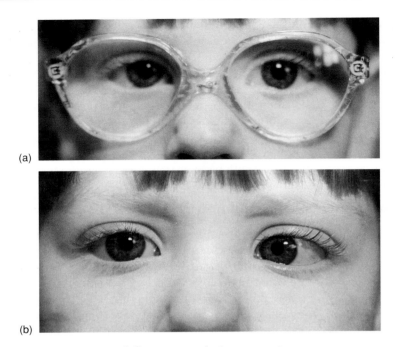

(a)

(b)

Figure 6.3   Intermittent fully accommodative esotropia.

Fully accommodative esotropia (Fig. 6.3)

Binocular single vision is present for all distances when the hypermetropia is corrected.

Investigation

Case history   An intermittent onset is usual between the age of two and five years. It may be precipitated by illness and there is often a positive family history for squint and/or hypermetropia.

Refraction   There is a moderate degree of hypermetropia and there may also be a degree of astigmatism and/or anisometropia. Ensure full prescription is given as deviation may remain intermittently manifest with glasses otherwise.

Visual acuity   Amblyopia is uncommon but may be present if the refractive correction is not worn until after a unilateral deviation has become well established.

Cover test   A manifest deviation is seen without the spectacle correction but is controlled to a latent deviation with the full hypermetropic correction.

Binocular function   Binocular single vision is demonstrated for near and distance fixation when fully corrected. Usually normal retinal correspondence is present unless the deviation is controlled to a microtropia where there is anisohypermetropia and a central suppression scotoma. Without glasses, there is suppression with the manifest esotropia. Older children may be aware of the esotropia without glasses and appreciate 'misty and clear'. Binocular visual acuity shows good control at near and distance with glasses but reduced without glasses.

AC/A ratio Normal.

Angle of deviation A slight convergent angle is measured with glasses, increasing without glasses and on accommodation.

Four dioptre prism test This demonstrates a central suppression scotoma when there is a microtropia with the spectacles. Where there is a latent deviation with the spectacles, there is bifoveal fixation.

Management

Give the full refractive correction after cycloplegic refraction. Hypermetropia may be seen to have increased on the second refraction and the deviation often will have become more noticeable when the spectacles are removed. Treat amblyopia if present. Orthoptic exercises may be indicated with older children to control the manifest deviation. It is important to take into account the strength of the correction.

Treatment for patients with a spectacle correction of < +3.0 DS and +1.0 cyl. Aim to have good binocular single vision and binocular visual acuity, and normal accommodation and convergence without the spectacle correction. Antisuppression exercises may be indicated initially to allow appreciation of pathological diplopia without glasses. Teach the patient to relax accommodation to gain one blurred image without the spectacles (misty). Then gradually encourage accommodation while maintaining the one image (clear). Concave lenses and bar reading may be used to improve negative relative convergence with stereograms (distance fixation). Fusion and synoptophore exercises may be used in addition in the clinical setting. Spectacles may be left off under supervision at a later stage, but prior to that, the strength of the correction may be gradually reduced.

Treatment for patients with a spectacle correction of > +3.0 DS and +1.0 cyl. The patient will always need some hypermetropic correction, particularly for close work.

Exercises may be given to achieve 'social' control of the deviation for sports and photographs but not for close work, etc. The aim is to obtain one misty, blurred image with relaxed accommodation. Two clear images will be seen on accommodation. Exercises may also be given to improve control of the deviation in order to reduce the strength of correction in spectacles for cosmetic reasons.

Surgery is not indicated in this type of deviation. It may rarely be considered if there is a persistent large angle deviation despite wearing the full correction, with a risk of decompensation.

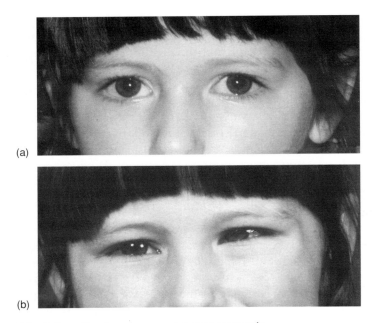

(a)

(b)

Figure 6.4   Intermittent convergence excess esotropia.

Convergence excess esotropia (Fig. 6.4)

There is binocular single vision for distant fixation, but esotropia on accommodation for near fixation.

Investigation

Case history   Onset is usually between the age of two and five years and is noticed when the patient is looking at close objects. However, if this type of squint is associated with hypermetropia which has not been corrected, the deviation will have been noticed for both near and distance. There is often a positive family history.

Refraction   The deviation may be associated with hypermetropia and occasionally a myopic refractive error is detected (Calcutt 1984, 1989).

Cover test   A manifest deviation is present for near fixation on accommodation but control may be demonstrated with a light target as less or no accommodation is exerted. A latent deviation is present for distance fixation.

Convergence   May be binocular to a light target but not to an accommodative target. Overconvergence may occur.

Binocular function   Binocular single vision is present on distance fixation and can be assessed using the synoptophore or free space distance tests. A light target and non-dissociative tests may demonstrate binocularity for near fixation. Normal retinal correspondence is usually present unless the deviation is controlled to a microtropia. Binocular visual acuity is normal for distance and reduced or absent for near fixation.

Angle of deviation	A slight convergent deviation is measurable at distance fixation with a larger manifest angle at near fixation.
+3.0 DS	The deviation is reduced by eliminating the need to accommodate for near fixation – esophoria is seen. Binocular single vision may be proved at this stage with Bagolini glasses and stereotests.
AC/A ratio	A high ratio at greater than 5:1 is expected.
Differential diagnosis	It is necessary to ensure the deviation is not an intermittent near type esotropia, intermittent fully accommodative esotropia with uncorrected or undercorrected hypermetropia or due to superior oblique under-action with a V eso pattern.

Hypoaccommodative esotropia is greater at near than distance fixation, is unrelated to an uncorrected hypermetropic refractive error and is caused by excessive convergence from an increased accommodative effort to overcome a primary or secondary weakness of accommodation. It is due to a remote near point of accommodation (Calcutt & Kinnear 1997; James 1997).

Management

Correct any refractive error and treat amblyopia if present.

Surgery is required in many cases, particularly if there is a high AC/A ratio.

The aim is to reduce the near angle of deviation so that binocular single vision is achieved, without overcorrecting the smaller distance angle, thus affecting binocularity for distance. The procedure usually involves bilateral medial rectus recessions and/or medial rectus posterior fixation sutures (Fadens) depending on the size of the deviation (Leitch *et al.* 1990).

Orthoptic exercises may be used with older co-operative children. The deviation should be less than 15 prism dioptres in angle with an AC/A ratio of no more than 8:1 and some appreciation of control for near fixation already. Antisuppression exercises may be necessary to allow appreciation of pathological diplopia. Accommodation is relaxed to obtain one misty image and then gradually encouraged while maintaining one clear image. Accommodation and negative relative convergence are further improved to achieve good binocularity for near fixation.

Bifocals may be used with older children (usually over five years of age). Executive bifocals are used ensuring that the near segment bisects the pupil. The weakest addition (up to +3.0) is given to allow comfortable binocular single vision and good binocular visual acuity. The aim is to restore to single vision lenses as soon as possible by reducing the bifocal segment strength over the follow-up period (Burian 1956).

Miotics act directly on the ciliary muscles. Miosis gives an increased depth of focus so that less accommodation is required. Phospholine-iodide 0.06/0.125% has been used in past years. This is no longer available on the UK market but may be available on a named patient basis from pharmacy departments for use under expert supervision. Generalised parasympathomimetic side effects such as sweating, bradycardia and intestinal colic may follow systemic absorption of these eye drops. Other effects may include hypersalivation and bronchospasm (Abraham 1961; Decker 1972). Pilocarpine 4.0% may also be used but is not as satisfactory as it has to be instilled on a more frequent basis. If after one month there is no improvement of control, the miotics are discontinued. If improvement has occurred, continue for 2–3 months and then gradually wean off over several weeks.

Contact lenses. Contact lenses of equivalent strength to the spectacle correction are given initially. An additional 1 D may be given if the esotropia persists. These are useful with patients with high AC/A ratios and those with associated myopia (Calcutt 1984, 1989).

RELATING TO FIXATION DISTANCE

Near esotropia

Binocular single vision is present for distance fixation and esotropia for near fixation even when the accommodative effort is relieved.

Investigation

Case history   An early onset is usual. Diplopia is noted if occurring in older patients. Patients may complain of asthenopic symptoms if trying to maintain control.

Refraction   There may be associated hypermetropia.

Visual acuity   Patients tend not to be amblyopic as there is no manifest deviation at distance.

Cover test   A manifest deviation for near fixation is present both with and without accommodative stimulus. A latent deviation is present for distance fixation.

Ocular motility   Bilateral superior oblique weaknesses may be noted.

Convergence   Absent or reduced convergence is recorded unless there is intersection of the visual axes followed by symmetrical convergence.

Binocular function   Normal retinal correspondence is demonstrable but binocular functions are weak. Binocular visual acuity is normal for distance and reduced or absent for near fixation.

Angle of deviation   Slight convergent deviation at distance and larger manifest angle at near fixation.

AC/A ratio   Normal. The deviation is unaffected by +3.0 DS lenses and there is a normal accommodative near point.

Differential diagnosis   A bilateral IV nerve weakness should be excluded by careful examination of the ocular movements.

Management

Correct any refractive error and treat amblyopia if present. Orthoptic exercises are contraindicated as it is not an accommodative deviation and lenses and miotics are of no help. Surgery, if indicated, usually involves bilateral medial recti recessions or Fadens depending on the angle of deviation.

Distance esotropia

Esotropia is present on distant fixation with binocular single vision present on near fixation.

Investigation

Case history   Diplopia is noted by older patients.

Visual acuity   Amblyopia is uncommon.

Cover test   A manifest deviation is present for distance and a latent deviation for near fixation.

Ocular motility   It is important to rule out lateral rectus weakness.

Binocular function   Suppression responses are recorded at distance fixation but binocular single vision when the angle is corrected on the synoptophore. Good fusion and stereopsis responses are recorded at near fixation using free space tests.

Binocular visual acuity is normal for near and reduced for distance fixation.

Angle of deviation   Slight convergent deviation at near and larger manifest angle at distance fixation.

Differential diagnosis   Ensure the deviation is not due to mild VI nerve paresis, thyroid eye disease with slightly limited abduction, convergence and accommodative spasm or divergence palsy.

Management

Treat amblyopia if present.

Prisms may be used with adult patients where a small angle of deviation less than 10 prism dioptres is present for distance and the patient wears spectacles.

Surgery, if indicated, usually involves bilateral lateral recti resections of equal but small amount.

Cyclic esotropia

This deviation relates to time with the deviation occurring at regular intervals.

Investigation

Case history   There is usually a late onset from four to five years. The most common pattern is an alternate day deviation. After a variable period of time the alternate day pattern may alter and the deviation eventually becomes constant (Rowe 1995).

Visual acuity   Amblyopia is uncommon.

Cover test   On the squinting day a marked deviation for near and distance fixation is present. On the straight day a latent deviation for near and distance fixation is present which is usually esophoria.

Binocular function   Suppression is present on the squinting day with normal binocular single vision present on the straight day. On a straight day, there is normal retinal correspondence with good fusion and stereopsis. On a squinting day, there is suppression but normal retinal correspondence is evident on correcting the angle of deviation in free space or using the synoptophore.

Management

Surgery is usually indicated for the manifest deviation. This may be performed once the deviation has become constant but may also be performed before the deviation has altered its cyclical pattern. As the deviation is often unilateral, a medial rectus recession and lateral rectus resection procedure on the deviating eye is usual. There is a good prognosis for restoration of binocular single vision.

Non-specific esotropia

An intermittent esotropia not conforming to any pattern.

Investigation

Case history   Older patients may be symptomatic and complain of headaches and intermittent diplopia.

Cover test   The deviation is intermittently manifest at any fixation distance and there is no significant change in the angle of deviation for near or distance fixation or with accommodation exerted.

Binocular function   Normal retinal correspondence is present but weak.

Differential diagnosis   Decompensating esophoria.

Secondary esotropia

Esotropia which follows loss or impairment of vision.

Investigation

Fundus and media examination   Retinal changes related to the cause of impaired vision may be evident.

Case history   Children who present with secondary esotropia indicate an onset of the visual loss or impairment from the age of six months to seven years

(Havertape *et al.* 2001). Adults who present with secondary esotropia indicate the presence of a pre-existing esophoria.

Visual acuity   Severe visual loss is present which may be unilateral or bilateral.

Cover test   Unilateral esotropia with poor fixation is usual.

Ocular motility   Limitations of motility may be noted if there is associated damage to the globe and extraocular muscles.

Angle of deviation   This is usually measured using corneal reflections as visual acuity is too poor to fixate.

Visuscope   Poor fixation is noted.

Binocular function   This is absent or reduced dependent on the extent of visual loss.

Suppression   Post-operative diplopia risk must be evaluated in patients over seven years of age.

Management

Treat the cause of visual loss if possible. Surgery is usually performed for cosmetic reasons. The aim is to leave the deviation slightly under-corrected as it should further decrease with time and this may guard against a later onset of consecutive exotropia.

Consecutive esotropia

Esotropia in a patient who has previously had exotropia or exophoria.

Investigation

Refraction   There may be under- or uncorrected hypermetropia which may be beneficial to the esotropia when corrected fully.

Case history   There is often a history of previous surgery which may have been deliberate to prevent redivergence in certain cases. The patient may appreciate diplopia immediately postoperatively, which usually resolves. Spontaneous onset of consecutive esotropia is rare (Fitton & Jampolsky 1964).

Visual acuity   Patients may be amblyopic if unilateral esotropia has developed or if amblyopic from previous exotropia.

Ocular motility   There may be a limitation of ocular movements, particularly in cases of unplanned surgical overcorrection.

Binocular function   Where binocular function was previously demonstrated pre-operatively, this should remain immediately postoperative. However, suppression is more often detected.

Management

When aiming for a functional response, if the deviation has not resolved within two weeks of surgery, postoperative treatment should be undertaken. Amblyopia may develop which requires treatment.

Convex lenses. Small angle deviations may respond to the use of convex lenses, particularly if there is a high AC/A ratio.

Orthoptic exercises may be given to improve negative relative convergence.

Prisms may be used to achieve binocular single vision and are gradually reduced at a later stage while maintaining binocularity.

Miotics may be used in cases of accommodative esotropia to reduce accommodation by increasing the depth of focus.

Surgery is indicated with larger angle deviations with the aim being parallel visual axes.

When a cosmetic result is required surgery may be indicated depending on the angle of deviation and the cosmetic appearance.

Exotropia

A condition in which one or other eye deviates outwards.

Classification

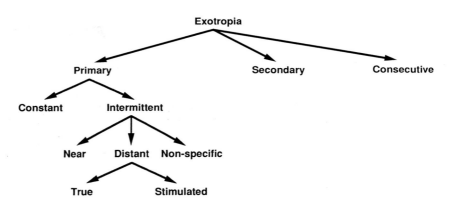

Figure 6.5 Classification of exotropia.

Aetiology

Primary exotropia

Constant
- Anatomical (wide IPD, exophthalmos, orbital asymmetry, muscle anomalies, craniofacial abnormalities), hereditary, myopia

Intermittent
- Near: acquired myopia, presbyopia
- Distant: high AC/A ratio, anatomical
- Non-specific: any of the above, weak fusion

Secondary
- Loss or impairment of vision (birth or > 8 years)

Consecutive
- Surgical overcorrection, passage of time

Primary exotropia

The divergent deviation constitutes the initial defect.

CONSTANT EXOTROPIA (Fig. 6.6)

The exotropia is present under all conditions.

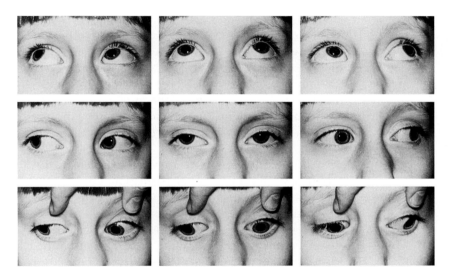

Figure 6.6   Constant exotropia.

Investigation

Case history   The deviation may have been intermittent first and then became constant; older children and adults may present like this. With early onset exotropia in children there may be a history of closing one eye in sunlight. The patient may be aware of panoramic vision.

Exotropia may be present in young children with slow mental and physical development and may decrease as general development improves.

Visual acuity   This is often equal if the deviation is alternating.

Cover test   There is a moderate angle exotropia at all distances which often alternates. DVD may be noted if infantile in onset.

Ocular motility   A V exo pattern may be documented.

Convergence   Convergence to 6 cm with the same angle of deviation indicates abnormal retinal correspondence. Convergence with reducing angle of deviation to intersection of the visual axes followed by symmetrical convergence of either eye indicates normal retinal correspondence. Further divergence following intersection of the visual axes indicates absence of retinal correspondence. Retinal correspondence cannot be estimated where there is convergence to 6 cm with reducing angle of deviation as intersection of the visual axes does not occur.

Accommodation   This may be reduced, particularly if there is a late onset exotropia. The decreased amplitude of accommodation may contribute to the decompensation of the deviation.

Binocular function   Free space tests may be used to assess the presence of abnormal retinal correspondence. A binocular response to Bagolini glasses or Worth's four lights test is indicative of normal or abnormal retinal correspondence but abnormal retinal correspondence will be seen in small angle deviations rather than large angles. Presence of abnormal retinal correspondence is unusual in exotropia but may develop in early onset exotropia, e.g. infantile. Normal retinal correspondence is noted in later onset exotropia. Free space fusion and stereopsis may be further tested to examine the quality of abnormal retinal correspondence if present. Suppression responses on free space tests do not give an indication of retinal correspondence. Suppression is often quite dense.

Retinal correspondence may be evaluated in full using the synoptophore. Normal retinal correspondence is present where superimposition is achieved at the full corrected angle of deviation. Abnormal retinal correspondence is present where superimposition is achieved at the angle of deviation. Quality of retinal correspondence, whether normal or abnormal, may be determined by assessing the fusion and stereopsis responses at these angles (Burian 1947; Moore & Cohen 1985).

Where suppression responses are obtained it is not possible to determine retinal correspondence. Further assessments may therefore be undertaken, including after-images and using vertical prisms to move the image out of the suppression area and align the vertically displaced images using horizontal prisms. Where there is suppression and the patient is aged seven years or greater, the depth and area of suppression should be measured in order to assess the risk of postoperative diplopia.

Angle of deviation   This should be measured for near and distance fixation.

Management

Classically, correcting hypermetropia will improve an esodeviation and worsen an exodeviation (Swan 1983). If there is significant blurring of vision, correcting hypermetropia will improve fusional convergence and lessen the amount of exodeviation (Iacobucci *et al.* 1993). Treat amblyopia if present.

Cosmetic result

Use of botulinum toxin A may be considered if there is a possibility of postoperative diplopia. This enables the deviating eye to take up a straighter position by temporarily paralysing the lateral rectus muscle and allowing a full assessment to be made of potential binocular function or the postoperative risk of diplopia. Some patients prefer to undertake repeated botulinum toxin A injections in preference to undergoing corrective surgery.

Surgery, if indicated, is usually a unilateral recession and resection procedure, using adjustable sutures with older patients. The aim is for parallel visual axes or a slight overcorrection.

Functional result

Use of adjustable suture surgery is again preferable with the older patient with the aim being parallel visual axes or a slight undercorrection.

INTERMITTENT EXOTROPIA

The exotropia is only present under certain conditions.

Near exotropia

Exotropia is present on near fixation and binocular single vision on distant fixation.

Investigation

Refraction	Patients may be myopic. If hypermetropia is present, order only the minimum prescription to maintain adequate visual acuity.
Case history	A later onset is common, usually with onset of myopia or presbyopia. Diplopia and asthenopic symptoms may be appreciated.
Visual acuity	Corrected acuity is usually equal.
Cover test	A manifest deviation is present for near fixation and a latent deviation for distance. Patients may have an exophoria to accommodative target at near fixation but exotropia to a light source.
Convergence	The level of convergence is poor or absent as a result of the divergent angle at near.
Binocular function	This can be assessed using the synoptophore or free space tests at distance. Normal retinal correspondence with demonstrable fusion involving a poor positive range is noted. For near, there may be suppression or crossed pathological diplopia which is joined with the appropriate prismatic correction.

Angle of   Slight divergent angle for distance increasing for near fixation.
deviation
Differential   It is necessary to ensure the deviation is not due to convergence palsy or
diagnosis   convergence insufficiency.

Management

Correct the refractive error as appropriate.

Orthoptic exercises may be used in cases where the angle of deviation measures less than 20 prism dioptres. Antisuppression exercises may be necessary to enable appreciation of pathological diplopia. The positive fusional range is improved with prism and synoptophore exercises and the positive relative convergence is improved with stereograms (near fixation). Binocular convergence is improved with convergence exercises.

Base-in prisms and/or concave lenses may be used as a support to orthoptic treatment. The minimum strength of prism to control the deviation is given and the aim is to reduce the strength as soon as possible (Hardesty 1972). Concave lenses are seldom useful for long-term wear as they blur visual acuity.

Surgery, if indicated, may involve bilateral medial rectus resections. It is advisable to do a small amount bilaterally than a large unilateral resection.

Diagnostic corrective prisms may be used to assess the effect on distance fixation pre-operatively.

Orthoptic exercises to improve positive relative convergence may be given post-operatively to consolidate the result.

Distance exotropia (Fig. 6.7)

Exotropia is present on distant fixation and binocular single vision on near fixation. The angle of deviation for near fixation may increase on prolonged disruption of fusion or elimination of accommodation. Cases which show such increase for near fixation are simulated distance types.

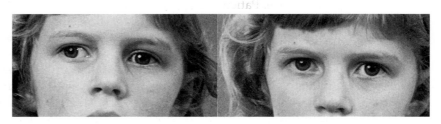

Figure 6.7   Intermittent distance exotropia.

Investigation

Refraction   May be myopic. If hypermetropic, the minimum correction should be ordered.

Case history   The age of onset of many exodeviations (constant and intermittent) is early and usually before the age of two years (Hall 1961; Biglan *et al.* 1996). Small angle deviations may not present until later because of the intermittent nature of the deviation. The deviation is noticed when daydreaming or tired. The patient is usually asymptomatic but may be aware of the divergence from the feel of the eye or increase in the visual field. The deviation is often worse during the summer and photophobia may be appreciated. The eyes may also tend to diverge in bright sunlight and the patient may close one eye in such circumstances (Holt 1951; Berg 1982). This is due to the increased depth of focus which is known to occur with miosed pupils. As a result less accommodation and therefore less accommodative convergence is required, resulting in decompensation of the exodeviation. The deviation tends to occur more frequently with poor health.

The patient may complain of blurred vision if using accommodation to control the deviation in the distance and may be aware of micropsia if using excessive accommodation to control the deviation. Control may vary throughout the day, being better in the morning, so it is useful to vary appointment times to assess overall ability to control the deviation.

Visual acuity   This is usually equal.

Cover test   There is a latent exodeviation on near fixation with a manifest deviation for distance and far distance. The deviation may appear controlled initially for distance but decompensates quickly on dissociation.

Ocular motility   Motility is often full but patients may have a V exo pattern with slight bilateral superior recti underactions. Lateral incomitance may be measured whereby the divergent angle of deviation reduces on lateral gaze (Moore 1969; Caldeira 1992). Compare the alternate cover test in primary position with right and left gaze positions. A reduction of more than 20% of the deviation is regarded as significant (von Noorden 1995). With lateral gaze incomitance, a decrease in the amount of lateral rectus recession is required (Moore 1969; Meyer *et al.* 1981).

Convergence   This is usually good, but if reduced, this may be an early sign of decompensation.

Accommodation Monocular and binocular near points may be measured.

Binocular   Normal retinal correspondence with fusion and stereopsis is present
function   at near fixation. Note the base-out range as fusional convergence is important in maintaining control for near.

Suppression or pathological crossed diplopia is present for distance which is joined with the appropriate prismatic correction. Suppression may be a hemiretinal suppression (Jampolsky 1955) or a less extensive suppression scotoma extending over the nasal and temporal retina similar to suppression in esotropia (Pratt-Johnson & Tillson 1984).

Binocular visual acuity is good for near acuity and reduced for distance. The near binocular visual acuity may be reduced in cases of simulated distance exotropia due to accommodative convergence control. The eyes may tend to diverge when accommodation is relaxed in order to see the smaller letters during the test.

Angle of deviation
A slight divergent angle is measured for near fixation which may increase on dissociation. A larger angle is measured for distance and far distance fixations. The deviation should be measured for near, distance, far distance, in lateral gaze and vertical gaze positions.

AC/A ratio and +3.0 DS
If simulated due to accommodative convergence, the angle of deviation will increase to equal or more than the distance measurement when measured for near fixation with +3.0 DS lenses in place. The AC/A ratio will be high if the deviation is controlled by accommodative convergence, indicating a simulated distance exotropia. Check to ensure that the target can be seen clearly with the lenses in place.

An increase in angle greater than 10 prism dioptres will differentiate between true and simulated distance exotropia in cases associated with accommodation.

Diagnostic occlusion
If simulated due to strong fusional convergence hold, the angle of deviation will increase for near fixation after a period of monocular occlusion (at least 30 minutes). The deviation should increase to equal or near equal to the distance measurement. It is important to ensure the patient never has a chance to regain binocular single vision when removing the occlusion to perform the prism cover test.

Management

Correct the refractive error. Correcting a myopic error is particularly useful in aiding control of the exodeviation. A hypermetropic error is under-corrected where possible but ensuring good visual acuity is maintained.

Orthoptic exercises may be useful in small angle deviations less than 15 prism dioptres. Antisuppression exercises may be required initially to demonstrate pathological diplopia (Luke 1970). It is necessary to improve binocular convergence, fusional amplitudes and positive relative convergence. Orthoptic treatment is contraindicated in cases where there is a possibility of surgery at a later stage as there would be a risk of overconvergence post-operatively.

Concave lenses up to −3.0 DS may be used in cases with high AC/A ratio to stimulate accommodative convergence and lenses are often combined with orthoptic exercises (Caltrider & Jampolsky 1983; Kushner 1999).

Base-in prisms may be used pre-operatively to obtain control and are often combined with orthoptic exercises. The aim is to reduce the strength of prism as soon as possible.

Alternating occlusion. Full time occlusion of either eye alternately for 3−6 months may improve sensory function and motor control.

Tinted spectacles. These are useful if bright light constitutes a major dissociative factor and may enable the patient to maintain control of the deviation in bright light (Eustace *et al.* 1973).

Surgery is required for large angle deviations and when decompensation of the deviation occurs for near fixation. Indications for delaying surgery include the following:

- Observe progress of the deviation, particularly variable control of a distance deviation.
- Allow for full facial development.
- More accurate measurements may be obtained when older.
- Post-operative treatment may be carried out.

Reasons for early surgery include the following:

- Prevents sensory changes.
- Minimises the development of a constant manifest deviation and deterioration of binocular single vision.
- The cosmetic appearance may be poor.

Surgery should not be delayed if the deviation begins to decompensate for near and there is development of secondary convergence insufficiency (Pratt-Johnson *et al.* 1977). The aim of surgery is to achieve parallel visual axes or a slight overcorrection. It is important to take into account the presence of lateral incomitance as this may lead to over-correction post-operatively should lateral rectus restrictions occur. Surgery usually involves bilateral lateral rectus recessions for true distance exotropia and unilateral lateral rectus recession/medial rectus resection for simulated distance exotropia (Burian & Spivey 1965; von Noorden 1969; Kushner 1998). Bilateral lateral recti recessions may also be considered whatever the type of distance exotropia (Kushner 1998).

Non-specific exotropia

Exotropia which shows intermittent binocular single vision not conforming to any pattern.

Investigation

Case history   Symptoms of headache, asthenopia and intermittent diplopia may be appreciated by older patients.

Visual acuity   This is usually equal as the deviation is intermittent.

Cover test   The deviation is intermittently manifest at any fixation distance and there is no significant change in the angle of deviation for near or distance fixation.

Binocular function   Normal retinal correspondence but with weak control.

Differential diagnosis   Decompensating exophoria.

Management

These deviations often require surgery and may need post-operative treatment to consolidate the result. Surgery usually involves unilateral lateral rectus recession and medial rectus resection procedure.

Secondary exotropia

Exotropia which follows loss or impairment of vision.

Investigation

Fundus and media   Retinal changes relating to the cause of impaired vision may be evident.

Case history   Loss of vision at birth or after the age of 7–8 years is often reported (Havertape *et al.* 2001).

Cover test   A moderate angle exotropia is present for all fixation distances.

Visual acuity   A severe visual deficit is observed and may be unilateral or bilateral.

Ocular motility   Limitations of ocular motility will be noted if there is associated damage to the globe.

Binocular function   This will be absent or reduced dependent on the extent of visual loss.

Suppression   Postoperative diplopia risk must be evaluated in patients over seven years of age.

Angle of deviation   The deviation is assessed by corneal reflections if there is poor fixation due to reduced visual acuity.

Management

Treat the cause of visual loss if possible.

Surgery. It is important to take into account the results of the postoperative diplopia test as the aim is for parallel visual axes or a slight overcorrection.

Contact lens. If surgery is contraindicated due to the physical state of the eye, a painted contact lens may be used to mask the appearance of the eye.

Consecutive exotropia

Exotropia in a patient who has previously had esotropia or esophoria.

Investigation

Case history   The consecutive deviation may occur spontaneously with the passage of time but may also be iatrogenic, when there will be a history of prior surgical procedures for a convergent deviation.

Symptoms of diplopia may be appreciated, particularly immediately postoperatively and in older patients. Surgery with overcorrection may be deliberate, particularly for esotropia, with an expected functional result. In cosmetic cases, overcorrection would be unplanned. Spontaneous cases occur in weak or absent fusion.

There is a gradual onset with no symptoms and it is commonly seen in older children and adults with a history of strabismus from early childhood and often associated with amblyopia.

Visual acuity   The patient is often amblyopic, particularly in cases of spontaneous unilateral exotropia.

Cover test   A manifest divergent deviation may be present either intermittently or constantly.

Ocular motility   Limitations may exist from strabismus surgery, e.g. lost muscle, maximum recessions.

Binocular function   Absent or weak binocular function will be demonstrated. Assess the potential for retinal correspondence particularly if the deviation was intermittent previously. The angle of deviation may be corrected in free space with prisms or on the synoptophore and the quality of binocular function evaluated.

Angle of deviation   Measure at near and distance fixation and with/without spectacle correction.

Management

When considering a cosmetic result, surgery is indicated if the appearance is poor with the aim being slight overcorrection. When considering a functional result, treatment is indicated if the deviation has not resolved.

Concave lenses may be used in cases with a high AC/A ratio to induce accommodative convergence and thereby reduce the angle of divergent deviation.

Base-in prisms. The lowest strength needed to control the deviation is given and then decreased gradually over a period of time.

Orthoptic exercises to improve positive relative convergence will aid control of the deviation.

Surgery should be considered for larger angles unresponsive to conventional therapy. The aim is for parallel visual axes as there is a good binocular prognosis.

Hypertropia

One eye is rotated upwards.

Hypotropia

One eye is rotated downwards.

Heavy eye phenomenon

Aetiology

This rare form of strabismus is due to a high degree of anisomyopia. The lateral rectus muscle is often displaced (Krzizok & Schroeder 1999).

Investigation

Cover test   This demonstrates a hypodeviation in the primary position.

Abnormal head   There is often a head tilt to the side of the hypo eye (the more myopic
posture   eye).

Binocular   Binocular single vision may be maintained by the use of the abnormal
function   head posture and a good fusional range is usually noted.

Cyclotropia

One eye is wheel rotated so that the upper end of its vertical axis is nasal (incyclotropia) or temporal (excyclotropia).

Dissociated vertical deviation (DVD)

When the vision of either eye is embarrassed, that eye deviates progressively upwards but reverts to its original position when the embarrassment ceases. It may sometimes be so asymmetrical as to be virtually unilateral and may be associated with binocular single vision or a manifest deviation.

Aetiology

The aetiology of DVD is obscure. Some theories include the following:

- DVD may be considered to be a movement towards the position of absolute rest when fusion is disrupted.
- There may be a paretic element involving bilateral paresis of the depressor muscles.
- DVD may be due to a variety of associated factors, including a return to the position of rest, relapse of peripheral fusion, unequal retinal stimulation and imbalance of the oblique muscles.
- Studies of monocular OKN have been found to be abnormal in normal infants up to a few months of age. The eyes respond to image movement from temporal to nasal but not from nasal to temporal. With increasing age OKN becomes bidirectional. Asymmetry of monocular horizontal OKN persists in patients with strabismus associated with DVD. This asymmetry in monocular

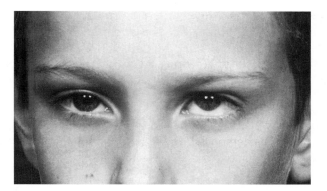

Figure 6.8   Hypertropia.

OKN is thought to be due to an abnormality of some of the temporal retinal fibres which are misdirected through the chiasm (Mein 1983).

Investigation

Case history   There is usually a history of manifest deviation from an early age. The parents may have noticed DVD when the patient looks to one side when it resembles an inferior oblique overaction. They may also notice spontaneous elevation (Fig. 6.8) which tends to occur if the patient is daydreaming or is excessively fatigued. An abnormal head posture is present in some cases with tilt usually to the side of the fixing eye (Crone 1954; Bechtel *et al.* 1996; Santiago & Rosenbaum 1998). Symptoms are rare.

DVD is part of the infantile squint syndrome where patients have infantile esotropia with manifest nystagmus. The nystagmus is manifest latent in type. DVD is usually demonstrated around the age of two years.

Visual acuity   Amblyopia may be present if there is a unilateral manifest deviation. Vision may be reduced uniocularly compared to binocularly due to manifest latent nystagmus.

Cover test   A manifest deviation is typically present which is often esotropic. Nystagmus is usually horizontal, but may have a vertical or rotational component. Progressive elevation of either eye is seen under cover and a slow downward movement when the cover is removed. The upward movement of the eye is slow, more marked on distance fixation and on prolonged dissociation. When the occluder is removed, the eye drifts down to the midline and occasionally may move below the midline before moving up again to refixate. DVD is often more marked on distance fixation.

Ocular motility   DVD is a bilateral condition but may be asymmetric (von Noorden 1988b). There may be apparent or true inferior oblique overactions (Helveston 1969; McCall & Rosenbaum 1991). In cases with inferior oblique overactions, a V eso pattern is expected.

Binocular function   Absent or defective fusion is detected. Normal binocular single vision is rare.

Monocular OKN testing   This is useful in young children with infantile esotropia in whom DVD is suspected but not confirmed on cover test. A defective nasal to temporal response is expected (Fitzgerald & Billson 1984).

Differential diagnosis

	DVD	Inferior oblique overaction
Cover test	Hyperdeviation remains the same in primary position and contralateral versions	Hyperdeviation increases on contralateral versions
Ocular motility	Sudden upshoot on contralateral versions when nose intervenes	Gradual updrift on contralateral versions
A/V pattern	Mainly A pattern	V pattern
Bielchowsky phenomenon	Positive	Negative

Dark wedge test   This is also know as the Bielchowsky phenomenon and differentiates between DVD and alternating hyperphoria. This is described in Chapter 4.

Management

Correct the refractive error and treat amblyopia if present. Manifest strabismus is treated according to the type and size of deviation.

DVD is managed surgically when indicated by spontaneous elevation which is cosmetically unacceptable. Surgery may involve a recession or a Faden procedure to the superior recti muscles (Esswein *et al.* 1992). The amount of recession may be varied when asymmetrical. A Faden procedure may be combined with superior recti recessions if there is a significant vertical deviation associated with the spontaneous elevation (Duncan & von Noorden 1984). Anterior displacement of the inferior oblique may also be considered (Kratz *et al.* 1989; Burke *et al.* 1993; Seawright & Gole 1996; Varn *et al.* 1996; Black 1997; Ruttum 1997). Surgery for residual deviations may involve inferior rectus resection as a second procedure (Esswein & von Noorden 1994).

Where DVD is associated with inferior oblique overaction, a combined inferior oblique resection and anterior transposition can be beneficial (Farvardin & Attarzadeh 2002).

Dissociated horizontal deviation (DHD)

Investigation

Cover test   There is intermittent asymmetrical abduction and elevation of the dissociated eye (Zubcov *et al.* 1990; Wilson & McClatchey 1991). Patients may have an associated vertical element and there may be latent nystagmus and excyclotropia (Wilson *et al.* 1995).

Sbiza bar   The deviation decreases with neutral density filters (Wilson & McClatchey 1991).

Management

Surgical treatment, if required, is with lateral rectus recessions (Wilson *et al.* 2000) and may be combined with superior rectus recession if there is an associated vertical element.

Pseudostrabismus

This is an appearance of strabismus when no manifest deviation of the visual axes is actually present.

Aetiology

(1) Epicanthus may give a convergent appearance where skinfolds are prominent between the medial canthi and the nose (Fig. 6.9). Lateral canthus may give a divergent appearance but this is relatively rare.

(2) Angle kappa is the angle between the pupillary axis and the visual axis. The corneal reflections may appear slightly nasal, producing a positive angle kappa. A large angle kappa gives an appearance of a divergent deviation. If both axes coincide, corneal reflections appear right in the centre of the pupil, producing a negative angle kappa and giving an appearance of a convergent deviation.

Synoptophore slides may be used to measure the degree of angle kappa (see Chapter 4).

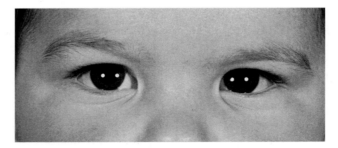

Figure 6.9   Pseudostrabismus.

(3) Interpupillary distance. A wide IPD gives the appearance of a divergent deviation. A narrow IPD gives the appearance of a convergent deviation.

(4) Enophthalmos gives the appearance of a convergent deviation and exophthalmos, a divergent deviation.

(5) Ptosis may give the appearance of a vertical deviation.

(6) Asymmetry of the palpebral fissure.

(7) Facial asymmetry.

(8) Ill fitting spectacles.

(9) Presence of an abnormal head posture.

(10) Heterochromia iridies – a difference in the iris colour of either eye.

(11) Iris coloboma – a fissure or gap in the iris.

(12) Anisocoria – a difference in the pupil size of either eye.

Management

Orthoptic investigation will establish the presence of binocular single vision and fusional control in cases of pseudostrabismus. If it is found to be associated with true strabismus, however, further treatment should be given as indicated.

REFERENCES

Abraham S. (1961) Present status of miotic therapy in nonparalytic convergent strabismus. *American Journal of Ophthalmology*, 51: 1249

Bechtel RT, Kushner BJ & Morton GV. (1996) The relationship between dissociated vertical deviation (DVD) and head tilts. *Journal of Pediatric Ophthalmology and Strabismus*, 33: 303

Berg PH. (1982) Effect of light intensity on the prevalence of exotropia in strabismus populations. *British Orthoptic Journal*, 39: 55

Biglan AW, Davis JS, Cheng KP & Pettapiece MC. (1996) Infantile exotropia. *Journal of Pediatric Ophthalmology and Strabismus*, 33: 79

Black BC. (1997) Results of anterior transposition of the inferior oblique muscle in incomitant dissociated vertical deviation. *Journal of the American Association of Pediatric Ophthalmology and Strabismus*, 1: 83

Burian HM. (1947) The sensorial retinal relationship in comitant strabismus. *Archives of Ophthalmology*, 37: 336

Burian HM. (1956) Use of bifocal spectacles in the treatment of accommodative esotropia. *British Orthoptic Journal*, 13: 3

Burian HM & Spivey BE. (1965) The surgical management of exodeviations. *American Journal of Ophthalmology*, 59: 603

Burke JP, Scott WE & Kutschke PJ. (1993) Anterior transposition of the inferior oblique muscle for dissociated vertical deviation. *Ophthalmology*, 100: 245

Calcutt C. (1984) The use of contact lenses in the treatment of accommodative esotropia. In: Ravault AP & Lenk M (eds) *Transactions of the Fifth International Orthoptic Congress*, LIPS, Lyon, p. 311

Calcutt C. (1989) Contact lenses in accommodative esotropia therapy. *British Orthoptic Journal*, 46: 59

Calcutt C & Kinnear P. (1997) Anomalous accommodative response in high AC/A ratio convergence excess esotropia. *British Orthoptic Journal*, 54: 51

Calcutt C & Murray A. (1998) Untreated essential infantile esotropia: factors affecting the development of amblyopia. *Eye*, 12: 167

Caldeira AAF. (1992) Lateral gaze incomitance in surgical exodeviations: clinical features. *Binocular Vision*, 7: 75

Caltrider N & Jampolsky A. (1983) Overcorrecting minus lens therapy for treatment of intermittent exotropia. *Ophthalmology*, 90: 1160

Campos EC, Schiavi C & Bellusci C. (2000) Critical age of botulinum toxin treatment in essential infantile esotropia. *Journal of Pediatric Ophthalmology and Strabismus*, 37: 328

Costenbader FD. (1961) Infantile esotropia. *Transactions of the American Ophthalmological Society*, 59: 397

Crone RA. (1954) Alternating hyperphoria. *British Journal of Ophthalmology*, 38: 591

Decker JH. (1972) Shallowing of the anterior chamber following the use of echothiopate (phospholine) iodide. *Journal of Pediatric Ophthalmology*, 9: 16

Dell'Osso LF, Ellenberger C, Abel LA & Flynn JT. (1983) The nystagmus blockage syndrome. *Investigative Ophthalmology and Visual Science*, 24: 1580

Demer JL & von Noorden GK. (1988) Optokinetic asymmetry in esotropia. *Journal of Pediatric Ophthalmology and Strabismus*, 25: 286

Duncan L & von Noorden GK. (1984) Surgical results in dissociated vertical deviation. *Journal of Pediatric Ophthalmology and Strabismus*, 21: 25

Esswein MB & von Noorden GK. (1994) Treatment of residual DVD with inferior rectus resection. *Journal of Pediatric Ophthalmology and Strabismus*, 31: 262

Esswein MB, von Noorden GK & Coburn A. (1992) Comparison of surgical methods in the treatment of dissociated vertical deviation. *American Journal of Ophthalmology*, 113: 287

Eustace P, Wesson ME & Druby DJ. (1973) The effect of illumination on intermittent divergent squint of the divergence excess type. *Transactions of the Ophthalmological Society of the United Kingdom*, 93: 559

Farvardin M & Attarzadeh A. (2002) Combined resection and anterior transposition of the inferior oblique muscle for the treatment of moderate to large dissociated vertical deviation associated with inferior oblique muscle overaction. *Journal of Pediatric Ophthalmology and Strabismus*, 39: 268

Fitton MH & Jampolsky A. (1964) A case report of spontaneous consecutive esotropia. *American Orthoptic Journal*, 14: 144

Fitzgerald BA & Billson FA. (1984) Evidence of abnormal optic nerve fiber projection in patients with dissociated vertical deviation (DVD). In: Ravault AP & Lenk M (Eds) *Transactions of the Fifth International Orthoptic Congress*. LIPS, Lyon, p. 161

Friedman Z, Neumann E, Hyams SW & Peleg B. (1980) Ophthalmic screening of 38,000 children, aged 1 to $2^{1}/_{2}$ years, in child welfare clinics. *Journal of Pediatric Ophthalmology and Strabismus*, 17: 261

Friedrick D & de Decker W. (1987) Prospective study of the development of strabismus during the first 6 months of life. In: Lenk-Schafer M, Calcutt C, Doyle M & Moore S (eds) *Transactions of the Sixth International Orthoptic Congress*. British Orthoptic Society, London, p. 21

Graham RA. (1974) Epidemiology of strabismus. *British Journal of Ophthalmology*, 58: 224

Hall IB. (1961) Primary divergent strabismus. Analysis of aetiological factors. *British Orthoptic Journal*, 18: 106

Hardesty HH. (1972) Prisms in the management of intermittent exotropia. *American Orthoptic Journal*, 22: 22

Havertape SA, Cruz OA & Chu FC. (2001) Sensory strabismus – eso or exo? *Journal of Pediatric Ophthalmology and Strabismus*, 38: 327

Helveston EM. (1969) A-exotropia, alternating circumduction and superior oblique overaction. *American Journal of Ophthalmology*, 67: 377

Helveston EM. (1993) Frank Costenbader lecture – the origins of congenital esotropia. *Journal of Pediatric Ophthalmology and Strabismus*, 30: 215

Helveston EM, Ellis FD, Schott J, Mitchelson J, Weber JC, Taube S & Miller K. (1983) Surgical treatment of congenital esotropia. *American Journal of Ophthalmology*, 96: 218

Holt R. (1951) A study of divergent strabismus in Australia. *British Orthoptic Journal*, 8: 95

Hugonnier R & Clayette-Hugonnier S. (1969) *Strabismus, Heterophoria, Ocular Motor Paralysis: Clinical Muscle Imbalance* (trans. Veronneau-Troutman S). Mosby, St Louis

Iacobucci IL, Archer SM & Giles CL. (1993) Children with exotropia responsive to spectacle correction of hyperopia. *American Journal of Ophthalmology*, 116: 79

Ing MR. (1983) Early surgical alignment for congenital esotropia. *Ophthalmology*, 90: 132

Ing M, Costenbader FD, Parks MM & Albert DG. (1966) Early surgery for congenital esotropia. *American Journal of Ophthalmology*, 61: 1419

James EL. (1997) Hypo-accommodative esotropia. *British Orthoptic Journal*, 54: 54

Jampolsky A. (1955) Characteristics of suppression in strabismus. *Archives of Ophthalmology*, 54: 683

Kratz RE, Rogers GL, Bremer DL & Leguire LE. (1989) Anterior tendon displacement of the inferior oblique for DVD. *Journal of Pediatric Ophthalmology and Strabismus*, 26: 212

Krzizok TH & Schroeder BU. (1999) Measurement of recti eye muscle paths by magnetic resonance imaging in highly myopic and normal subjects. *Investigative Ophthalmology and Visual Science*, 40: 2554

Kushner BJ. (1998) Selective surgery for intermittent exotropia based on distance/near differences. *Archives of Ophthalmology*, 116: 324

Kushner BJ. (1999) Does overcorrecting minus lens therapy for intermittent exotropia cause myopia? *Archives of Ophthalmology*, 117: 638

Kushner BJ & Morton GV. (1984) A randomised comparison of surgical procedures for infantile esotropia. *American Journal of Ophthalmology*, 98: 50

Lang J. (1968) Squint dating from birth or with early onset. In: *Transactions of the First International Congress of Orthoptists*. Kimpton, London, p. 231

Lang J. (1981) Normo-sensorial late convergent squint. In: Mein J & Moore S (eds) *Orthoptics, Research and Practice*. Kimpton, London, p. 230

Lang J. (1986) Normosensorial late convergent strabismus. In: Campos E (Ed) *Transactions of the Fifth International Strabismological Association*. Rome, p. 536

Leitch RJ, Burke JP & Strachan IM. (1990) Convergence excess esotropia treated surgically with fadenoperation and medial rectus muscle recessions. *British Journal of Ophthalmology*, 74: 278

Luke NE. (1970) Antisuppression exercises in exodeviations. *American Orthoptic Journal*, 20: 100

McCall LC & Rosenbaum AL. (1991) Incomitant dissociated vertical deviation and superior oblique overaction. *Ophthalmology*, 98: 911

McNeer KW, Tucker MG & Spencer RF. (2000) Management of essential infantile esotropia with botulinum toxin A: review and recommendations. *Journal of Pediatric Ophthalmology and Strabismus*, 37: 63

Mein J. (1983) The asymmetrical optokinetic response. *British Orthoptic Journal*, 40: 1

Meyer E, von Noorden GK & Avilla CW. (1981) Management of consecutive esotropia. In: Mein J & Moore S (eds) *Orthoptics: Research and Practice*. Kimpton, London, p. 236

Moore D. (1990) Back to basics; assessment of binocular convergence in esotropia. *British Orthoptic Journal*, 47: 67

Moore S. (1969) The prognostic value of lateral gaze measurements in intermittent exotropia. *American Orthoptic Journal*, 19: 69

Moore S & Cohen RL. (1985) Congenital exotropia. *American Orthoptic Journal*, 35: 68

Nixon RB, Helveston EM, Miller M, Archer SM & Ellis FD. (1985) Incidence of strabismus in neonates. *American Journal of Ophthalmology*, 100: 798

Parks MM. (1984) Congenital esotropia with a bifixational result. Report of a case. *Documenta Ophthalmologica*, 58: 109

Pratt-Johnson JA & Tillson G. (1984) Suppression in strabismus, an update. *British Journal of Ophthalmology*, 68: 174

Pratt-Johnson J, Barlow JM & Tillson G. (1977) Early surgery for intermittent exotropia. *American Journal of Ophthalmology*, 84: 689

Prieto-Diaz J. (1980) Large bilateral medial rectus recessions in early esotropia with bilateral limitation of abduction. *Journal of Pediatric Ophthalmology and Strabismus*, 17: 101

Prieto-Diaz J. (1985) Five year follow-up of large (6–9) bimedial recession in the management of early onset essential infantile esotropia with Ciancia syndrome. *Binocular Vision*, 1: 209

Rizk A. (1999) Bilateral posterior fixation sutures on the medial rectus muscles for correction of non-accommodative esotropia with infantile onset criteria. *Journal of Pediatric Ophthalmology and Strabismus*, 36: 320

Rowe FJ. (1995) Cyclic (alternate day) esotropia. Case report and literature review. In: Spiritus M (ed) *Transactions of the 22nd Meeting of the European Strabismological Association*. Cambridge, United Kingdom, p. 118

Ruttum MS. (1997) Anterior transposition of the inferior oblique muscles. *American Orthoptic Journal*, 47: 118

Santiago AP & Rosenbaum AL. (1998) Dissociated vertical deviation and head tilt. *Journal of the American Association for Pediatric Ophthalmology and Strabismus*, 2: 5

Schor CM, Fusaro RE, Wilson N & McKee SP. (1997) The prediction of onset esotropia from components of the infantile squint syndrome. *Investigative Ophthalmology and Visual Science*, 38: 719

Seawright AA & Gole GA. (1996) Results of anterior transposition of the inferior oblique. *Australian and New Zealand Journal of Ophthalmology*, 24: 339

Shauly Y, Prager TC & Mazow ML. (1994) Clinical characteristics and long-term postoperative results of essential infantile esotropia. *American Journal of Ophthalmology*, 117: 183

Swan KC. (1983) Accommodative esotropia long range follow-up. *Ophthalmology*, 90: 1141

Varn MM, Saunders RA & Wilson ME. (1996) Combined bilateral superior rectus muscle recession and inferior oblique muscle weakening for dissociated vertical deviation. *Journal of the American Association for Pediatric Ophthalmology and Strabismus*, 1: 134

von Noorden GK. (1969) Divergence excess and simulated divergence excess: diagnosis and surgical management. *Ophthalmologica*, 26: 719

von Noorden GK, Isaza A & Parks MM. (1972) Surgical treatment of congenital esotropia. *Transactions of the American Academy of Ophthalmology and Otolaryngology*, 76: 1465

von Noorden GK & Wong SY. (1986) Surgical results in nystagmus blockage syndrome. *Ophthalmology*, 93: 1028

von Noorden GK. (1988a) Current concepts of infantile esotropia. *Eye*, 2: 343

von Noorden GK. (1988b) A reassessment of essential infantile esotropia (XLIV Edward Jackson Memorial Lecture). *American Journal of Ophthalmology*, 105: 1

von Noorden GK. (1995) *Binocular Vision and Ocular Motility. Theory and Management of Strabismus*, 5th edn. Mosby, St Louis

Weakley DR, Stager DR & Everett ME. (1991) Seven-millimeter bilateral medial rectus recessions in essential infantile esotropia. *Journal of Pediatric Ophthalmology and Strabismus*, 28: 113 ·

Wilson ME & McClatchey SK. (1991) Dissociated horizontal deviation. *Journal of Pediatric Ophthalmology and Strabismus*, 28: 90

Wilson ME, Saunders RA & Berland JE. (1995) Dissociated horizontal deviation and accommodative esotropia: treatment options when an eso- or exo-deviation co-exists. *Journal of Pediatric Ophthalmology and Strabismus*, 32: 228

Wilson ME, Hutchinson AK & Saunders R. (2000) Outcomes from surgical therapy for dissociated horizontal deviations. *Journal of the American Association for Pediatric Ophthalmology and Strabismus*, 4: 94

Zubcov A, Reinecke RD & Calhoun JH. (1990) Asymmetrical horizontal tropias, DVD and manifest latent nystagmus: an explanation of dissociated horizontal deviation. *Journal of Pediatric Ophthalmology and Strabismus*, 27: 59

FURTHER READING

Abrahamson M, Fabian G & Sjostrand J. (1992) Refraction changes in children developing convergent or divergent strabismus. *British Journal of Ophthalmology*, 76: 723

Abrahamson M, Magnusson G & Sjostrand J. (1999) Inheritance of strabismus and the gain of using heredity to determine populations at risk of developing strabismus. *Acta Ophthalmologica Scandinavica*, 77: 653

Adler FH. (1945) Pathologic physiology of convergent strabismus. Motor aspects of the non-accommodational type. *Archives of Ophthalmology*, 33: 362

Adler FH & Jackson FE. (1947) Correlations between sensory and motor disturbances in convergent squint. *Archives of Ophthalmology*, 38: 289

Albert DG & Hiles DA. (1969) Myopia, bifocals and accommodation. *American Orthoptic Journal*, 19: 59

Altizer LB. (1972) The nonsurgical treatment of exotropia. *American Orthoptic Journal*, 22: 71

Alvara ME. (1950) Simultaneous surgical correction of vertical and horizontal deviations. *Ophthalmologica*, 120: 191

Anst W & Welge-Lussen L. (1971) Effect of prolonged use of prisms on the operative results of strabismus. *Annals of Ophthalmology*, 3: 571

Apt L & Call NB. (1978) Inferior oblique muscle recession. *American Journal of Ophthalmology*, 85: 95

Apt L & Isenberg S. (1977) Eye position of strabismus patients under general anaesthesia. *American Journal of Ophthalmology*, 84: 574

Archer SM, Helveston EM, Miller KK & Ellis FD. (1986) Stereopsis in normal infants and infants with congenital esotropia. *American Journal of Ophthalmology*, 101: 591

Awaya S, Nozaki H, Itoh T & Harada K. (1976) Studies of suppression in alternating constant exotropia and intermittent exotropia: with reference to the effects of fusional background. In: Moore S, Mein J & Stockbridge L (eds) *Orthoptics, Past, Present and Future.* Symposia Specialists, Miami, p. 531

Bagolini B. (1966) Postsurgical treatment of convergent strabismus with a critical evaluation of various tests. *International Ophthalmology Clinics*, 6: 633

Bagshaw J. (1961) Convergence excess. *British Orthoptic Journal*, 18: 95

Bagshaw J. (1966) Heavy eye phenomenon. *British Journal of Ophthalmology*, 23: 73

Baker JD & Parks MM. (1980) Early onset accommodative esotropia. *American Journal of Ophthalmology*, 90: 11

Beneish R & Flanders M. (1994) The role of stereopsis and early postoperative alignment in long-term results of intermittent exotropia. *Canadian Journal of Ophthalmology*, 29: 119

Bielchowsky A. (1934) Divergence excess. *Archives of Ophthalmology*, 12: 157

Breinen GM. (1974) Accommodative strabismus and the AC/A ratio. *American Journal of Ophthalmology*, 1: 303

Breinin GM, Chin NB & Ripps H. (1966) A rationale for therapy of accommodative strabismus. *American Journal of Ophthalmology*, 61: 1030

Bremer DL, Palmer EA, Fellows RR, Baker JD, Hardy RJ, Tung B & Rogers GL. (1998) Strabismus in premature infants in the first year of life. Cryotherapy for Retinopathy Co-operative Group. *Archives of Ophthalmology*, 116: 329

Broendstrup P. (1944) The squinting position of weak-sighted eyes. *Acta Ophthalmologica*, 20: 386

Bruce CJ, Isley MR & Shinkman PG. (1981) Visual experience and development of interocular orientation disparity in visual cortex. *Journal of Neurophysiology*, 46: 215

Buckley EG & Flynn JT. (1983) Superior oblique recession versus tenotomy: a comparison of surgical results. *Journal of Pediatric Ophthalmology and Strabismus*, 20: 112

Burian HM. (1945) Motility clinic; sudden onset of concomitant convergent strabismus. *American Journal of Ophthalmology*, 28: 407

Burian HM & Miller JE. (1958) Concomitant convergent strabismus with acute onset. *American Journal of Ophthalmology*, 45: 55

Burian HM. (1966) Exodeviations: their classification, diagnosis and treatment. *American Journal of Ophthalmology*, 62: 1161

Burian HM. (1972) Hypermetropia and esotropia. *Journal of Pediatric Ophthalmology*, 9: 135

Caldeira JA. (1975) Graduated recession of the superior oblique muscle. *British Journal of Ophthalmology*, 59: 553

Campos EC. (1982) Binocularity in comitant strabismus; binocular visual field studies. *Documenta Ophthalmologica*, 53: 249

Chamberlain W. (1968) Cyclic esotropia. *American Orthoptic Journal*, 18: 31

Chew E, Remaley NA, Tamboli A, Zhao J, Podgor MJ & Klebanoff M. (1994) Risk factors for esotropia and exotropia. *Archives of Ophthalmology*, 112: 1349

Chin NB, Gold AA & Breinin GM. (1964) Iris cysts and miotics. *Archives of Ophthalmology*, 71: 611

Clark AC, Nelson LB, Simon JW, Wagner R & Rubin SE. (1989) Acute acquired comitant esotropia. *British Journal of Ophthalmology*, 73: 636

Clark RA, Miller JM, Rosenbaum AL & Demer JL. (1998) Heterotopic muscle pulleys or oblique muscle dysfunction? *Journal of the American Association of Pediatric Ophthalmology and Strabismus*, 2: 17

Cohen RL & Moore S. (1980) Primary dissociated vertical deviation. *American Orthoptic Journal*, 30: 107

Cooper E. (1961) The surgical management of secondary exotropia. *Transactions of the American Academy of Ophthalmology and Otolaryngology*, 65: 595

Dahan A & Spielmann A. (1985) Double torticollis and surgical artificial divergence. In: *Acta Strabologica*. CERES, Paris, p. 187

Dankner SR, Mash AJ & Jampolsky A. (1978) Intentional surgical overcorrection of acquired esotropia. *Archives of Ophthalmology*, 96: 1848

Diamond GR, Katovitz JA, Whitaker LA, Quinn GE & Schaffer DB. (1980) Variations in extraocular muscle number and structure in craniofacial dysotosis. *American Journal of Ophthalmology*, 90: 416

Ellis PP. (1966) Systemic effects of locally applied anticholinesterase agents. *Investigative Ophthalmology*, 51: 146

Elsas FJ & Witherspoon CD. (1987) Anterior segment ischemia after strabismus surgery in a child. *American Journal of Ophthalmology*, 103: 833

Gage J. (1996) A comparison of AC/A ratio measurement using the gradient method at near and distance fixation. *British Orthoptic Journal*, 53: 25

Goldstein JH. (1968) The role of miotics in strabismus. *Survey of Ophthalmology*, 13: 31

Greenstein V, Goldstein J, Adler R & Karp E. (1976) Prognosis for binocular vision in monocular trauma. *British Orthoptic Journal*, 33: 44

Hart CT. (1969) Disturbances of fusion following head injury. *Proceedings of the Royal Society of Medicine*, 62: 704

Helveston EM. (1973) Cyclic strabismus. *American Orthoptic Journal*, 23: 48

Helveston EM. (1980) Dissociated vertical deviation: a clinical and laboratory study. *Transactions of the American Ophthalmological Society*, 78: 734

Helveston EM. (1990) The value of strabismus surgery. *Ophthalmic Surgery*, 21: 311

Helveston EM & Cofield DD. (1970) Indications for marginal myotomy and technique. *American Journal of Ophthalmology*, 70: 574

Hiles DA, Watson A & Biglan AW. (1980) Characteristics of infantile esotropia following early bimedial rectus recession. *Archives of Ophthalmology*, 98: 697

Horwood A. (1993) The early development of binocular single vision in normal infants. *British Orthoptic Journal*, 50: 42

Ing MR. (1991) Infection following strabismus surgery. *Ophthalmic Surgery*, 22: 41

Jampolsky A. (1958) Surgical management of exotropia. *American Journal of Ophthalmology*, 46: 646

Jampolsky A. (1986), Management of vertical strabismus. In: Allen JH (ed) *Pediatric Ophthalmology and Strabismus. Transactions of the New Orleans Academy of Ophthalmology*. Raven Press, New York, p. 141

Jenkins R. (1992) Demographics; geographic variations in the prevalence and management of exotropia. *American Orthoptic Journal*, 42: 82

Keech RV, Scott WE & Baker JD. (1990) The medial rectus muscle insertion site in infantile esotropia. *American Journal of Ophthalmology*, 109: 79

Keenan JM & Willshaw HE. (1992) Outcome of strabismus surgery in congenital esotropia. *British Journal of Ophthalmology*, 76: 342

Knapp P. (1975) The use of membrane prisms. *Transactions of the American Academy of Ophthalmology and Otolaryngology*, 79: 718

Kushner BJ. (2001) Functional benefits of strabismus surgery. *Binocular Vision Strabismus Quarterly*, 16: 11

Kushner BJ, Lucchese NJ & Morton GV. (1991) Variation in axial length and anatomical landmarks in strabismus patients. *Ophthalmology*, 98: 400

Lorenz B, Raab I & Boergen KP. (1992) DVD: what is the most effective surgical approach? *Journal of Pediatric Ophthalmology and Strabismus*, 29: 21

Ludwig IH, Parks MM & Jetson PP. (1989) Long-term results of bifocal therapy for accommodative esotropia. *Journal of Pediatric Ophthalmology and Strabismus*, 26: 264

MacEwen CJ, Lee JP & Fells P. (1992) Aetiology and management of the 'detached' rectus muscle. *British Journal of Ophthalmology*, 76: 131

Maumenee IH, Alston A, Mets MB, Flynn JT, Mitchell TN & Beaty TH. (1985) Inheritance of congenital esotropia. *Transactions of the American Ophthalmological Society*, 84: 85

McIntyre A & Fells P. (1996) Bangerter foils: a new approach to the management of pathological intractable diplopia. *British Orthoptic Journal*, 53: 43

McKeown K. (1982) An interesting case of intermittent esotropia. *British Orthoptic Journal*, 39: 64

Milot J, Jacob JL, Blanc VF & Hardy JF. (1983) The oculocardiac reflex in strabismus surgery. *Canadian Journal of Ophthalmology*, 18: 314

Moore S. (1963) Orthoptic treatment for intermittent exotropia. *American Orthoptic Journal*, 13: 14

Neikter B. (1994) Effects of diagnostic occlusion on ocular alignment in normal subjects. *Strabismus*, 2: 67

Nordlow W. (1953) Age distribution at the onset of esotropia. *British Journal of Ophthalmology*, 37: 593

Olitsky SE, Sudesh S, Graziano A, Hamblen J, Brooks SE & Shaha SH. (1999) The negative psychosocial impact of strabismus in the adult. *Journal of the American Association for Pediatric Ophthalmology and Strabismus*, 3: 209

Olivier R & von Noorden GK. (1982) Excyclotropia of the nonparetic eye in unilateral superior oblique muscle paralysis. *American Journal of Ophthalmology*, 93: 30

Parks MM. (1958) Abnormal accommodative convergence in squint. *Archives of Ophthalmology*, 59: 364

Parks MM. (1974) The overacting inferior oblique muscle. *American Journal of Ophthalmology*, 77: 787

Parks MM. (1975) *Ocular Motility and Strabismus*. Harper and Row, New York

Plenty J. (1988) A new classification for intermittent exotropia. *British Orthoptic Journal*, 45: 19

Podger MJ, Remaley NA & Chew E. (1996) Associations between siblings for esotropia and exotropia. *Archives of Ophthalmology*, 114: 739

Pott JWR, Sprunger DT & Helveston EM. (1999) Infantile esotropia in very low birth weight (VLBW) children. *Strabismus*, 7: 97

Pratt-Johnson JA. (1973) Central disruption of fusional amplitude. *British Journal of Ophthalmology*, 57: 347

Pratt-Johnson JA & Tillson G. (1979) Acquired central disruption of fusional amplitude. *Ophthalmology*, 86: 2140

Pratt-Johnson J & Wee HS. (1969) Suppression associated with exotropia. *Canadian Journal of Ophthalmology*, 4: 136

Pratt-Johnson JA, Pop A & Tillson G. (1981) The complexities of suppression in intermittent exotropia. In: Mein J & Moore S (eds) *Orthoptics, Research and Practice*. Kimpton, London, p. 172

Raab EL. (1982) Etiologic factors in accommodative esotropia. *Transactions of the American Ophthalmological Society*, 80: 657

Ravault AP, Bongrand M & Bonamour G. (1972) The utilisation of prisms in the treatment of divergent strabismus. In: Mein J, Bierlaagh JJM & Brummelkamp-Dons TEA (eds) *Orthoptics*. Excerpta Medica, Amsterdam, p. 77

Repka MX & Arnoldi KA. (1991) Lateral incomitance in exotropia: fact or artifact? *Journal of Pediatric Ophthalmology and Strabismus*, 28: 125

Rosenbaum AL. (1999) Adult strabismus surgery: the rehabilitation of a disability. *Journal of American Association for Pediatric Ophthalmology and Strabismus*, 3: 193

Ruttum M & von Noorden GK. (1983) Adaptation to tilting of the visual environment in cyclotropia. *American Journal of Ophthalmology*, 96: 229

Scobee RG. (1948) Anatomic factors in the etiology of heterotropia. *American Journal of Ophthalmology*, 31: 781

Scott AB. (1980) Botulinum toxin injection into extraocular muscles as an alternative to strabismus surgery. *Ophthalmology*, 87: 1044

Scott AB. (1981) Botulinum toxin injection of the eye muscles to correct strabismus. *Transactions of the American Ophthalmological Society*, 79: 734

Scott WE & Thalacker A. (1984) Preoperative prism adaptation in acquired esotropia. *Ophthalmologica*, 189: 49

Sidikaro Y & von Noorden GK. (1982) Observations in sensory heterotropia. *Journal of Pediatric Ophthalmology and Strabismus*, 19: 12

Spielmann A. (1987) The oblique Kestenbaum procedure revisited (sloped recession of the recti). In: Lenk-Schafer M, Calcutt C, Doyle M & Moore S (eds) *Transactions of the Sixth International Orthoptic Conference*. British Orthoptic Society, London, p. 433

Veronneau-Troutman S. (1971) Fresnel prism membrane in the treatment of strabismus. *Canadian Journal of Ophthalmology*, 6: 249

von Noorden, Brown DJ & Parks MM. (1973) Associated convergence and accommodative insufficiency. *Documenta Ophthalmologica*, 34: 393

von Noorden GK, Morris J & Edelman P. (1978) Efficacy of bifocals in the treatment of accommodative esotropia. *American Journal of Ophthalmology*, 85: 830

von Noorden GK. (1978) Indications of the posterior fixation operation in strabismus. *Ophthalmology*, 85: 512

von Noorden GK & Avilla C. (1986) Non-accommodative convergence excess. *American Journal of Ophthalmology*, 100: 70

von Noorden & Munoz M. (1988) Recurrent esotropia. *Journal of Pediatric Ophthalmology and Strabismus*, 25: 275

Wang FM & Chryssanthou G. (1988) Monocular eye closure in intermittent exotropia. *Archives of Ophthalmology*, 106: 941

Chapter 7
Microtropia

Microtropia is a small angle heterotropia (usually of 10 prism dioptres or less) in which a form of binocular single vision occurs. When there is an associated heterophoria it is known as microtropia with a latent component. The incidence of microtropia is 2–3%, of which most cases are microesotropia with microexotropia occurring less commonly.

Terminology

Fixation disparity, fusion disparity, convergence fixation disparity, pathologic fixation disparity and fixation disparity with neuroanomalous correspondence are terms that have been used to describe a physiological disparity occurring in Panum's area in cases of heterophoria with foveal suppression. Jampolsky (1951, 1956) commented on the presence of central suppression and peripheral fusion in small angle deviations. The central suppression prevents diplopia of the fixation object. Peripheral fusion with normal retinal correspondence is achieved as Panum's fusional space is large enough to compensate for the small angle deviation.

Eso flick, flicker cases and ultra small angles are terms that have been used to describe cases of minimal manifest deviation detectable on cover test (Bryer 1953).

Parks & Eustis (1961) used the term monofixation phoria to describe deviations less than 8 prism dioptres which exhibited characteristics of a phoria and a tropia and which might occur primarily due to an inability to fuse macular images, secondary to treatment of large angle strabismus, secondary to anisometropia or secondary to a unilateral macular lesion. Peripheral fusion with normal retinal correspondence in the presence of a foveal suppression scotoma was thought possible due to a stretched Panum's area (Jampolsky 1956). Bagolini glasses and after-image testing suggested that abnormal retinal correspondence was present rather than normal. Bagolini & Capobianco (1965) demonstrated an enlarged Panum's area with abnormal retinal correspondence.

The terms microstrabismus and microtropia were introduced by Lang (1968). This emphasises the manifest part of the condition and is therefore considered to be most appropriate. The term describes cases of small angle tropia with harmonious abnormal retinal correspondence, gross stereopsis and slight amblyopia. Helveston & von Noorden (1967) used the term to describe a condition with amblyopia, suppression scotoma, abnormal retinal correspondence, an absence of movement on cover test and parafoveal eccentric fixation (microtropia with identity).

In addition to the term microtropia, the term subnormal binocular vision was used by von Noorden as a category to describe binocular co-operation. Subnormal binocular vision included orthotropia or heterophoria, normal visual acuity in both eyes, fusional amplitudes, normal retinal correspondence, foveal suppression in one eye in binocular vision, reduced or absent stereopsis.

Most authors now use the term microtropia for both positive and negative cover test findings (with and without identity).

Classification

Microtropia is usually associated with abnormal retinal corresondence (Lang 1969) but also with normal retinal correspondence with an expanded Panum's fusional area (Gittoes-Davies 1951; Jampolsky 1956). Microtropia may be:

- **with identity**, which occurs when there is harmonious abnormal retinal correspondence and absolute eccentric fixation, and the angle of anomaly equals the angle of eccentricity. A manifest deviation is not seen on cover test
- **without identity**, which may have central or non-absolute eccentric fixation and the retinal correspondence may be:
  — abnormal retinal correspondence
  — normal retinal correspondence with central suppression and peripheral fusion.
  A manifest deviation will be seen on cover test.

Microtropia may be further classified as follows.

- **Primary microtropia.** There is no history of previous large angle strabismus. Microtropia is usually stable and deterioration into a large angle is not common (Arthur *et al.* 1989).
- **Primary decompensating microtropia.** These cases have an accommodative element with hypermetropia. Onset is between one and three years usually where the deviation has decompensated into a larger angle.
- **Secondary microtropia.** This follows optical or surgical reduction of a primary concomitant larger angle deviation, e.g. fully accommodative esotropia controlled to microtropia.

Aetiology

A number of aetiological factors are associated with microtropia, the most common being anisometropia but also foveal pathology, hereditary factors and the presence of a congenital defect.

Anisometropia

The high incidence of anisometropia suggests a possible aetiological relationship (Helveston & von Noorden 1967; Setayesh *et al.* 1978). Microtropia may develop secondary to a foveal scotoma caused by uncorrected anisometropia during early infancy (Helveston & von Noorden 1967). It is proposed that uncorrected anisometropia presents a blurred image to the eye with the higher refractive error and a foveal suppression scotoma develops with subsequent development of parafoveal fixation and microtropia.

This may lead to eccentric fixation under monocular conditions and abnormal retinal correspondence under binocular conditions (von Noorden 1970). Anisometropia may decrease with age and therefore the refractive error may not be evident on examination of the child at older presentation to the clinic.

Foveal pathology

Microtropia resulting from foveal pathology may include cases of infection with scar formation (e.g. toxocara) or foveal haemorrhage at an early age.

Hereditary factors

There is a high incidence of associated anomalies of binocular vision in families of microtropic patients which suggests that it may be caused by multifactorial inheritance of refractive errors or motor and sensory anomalies of binocular vision (Cantolino & von Noorden 1969).

Congenital

There may be an inherent inability or loss of a prior ability for bifoveal fusion (Gittoes-Davies 1951; Parks 1974; Wilson *et al.* 1993). There may also be a variant in the fixation reflex feedback mechanism. Precision in the development of the fixation reflex is essential for the evolution of normal binocular single vision and an anomaly of this reflex has been postulated as an aetiological factor in microtropia and eccentric fixation (von Noorden 1970). A variation in the interaction between the feedback of uniocular fixation and the feedback of binocular fixation may exist.

Investigation

Refraction

Patients are often anisometropic which has been reported in up to 80% of cases. The amblyopic eye is commonly the more hypermetropic with or without astigmatism. With microtropia exo, anisometropia is usually of mixed astigmatism. With microtropia eso, anisometropia is usually spherical. If due to a macular lesion, this may be detected on fundoscopy.

Case history

Primary microtropes often present later with referral from school vision checks. Primary decompensating microtropes may present with symptoms if the latent component becomes decompensated. The previous treatment is particularly important and may have included optical correction, orthoptic treatment or surgery for a large deviation, anisometropia or an accommodative esotropia.

Visual acuity   Varying degrees of amblyopia of the deviating eye may be noted. The crowding phenomenon is a characteristic of microtropia. Since the fovea of the deviating eye is suppressed, the beginning of words may be blurred or absent in left microesotropia and the end of words blurred or absent in right microtropia. This is important to consider when testing linear visual acuity and may occasionally produce symptoms with difficulties in reading text. Separation difficulties tend to be more notable on near fixation.

Cover test   With identity there is no manifest deviation but a latent deviation may be present. The size of the very small angle of deviation equals the distance in the amblyopic eye between the fovea and the area used for eccentric fixation. Because of eccentric fixation the parafoveal area of the eye is used for binocular as well as monocular vision. Therefore, no refixation movement is required by the amblyopic eye when the foveally fixing eye is covered.

Without identity a slight manifest deviation is detected. There may also be an associated latent component which is usually but not invariably in the direction of the heterotropia. This will be detected by alternate cover test. Where there is an associated heterophoria the recovery is to the microtropia rather than the bifoveal fixation. The rate of recovery is very important since decompensation of the heterophoria may become symptom producing.

Vertical microtropia is rare but is sometimes seen in patients with congenital or long-standing vertical muscle palsies.

Bagolini glasses   A central scotoma may be detected. Under normal circumstances, a symmetrical cross is expected. A central or paracentral gap in the line seen by the affected eye is reported by some patients.

Four dioptre prism test   This is assessed base out and base in for microtropia with identity to differentiate from bifoveal fixation with heterophoria. If a base-out prism is placed before the unaffected eye, it will make a movement inwards to overcome the effect of the prism. By Hering's law the other eye will also move conjugately by the same amount. However, as the amount of movement is so small, the deviated image remains within the scotoma area of the affected eye and no disjugate recovery movement of the affected eye will be seen. When the base-out prism is placed before the affected eye, there will be no movement of that eye as the image remains within the scotoma area and, consequently, there is no associated movement of the other eye.

The base-in prism is used particularly for microextropia (Epstein & Tredici 1972).

Fixation   This should be assessed with a visuscope particularly if no deviation is seen on cover test.

Eccentric fixation will be seen in microtropia with and without identity with absolute and non-absolute eccentricity respectively. Eccentric fixation in microtropia occurs with sensorimotor adaptation of fixation at the edge of the foveal scotoma. Fixation is typically parafoveal or parafoveolar. In microesotropia the fixation is nasal and slightly superior to the fovea. In microexotropia, fixation is temporal and/or superior to the fovea (Johnson *et al.* 1981).

Binocular function

Microtropia with identity is associated with absolute eccentric fixation with abnormal retinal correspondence. Microtropia without identity may demonstrate harmonious abnormal retinal correspondence but some cases may have central suppression and peripheral fusion and normal retinal correspondence, particularly those with a flick and associated phoria. Cases of harmonious abnormal retinal correspondence that show an associated latent component do so because the abnormal retinal correspondence is so well developed that the latent element develops around the fixation point.

A good range of peripheral fusion may be demonstrated and the patient often appreciates diplopia when fusion fails.

Reduced stereoacuity is present but to a varying degree, dependent on the level of visual acuity. Random dot tests are reported as being more difficult to perceive.

In microtropia, suppression only involves the fovea and the diplopic fixation point of the deviating eye.

Angle of deviation

An alternate prism cover test will measure the total deviation. If an associated latent deviation is present, a simultaneous prism cover test will measure only the manifest portion of the deviation. This measurement must be less than 10 prism dioptres for a diagnosis of microtropia. The difference between the alternate prism cover test and simultaneous prism cover test is the amount of heterophoria kept latent by peripheral fusion. When performing the simultaneous prism cover test, the prisms are placed before the microtropic eye and a cover/uncover test used on the other eye until the movement of the affected eye is neutralised.

Synoptophore

In cases of central fixation, the synoptophore can be used to find an angle of anomaly, so proving the presence of abnormal retinal correspondence. In practice, this is very difficult to demonstrate as the angle of deviation is so small. Foveal slides are used. There will be no angle of anomaly in cases of normal retinal correspondence.

Management

Correct the refractive error and treat amblyopia to achieve optimum visual acuity. If there is low visual acuity, full time total occlusion may be recommended dependent on age. Otherwise, part time occlusion is suitable. Occlusion is continued until there is no further improvement in acuity. While occlusion treatment is undertaken, the orthoptic investigation must include assessment of fixation, suppression and fusional vergence to ensure adequate control of the deviation and guard against the possibility of intractable diplopia. The risk of intractable diplopia has been deemed a contraindication to treatment in some cases (Lang 1969). Decompensation of the angle of deviation is unlikely as patients usually have comfortable and near normal binocular function with good peripheral fusion.

There are reports of poor acuity levels in microtropia despite treatment (Everhard-Halm & Wenniger-Pick 1989) and it has been suggested that, with treatment, vision does not improve beyond 6/9 and there is at least one line difference in acuity between both eyes (Lithander & Sjostrand 1991). Amblyopia treatment should continue as long as visual acuity is improving and be stopped only when improvement in acuity ceases. It has been thought that the sensory status is irreversible but there are reports of elimination of microtropia and amblyopia following occlusion treatment (Houston *et al.* 1998; Cleary *et al.* 1998; Henshall & Rowe 1999). Fixation becomes foveal with improved stereoacuity and resolution of the microtropia.

It is usual to treat the microtropia as if there is normal single vision. Therefore, any associated heterophoria which seems to be decompensating can be treated with orthoptic exercises to improve the fusional range, or surgery, if there is a large angle which warrants surgical intervention.

REFERENCES

Arthur BW, Smith JT & Scott WE. (1989) Long-term stability of alignment in the monofixational syndrome. *Journal of Pediatric Ophthalmology and Strabismus*, 26: 224

Bagolini B & Capobianco NM. (1965) Subjective space in comitant squint. *American Journal of Ophthalmology*, 59: 430

Bryer J. (1953) Aetiology and treatment of small convergent deviations associated with a low degree of hypermetropia. *British Orthoptic Journal*, 10: 85

Cantolino SJ & von Noorden GK. (1969) Heredity in microtropia. *Archives of Ophthalmology*, 81: 753

Cleary M, Houston CA, McFadzean RM & Dutton GN. (1998) Recovery in microtropia; implications for aetiology and neurophysiology. *British Journal of Ophthalmology*, 82: 225

Epstein DL & Tredici TJ. (1972) Use of the 4 dioptre base-in prism test in microexotropia. *American Journal of Ophthalmology*, 73: 340

Everhard-Halm YS & Wenniger-Pick LJJM. (1989) Amblyopia in microtropia. *British Orthoptic Journal*, 46: 109

Gittoes-Davies R. (1951) An examination of the aetiology and treatment of small convergent deviations, associated with a low degree of hypermetropia with a new approach to the treatment of this condition. *British Orthoptic Journal*, 8: 71

Helveston EM & von Noorden GK. (1967) Microtropia. A newly defined entity. *Archives of Ophthalmology*, 78: 272

Henshall VS & Rowe FJ. (1999) Bifoveal binocular single vision following recovery of microtropia. *British Orthoptic Journal*, 56: 45

Houston CA, Cleary M, Dutton GN & McFadzean RM. (1998) Clinical characteristics of microtropia – is microtropia a fixed phenomenon? *British Journal of Ophthalmology*, 82: 219

Jampolsky A. (1951) Retinal correspondence in patients with small degree strabismus. *Archives of Ophthalmology*, 51:18

Jampolsky A. (1956) Esotropia and convergent fixation disparity of small degree; differential diagnosis and management. *American Journal of Ophthalmology*, 41: 825

Johnson F, Cunha LAP & Harcourt RB. (1981) The clinical characteristics of micro-exotropia. *British Orthoptic Journal*, 38: 54

Lang J. (1969) Microtropia. *Archives of Ophthalmology*, 81: 758

Lithander J & Sjostrand J. (1991) Anisometropic and strabismic amblyopia in the age group 2 years and above; a prospective study of the result of treatment. *British Journal of Ophthalmology*, 5: 111

Parks MM. (1974) Management of acquired esotropia. *British Journal of Ophthalmology*, 58: 240

Parks MM & Eustis AT. (1961) Monofixational phoria. *American Orthoptic Journal*, 11: 38

Setayesh AR, Khodadoust AA & Daryani SM. (1978) Microtropia. *Archives of Ophthalmology*, 96: 1842

von Noorden GK. (1970) Etiology and pathogenesis of fixation anomalies in strabismus. I Relationships between eccentric fixation and anomalous retinal correspondence. *American Journal of Ophthalmology*, 69: 210

Wilson ME, Bluestein EC & Parks MM. (1993) Binocularity in accommodative esotropia. *Journal of Pediatric Ophthalmology and Strabismus*, 30: 233

FURTHER READING

Banks MS, Aslin RN & Letson RD. (1975) Sensitive period for the development of human binocular vision. *Science*, 190: 675

Bishop PO. (1991) Control of eye vergence and anomalous retinal correspondence. *Binocular Vision*, 6: 75

Crone RA. (1981) Anomalous binocular vision. In: Mein J & Moore S (eds) *Orthoptics, Research and Practice*. Kimpton, London, p. 160

de Decker W, Scheffel T & Baenge J. (1976) Fixation disparity and the origin of microstrabismus. In: Moore S, Mein J & Stockbridge L (eds) *Orthoptics, Past, Present and Future*. Symposia Specialists, Miami, p. 155

Hardman Lea SJ, Snead MP, Loades J & Rubinstein MP. (1991) Microtropia versus bifoveal fixation in anisometropic amblyopia. *Eye*, 5: 576

Irvine SR. (1948) Amblyopia ex anopsia; observations on retinal inhibition, scotoma, projections, light difference discrimination and visual acuity. *Transactions of the American Ophthalmological Society*, 46: 527

Keiner EC. (1976) Spontaneous recovery in microstrabismus. *Ophthalmologica*, 177: 280

Lang J. (1968) Evaluation in small angle strabismus or microtropia. In: *International Strabismus Symposium*. Karger, Basle, p. 219

Lang J. (1969) Microtropia. *British Orthoptic Journal*, 26: 30

Lang J. (1974) Management of microtropia. *British Journal of Ophthalmology*, 58: 287

Parks MM. (1961) Monofixational phoria. *American Orthoptic Journal*, 11: 38

Parks MM. (1964) Second thoughts about the pathophysiology of monofixational phoria. *American Orthoptic Journal*, 14: 159

Parks MM. (1969) The monofixational syndrome. *Transactions of the American Ophthalmological Society*, 67: 609

Parks MM. (1971) The monofixation syndrome. In: Allen JH (ed) *Symposium on Strabismus. Transactions of the New Orleans Academy of Ophthalmology*. Mosby, St Louis, p. 121

von Noorden GK. (1970) The etiology and pathogenesis of fixation anomalies in strabismus. IV. Roles of suppression scotoma and of motor factors. *American Journal of Ophthalmology*, 69: 236

Chapter 8
Amblyopia

Amblyopia is a condition of diminished visual form sense which is not a result of any clinically demonstrable anomaly of the visual pathway and which is not relieved by the elimination of any defect which constitutes a dioptric obstacle to the formation of the foveal image.

Classification

- **Stimulus deprivation amblyopia**: amblyopia which is the result of lack of adequate visual stimulus in early life. This may be unilateral or bilateral and may be:
  — complete, where no light enters the eye
  — partial, where there is some passage of light into the eye.
- **Strabismic amblyopia**: amblyopia which is the result of manifest strabismus and is caused by constant unilateral strabismus in childhood.
- **Anisometropic amblyopia**: amblyopia which is the result of a significant difference in the refractive errors of the two eyes where one eye has the visual advantage at all distances.
- **Meridional amblyopia**: amblyopia which is the result of uncorrected astigmatism where one or both eyes are predominantly astigmatic.
- **Ametropic amblyopia**: bilateral amblyopia which is the result of a high degree of uncorrected bilateral refractive error.
- **Occlusion amblyopia**: amblyopia which may occur after use of total occlusion or atropine, particularly before the age of two years. Visual acuity is usually restored with careful treatment and monitoring.

Aetiology

Amblyopia is caused by inadequate stimulation of the visual system during the critical period of visual development in early childhood (< 8 years). This is most marked under the age of two years (Awaya *et al.* 1987). Amblyopia may be unilateral or bilateral and the cause may be any or a combination of the following factors.

- **Light deprivation**. There is no stimulus to the retina. This is uncommon as it is likely that some light enters the eye even in dense cataract (white noise).
- **Form deprivation**. The retina receives a defocused image as with refractive errors.
- **Abnormal binocular interaction**. Non-fusible images fall on each fovea, as with strabismus.

165

The prognosis for achieving good visual acuity decreases when more than one of these factors are present together in one case.

There has been a decrease in amblyopia over recent years which may be due to better screening and detection (Latvala *et al.* 1996; Kvarnstrom *et al.* 1998).

Investigation

Refraction   Anisometropia, high astigmatism and bilateral high refractive errors are aetiological factors.

Case history   Early onset, unilateral, constant strabismus with long duration without treatment predisposes to strabismic amblyopia. Congenital ocular abnormalities such as cataract and ptosis predispose to stimulus deprivation amblyopia (Anderson & Baumgartner 1980).

Visual acuity   Many aspects of visual function are adversely affected by the presence of amblyopia, including high contrast linear, single optotype, repeat letter and low contrast linear, Vernier and displacement thresholds (Simmers *et al.* 1999).

If possible, it is better to use a linear test type. The patient may demonstrate the crowding phenomenon where reduced visual acuity is detected on linear testing despite better visual acuity on single optotype testing. This is due to additional stimulation from contours of adjacent letters in a linear test type and a reduction in lateral retinal inhibition which produces confusion (Hess *et al.* 2000).

Assessment of fixation aids determination of visual acuity. Free alternation indicates equal visual acuity. Holding fixation beyond a blink indicates good visual acuity. Strong objection to occlusion of the good eye and no objection to occlusion of the deviating eye suggests severely reduced visual acuity. This is also indicated with searching eye movements of the deviating eye.

Visual acuity tends to be better at near rather than distance fixation (von Noorden & Frank 1976).

Cover test   There may be a unilateral constant strabismus. By observing fixation and reaction to occlusion, an estimate of visual acuity can be obtained as detailed above. There may be ptosis which can be unilateral or bilateral. Congenital ptosis is associated with amblyopia of strabismic, anisometropic and stimulus deprivation types (Dray & Leibovitch 2002).

Visuscope   Fixation may be eccentric or wandering, in a parafoveal, paramacular or peripheral retinal area. Generally the further from the fovea, the poorer the visual acuity.

Neutral density filter   This test makes use of the fact that amblyopic eyes perform relatively well under conditions of low illumination. The visual acuity when tested with the filter is not significantly reduced in the amblyopic eye when compared with visual acuity of the normal eye. This test differentiates between amblyopia and reduced visual acuity due to organic defects as organic amblyopia will have further reduction in visual acuity under poor illumination (Burian 1967). Neutral filters profoundly reduce vision in eyes with central retinal lesions and glaucoma whereas the vision of eyes with amblyopia is not reduced with filters (von Noorden & Burian 1959; Sloan 1969; Hess & Howell 1978; France 1984).

Management

Correct the refractive error as visual acuity may respond when the correct prescription is worn as in cases of ametropic amblyopia.

Occlusion is the most commonly used method of treating amblyopia. The normal eye is occluded and occlusion may be in the form of total light and form, total form or partial.

- *Total light and form*: Opticlude and Coverlet are most widely used. Elastoplast is also available.
- *Total form*: Blenderm, Micropore, frosted lens.
- *Partial*: Fablon, Sellotape.

Risks of occlusion

(1) Intractable diplopia may occur in patients with strabismus and should be carefully monitored if giving occlusion after the age of 6–7 years due to the risk of overcoming their suppression. Patients with anisometropic amblyopia usually have binocular single vision and therefore occlusion after the age of eight years is possible but binocular function must be monitored carefully to ensure that loss of good control of a latent deviation does not occur.

(2) Occlusion amblyopia.

(3) Dissociation of latent/intermittent deviation.

(4) An increase in angle of deviation may occur on removal of occlusion.

(5) DVD: the eye may elevate further.

(6) Allergic response.

(7) Infection may be incubated by the patch.

(8) Danger socially due to disorientation.

Aims of occlusion

(1) Equalise visual acuity.

(2) Achieve optimum visual acuity.

(3) Central fixation.

Occlusion should be continued until:

- equal visual acuity is achieved
- the optimum visual acuity is achieved
- there is no further increase in visual acuity with full time total occlusion.

Compliance issues

Success of occlusion treatment relates in part to the compliance of the patient and parents/guardian in undertaking the occlusion regime. Dose monitors and diaries of occlusion wear have been used to monitor occlusion compliance. It is generally agreed that thorough discussion of the occlusion regime backed up by written information has a positive impact on occlusion success (Newsham 2002).

The age of the patient, type of amblyopia, type of occlusion, length of time it must be worn each day and length of time over which occlusion treatment continues also play a part in the general compliance with and ultimate outcome of occlusion treatment.

Factors influencing outcome include the presence of anisometropia, visual acuity at the start of treatment and compliance with treatment. Poor acuity or fixation at the start of treatment is a significant factor in the outcome (Beardsell *et al.* 1999).

Cycloplegic drugs

Where occlusion is not tolerated, cycloplegic drugs may be used to blur the vision in the better eye, thereby giving the amblyopic eye more stimulus. Typically atropine 1% is used once daily.

Advantages

(1) The patient cannot cheat, as can occur with occlusion where the child peeps over the patch or where there is poor or non-compliance.
(2) The child and parent often prefer it to occlusion.
(3) There is little or no cosmetic problem.

Disadvantages

(1) Side effects of atropine.
(2) Visual acuity may not be reduced enough where there is dense amblyopia.
(3) Atropine takes a period of 10–14 days to wear off.
(4) Frequent visits are required to monitor fixation as an indicator of visual acuity.

Penalisation

This is a further option where occlusion treatment is not tolerated. Penalisation is the treatment of amblyopia by optical reduction of form vision of the non-amblyopic eye at one or all fixation distances. The effect may be achieved by the alteration of the spectacle correction and may be enhanced by the use of a cycloplegic drug (Gregersen *et al.* 1965; Repka & Ray 1993).

Total penalisation is the use of the amblyopic eye at all distances by using strong convex lenses before the better eye. Near penalisation is the use of the amblyopic eye for near fixation by using a cycloplegic drug in the better eye and adding a convex lens up to 3.0 DS before the amblyopic eye. Distance penalisation is the use of the amblyopic eye for distance fixation by using additional convex lenses before the better eye.

Other drugs

Levodopa and carbidopa have been used to improve visual acuity, often in conjunction with occlusion therapy (Nahata *et al.* 2000; Mohan *et al.* 2001). The improvement is believed to be due to the general role of dopamine in both the retina and visual pathway (Gottlob & Strangler-Zuschrott 1990; Harris *et al.* 1990; Gottlob *et al.* 1992; Leguire *et al.* 1993, 1995). An improvement in vision is dose dependent, with a higher dose showing a better response. Patients with very poor starting vision or sensory deprivation amblyopia respond poorly to treatment. Some reduction in vision is generally noted after treatment is stopped (Pandey *et al.* 2002).

Pleoptics

Pleoptics is a method of treatment which is now rarely used. It employs after-images and Haidinger's brushes to encourage foveal fixation with normal projection. Treatment sessions need to be carried out several times per day over a period of weeks and therefore usually entail hospital admission.

Pleoptics requires high motivation on the part of the patient and is used almost exclusively to treat adults with untreated functional amblyopia who have lost the use of the good eye (Bangerter 1969).

Improvement in acuity of the amblyopic eye is quite often noted after the loss of the better eye (Vereecken & Brabant 1984).

Eccentric fixation

This is a uniocular condition in which there is fixation of an object by a retinal point other than the fovea without change in the principal visual direction. Eccentric fixation is seen in long-standing esotropia and microtropia with identity. In cases of microtropia, the eccentric fixation should not be disrupted. However, eccentric fixation associated with large angle deviations may be treated with occlusion. In cases of non-absolute fixation, direct occlusion is used to treat the amblyopia.

With fixed eccentric fixation, indirect occlusion is commenced by occluding the amblyopic eye initially, which disrupts fixation in the eye. Direct occlusion is then implemented full time to take advantage of the disrupted fixation and promote foveal stimulation. Red filter occlusion directly stimulates the foveal cells and may be combined with indirect occlusion (Cowle *et al.* 1967; Malik *et al.* 1969).

REFERENCES

Anderson RL & Baumgartner SA. (1980) Amblyopia in ptosis. *Archives of Ophthalmology*, 98: 1068

Awaya S, Miyake S, Koizumi E & Hirai T. (1987) The sensitive period of visual system in humans. In: Lenk-Schafer M, Calcutt C, Doyle M & Moore S (eds) *Transactions of the Sixth International Orthoptic Congress*. British Orthoptic Society, London, p. 44

Bangerter A. (1969) The purpose of pleoptics. *Ophthalmologica*, 158: 334

Beardsell R, Clarke S & Hill M. (1999) Outcome of occlusion treatment for amblyopia. *Journal of Pediatric Ophthalmology and Strabismus*, 36: 19

Burian HM. (1967) The behaviour of the amblyopic eye under reduced illumination and the theory of functional amblyopia. *Documenta Ophthalmologica*, 23: 189

Cowle JB, Kunst JH & Philpotts AM. (1967) Trial with red filter in the treatment of eccentric fixation. *British Journal of Ophthalmology*, 51: 165

Dray J-P & Leibovitch I. (2002) Congenital ptosis and amblyopia; a retrospective study of 130 cases. *Journal of Pediatric Ophthalmology and Strabismus*, 39: 222

France TD. (1984) Amblyopia update: diagnosis and therapy. *American Orthoptic Journal*, 34: 4

Gottlob I & Strangler-Zuschrott E. (1990) Effect of levodopa on contrast sensitivity and scotomas in human amblyopia. *Investigative Ophthalmology and Visual Science*, 31: 776

Gottlob I, Charlier J & Reinecke RD. (1992) Visual acuities and scotomas after one week of levodopa administration in human amblyopia. *Investigative Ophthalmology and Visual Science*, 33: 2722

Gregersen E, Pontoppodian M & Rindziunski E. (1965) Optic and drug penalization and favouring in the treatment of squinting amblyopia. *Acta Ophthalmologica*, 43: 462

Harris JP, Calvert JE, Leendertz JA & Phillipson OT. (1990) The influence of dopamine on spatial vision. *Eye*, 4: 806

Hess RF & Howell ER. (1978) The luminance-dependent nature of the visual abnormality in strabismic amblyopia. *Vision Research*, 18: 931

Hess RF, Dakin SC & Kapoor N. (2000) The foveal 'crowding' effect: physics or physiology. *Vision Research*, 40: 365

Kvarnstrom G, Jakobsson P & Lennerstrand G. (1998) Screening for visual and ocular disorders in children. Evaluation of the system in Sweden. *Acta Paediatrica*, 87: 1173

Latvala M-L, Paloheimo M & Karma A. (1996) Screening of amblyopic children and long-term follow-up. *Acta Ophthalmologica Scandinavica*, 74: 488

Leguire LE, Rogers GL, Bremer DL, Walson PD & McGregor ML. (1993) Levodopa/carbidopa for childhood amblyopia. *Investigative Ophthalmology and Visual Science*, 34: 3090

Leguire LE, Walson PD, Rogers GL, Bremer DL & McGregor ML. (1995) Levodopa/carbidopa treatment for amblyopia in older children. *Journal of Pediatric Ophthalmology and Strabismus*, 32: 143

Malik SRK, Gupta AK & Choudry S. (1969) The red filter treatment of eccentric fixation. *American Journal of Ophthalmology*, 67: 586

Mohan K, Dhankar V & Sharma A. (2001) Visual acuities after levodopa administration in amblyopia. *Journal of Pediatric Ophthalmology and Strabismus*, 38: 62

Nahata MC, Morosco RS & Leguire LE. (2000) Development of two stable oral suspensions of levodopa-carbidopa for children with amblyopia. *Journal of Pediatric Ophthalmology and Strabismus*, 37: 333

Newsham D. (2002) A randomised controlled trial of written information: the effect on parental non-concordance with occlusion therapy. *British Journal of Ophthalmology*, 86: 787

Pandey PK, Chaudhuri Z, Kumar M, Satyabala K & Sharma P. (2002) Effect of levodopa and carbidopa in human amblyopia. *Journal of Pediatric Ophthalmology and Strabismus*, 39: 81

Repka MX & Ray JM. (1993) The efficacy of optical and pharmacological penalization. *Ophthalmology*, 100: 769

Simmers AJ, Gray LS, McGraw & Winn B. (1999) Functional visual loss in amblyopia and the effects of occlusion therapy. *Investigative Ophthalmology and Visual Science*, 40: 2859

Sloan L. (1969) Variations in acuity with luminance in ocular disease and anomalies. *Documenta Ophthalmologica*, 26: 384

Vereecken EP & Brabant P. (1984) Prognosis for vision in amblyopia after loss of the good eye. *Archives of Ophthalmology*, 102: 220

von Noorden GK & Burian HM. (1959) Visual acuity in normal and amblyopic patients under reduced illumination. I Behaviour of visual acuity with and without neutral density filter. *Archives of Ophthalmology*, 61: 533

von Noorden GK & Frank JW. (1976) Relationships between amblyopia and the angle of strabismus. *American Orthoptic Journal*, 26: 31

FURTHER READING

Attebo K, Mitchell P, Cumming R, Smith W, Jolly N & Sparkes R. (1998) Prevalence and causes of amblyopia in an adult population. *Ophthalmology*, 105: 154

Banks RV, Campbell F, Hess RF & Watson PG. (1978) A new treatment for amblyopia. *British Orthoptic Journal*, 35: 1

Blakemore C & Cooper G. (1970) Development of the brain depends on the visual environment. *Nature*, 228: 477

Calcutt C & Crook W. (1972) The treatment of amblyopia in patients with latent nystagmus. *British Orthoptic Journal*, 29: 70

Campos EC. (1995) Review of amblyopia. *Survey of Ophthalmology*, 40: 23

Cole RBW. (1959) The problems of unilateral amblyopia. A preliminary study of 10,000 National Health patients. *British Medical Journal*, 1(5116): 202

Crawford MLJ, Blake R, Cool SJ & von Noorden GK. (1975) Physiological consequences of unilateral and bilateral eye closure in macaque monkeys: some further observations. *Brain Research*, 84: 150

Dobson V & Teller DY. (1978) Visual acuity in human infants: a review and comparison of behavioural and electrical-physiological studies. *Vision Research*, 18: 1469

Friedman Z, Neumann E, Hyams SW & Peleg B. (1980) Ophthalmic screening of 38,000 children age 1 to $2^{1}/_{2}$ years, in child welfare clinics. *Journal of Pediatric Ophthalmology and Strabismus*, 17: 261

Gwiazda J, Bauer J, Thorn F & Held R. (1986) Meridional amblyopia does result from astigmatism in early childhood. *Clinical Visual Science*, 1: 145

Hardesty HH. (1959) Occlusion amblyopia. Report of a case. *Archives of Ophthalmology*, 62: 314

Harrad RA, Graham CM & Collin JR. (1988) Amblyopia and strabismus in congenital ptosis. *Eye*, 2: 625

Harrad R, Sengpiel F & Blakemore C. (1996) Physiology of suppression in strabismic amblyopia. *British Journal of Ophthalmology*, 80: 373

Harwerth RS, Smith EL, Duncan GC, Crawford ML & von Noorden GK. (1986) Multiple sensitive periods in the development of the primate visual system. *Science*, 232: 235

Held R. (1988) Normal visual development and its deviations. In: Lennerstrand G, von Noorden GK & Campos EC (eds) *Strabismus and Amblyopia*. Wenner Gren International Symposium Series No. 49. Macmillan Press, London, p. 247

Hubel DH & Wiesel TN. (1972) Laminar and columnar distribution of geniculo-cortical fibres in the macaque monkey. *Journal of Comparative Neurology*, 146: 421

Ikeda H & Tremain KE. (1978) Amblyopia resulting from penalisation: neurophysiological studies of kittens reared with atropinisation of one or both eyes. *British Journal of Ophthalmology*, 62: 21

Ikeda H & Wright MJ. (1974) Is amblyopia due to inappropriate stimulation of 'sustained' visual pathways during development? *British Journal of Ophthalmology*, 58: 168

Irvine RA. (1945) Amblyopia ex anopsia: observations on retinal inhibition, scotoma, projection, light difference, discrimination and visual acuity. *Transactions of the American Ophthalmic Society*, 66: 527

Jampolsky A. (1978) Unequal visual inputs and strabismus management: a comparison of human and animal strabismus. In: Allen JH (ed) *Symposium on Strabismus. Transactions of the New Orleans Academy of Ophthalmology*. Mosby, St Louis, p. 358

Keith CG, Howell ER, Mitchell DE & Smith S. (1980) Clinical trial of the use of grating patterns in the treatment of amblyopia. *British Journal of Ophthalmology*, 64: 8

Mehdorn E, Mattheus S, Schuppe A, Klein U & Kommerell G. (1981) Treatment for amblyopia with rotating gratings and subsequent occlusion; a controlled study. *International Ophthalmology*, 3: 161

Vinding T, Gregersen E, Jensen A & Rindzinnski E. (1991) Prevalence of amblyopia in old people without previous screening and treatment. *Acta Ophthalmologica*, 69: 796

von Noorden GK. (1985) Amblyopia, a multi-disciplinary approach. *Investigative Ophthalmology and Visual Science*, 26: 1704

von Noorden GK & Crawford MLJ. (1980) The sensitive period. *Transactions of the Ophthalmological Society of the United Kingdom*, 99: 442

von Noorden GK & Middleditch PR. (1975) Histology of the monkey lateral geniculate nucleus after unilateral lid closure and strabismus: further observations. *Investigative Ophthalmology*, 14: 674

Wiesel TN & Hubel DH. (1963) Single-cell responses in striate cortex of kittens deprived of vision in one eye. *Journal of Neurophysiology*, 26: 1003

Wiesel TN & Hubel DH. (1965) Comparison of the effects of unilateral and bilateral eye closure on cortical unit responses in kittens. *Journal of Neurophysiology*, 28: 1029

Chapter 9
Aphakia

Aphakia follows the treatment of congenital or acquired cataract and may occur at any age although patients are most likely to be rendered pseudophakic with the insertion of an intraocular lens following cataract extraction.

Investigation

Case history
Ascertain the cause and duration of the cataract, time of extraction and form of subsequent correction. With paediatric cases check how long the cataract has been present before treatment as this can help predict prognosis for visual outcome. Symptoms may include diplopia and blurred near vision. There may be a previous history of strabismus and positive family history. An additional +3.0 DS lens in front of the corrected aphakic eye should be used for near testing with older children and adults.

Visual acuity
Children will generally have severe amblyopia of stimulus deprivation type and often strabismic type in addition. However, good visual acuity can be maintained in some cataracts, e.g. anterior peripheral lens opacity.

Cover test
Adults may have latent, intermittent or manifest strabismus. Children frequently have manifest secondary strabismus (see Chapter 6).

Ocular motility
In cases of traumatic cataract, ocular motility may be limited where there has been associated globe and/or extraocular muscle damage.

Binocular function
Adults may demonstrate binocular single vision with latent or intermittent strabismus. If manifest strabismus is present, the angle is corrected to assess the state of binocularity. Children rarely demonstrate binocularity due to the presence of strabismus and dense amblyopia.

There may be loss of fusion in adults with cataract that has been left untreated over a period of years (Sloper & Collins 1995).

Aniseikonia
The presence and extent of aniseikonia can be assessed with Ruben's slides on the synoptophore.

Angle of deviation
This is measured using corneal reflections where the visual acuity is insufficient to obtain adequate fixation.

Problems with unilateral aphakia
- Insuperable aniseikonia
- Manifest strabismus:
    — secondary divergent deviation in adults
    — secondary convergent deviation in young children
- Stimulus deprivation amblyopia plus strabismus amblyopia

Management

Methods of correction may be:

- **unilateral**
  - intraocular lens implant
  - contact lenses
  - epikeratophakia
- **bilateral**
  - intraocular lens implant
  - spectacles – must be correctly centred and accurately fitted
  - contact lenses.

Intraocular lenses give the least increase in image size. Spectacles may be used with bilateral cases, but problems arise with aberrations, prismatic effects and weight and they must be a good fit to encourage tolerance with young children.

Adults

Symptomatic heterophoria is treated with orthoptic exercises (see Chapter 4). With intermittent deviations, orthoptic exercises are used to improve fusional reserves. Surgery may be required if a large angle is present and orthoptic exercises given post-operatively to consolidate the result. Manifest deviations may require surgery to correct the deviation, aiming for parallel visual axes with functional cases. In cosmetic divergent deviations, aim for a slight overcorrection. Where there has been a loss of fusion, occlusion, Bangerter filters or occlusive contact lenses may be required.

Children

There is often a poor prognosis for vision in unilateral cataracts. Contact lenses are fitted and occlusion is implemented to improve vision. These patients usually require full time total occlusion. Cosmetic surgery may be indicated for manifest strabismus.

The cataract can be removed within days of birth and intraocular lenses (Spierer *et al*. 1999) are implanted at increasingly earlier ages with a top-up correction obtained with a contact lens.

Posterior chamber intraocular lens implantation is a safe and effective method for treatment of cataracts in children over the age of two years. There is, however, considerable debate as to the safety and long term effects of intraocular lens implantation in neonates.

Early treatment is advisable as this results in fewer acuity deficits than later treatment. Treatment during the initial six weeks is maximally effective and effectiveness rapidly decreases from 12 weeks of age (Birch *et al*. 1998). Better results are also achieved with combined treatment (intraocular lens plus contact lens) rather than sole treatment regimes. Factors affecting visual outcome include amblyopia and antecedent posterior segment trauma (Simons *et al*. 1999).

REFERENCES

Birch EE, Stager D, Laffler J & Weakley D. (1998) Early treatment of congenital unilateral cataract minimises unequal competition. *Investigative Ophthalmology and Visual Science*, 39: 1560

Simons BD, Siatkowski RM, Schiffman JC, Flynn JT, Capo H & Munoz M. (1999) Surgical technique, visual outcome, and complications of pediatric IOL implantation. *Journal of Pediatric Ophthalmology and Strabismus*, 36: 118

Sloper JJ & Collins AD. (1995) Delayed visual evoked potentials in adults after monocular visual deprivation by a dense cataract. *Investigative Ophthalmology and Visual Science*, 36: 2663

Spierer A, Desatnik H & Blumenthal M. (1999) Refractive status in children after long-term follow up of cataract surgery with intraocular lens implantation. *Journal of Pediatric Ophthalmology and Strabismus*, 36: 25

FURTHER READING

Birch EE & Stager DR. (1996) The critical period for surgical treatment of dense congenital unilateral cataract. *Investigative Ophthalmology and Visual Science*, 37: 1532

Churchill AJ, Noble BA, Etchells DE & George NJ. (1995) Factors affecting visual outcome in children following uniocular traumatic cataract. *Eye*, 9: 285

Jampolsky A. (1978) Unequal visual inputs and strabismus management: a comparison of human and animal strabismus. In: Allen JH (ed) *Symposium on Strabismus. Transactions of the New Orleans Academy of Ophthalmology*. Mosby, St Louis, p. 358

Lloyd IC, Dowler JGF, Kriss A, Speedwell L, Thompson DA, Russell-Eggitt I & Taylor D. (1995) Modulation of amblyopia therapy following early surgery for unilateral congenital cataracts. *British Journal of Ophthalmology*, 79: 802

McElvvanney A, Moseley MJ & Jones HS. (1994) Binocular inhibition of visual performance in patients with cataract. *Acta Ophthalmologica*, 72: 606

Mills A. (1979) Aniseikonia in corrected anisometropia. *British Orthoptic Journal*, 36: 36

Pratt-Johnson JA & Tillson G. (1989) Unilateral congenital cataract: binocular status after treatment. *Journal of Pediatric Ophthalmology and Strabismus*, 26: 72

Robb RM. (1994) Strabismus and strabismic amblyopia before and after surgery for bilateral congenital cataracts. *Binocular Vision*, 9: 183

Wylie J, Henderson M, Doyle M & Hickey-Dwyer M. (1994) Persistent binocular diplopia following cataract surgery: aetiology and management. *Eye*, 8: 543

SECTION III

Chapter 10
Incomitant strabismus

Incomitant strabismus is strabismus in which the angle of deviation differs depending upon the direction of gaze or according to which eye is fixing and is associated with defective movement of the eye or with asymmetrical accommodative effort.

Ophthalmoplegia is a group of conditions which have a variety of causative factors, where there is a paresis of two or more of the extra-ocular muscles.

When examining these patients, the angle of deviation may be different depending on which eye is fixing and how long the deviation has been present.

- **Primary angle of deviation**. The deviation when fixing with the unaffected eye in paralytic incomitant deviation.
- **Secondary angle of deviation**. The deviation when fixing with the affected eye in paralytic incomitant deviation.

Generally, with more recently acquired palsies, the strabismus will be quite incomitant with a significant difference between the primary and secondary angles of deviation. With time, the strabismus becomes less incomitant and it is harder to assess whether it is congenital or long-standing. It is often difficult to differentiate between primary and secondary deviations, as relative concomitance usually only occurs following long-standing incomitance.

Aetiology

Incomitant strabismus may be found in association with many disorders. The list below is designed to give an overall idea of the types of condition which can cause incomitance.

Congenital

Neurogenic
- In association with other congenital developmental disorders
- As an isolated feature

Form
- Aplasia; hypoplasia of nerve/nucleus
- Abnormal innervation
- Trauma during gestation/delivery
- Inflammation: neonatal/antenatal

Mechanical
- Duane's retraction syndrome
- Brown's syndrome

Myogenic
- Developmental abnormality: hypoplasia/hyperplasia/aplasia of extraocular muscles
- Abnormal attachments, e.g. muscle insertions to the eyeball or to the orbital contents
- Fibrosis
- Adhesions: intermuscular, muscle to orbit

Acquired

Neurogenic
- Trauma
- Inflammation, e.g. multiple sclerosis
- Vascular, e.g. hypertension
- Space occupying lesions
- Metabolic disorder, e.g. diabetes

Mechanical
- Trauma: development of fibrous tethers, fractures
- Space occupying lesions
- Iatrogenic adhesions
- Secondary to myogenic inflammation, e.g. thyroid eye disease

Myogenic

Lesions at:
- neuromuscular junction, e.g. myasthenia gravis
- muscle fibre membrane, e.g. myotonia
- muscle fibre contents, e.g. dystrophies (chronic progressive external ophthalmoplegia), endocrine (dysthyroid eye disease), inflammatory (myositis)

Aid to diagnosis

Congenital and acquired defects often show different characteristics which help in making the diagnosis. Tables 10.1 and 10.2 opposite show the findings that might be expected when the patient is examined in the eye clinic.

Abnormal head posture

An abnormal head posture is any state in which the head is consistently not held in an upright position but adopts one or more of the following components:

- head tilt
- face turn
- chin elevation or depression.

Table 10.1   Differences between congenital and acquired defects.

	Congenital	Acquired

Presentation	Symptoms of decompensation
	Unaware of abnormal
	   head posture
	Unacceptable cosmetic appearance
		Diplopia and occasionally pain
		Aware of uncomfortable
		   abnormal head posture

Ocular motility	Often full muscle sequelae	Muscle sequelae not fully developed
Binocular function	Extended vertical fusion range	Normal fusion range

Table 10.2   Differences between neurogenic and mechanical defects.

	Neurogenic	Mechanical

Cover test	Deviation in primary position
	   reflects the extent of palsy
		Often only small deviation in
		   primary position

Ocular motility	Movement is greater on ductions
	   compared to versions
	No retraction of the globe
		Movement is the same on
		   ductions and versions
		Retraction may be noted

Hess chart	Space between inner and outer
	   fields is equal and proportional
	Fields are displaced away from
	   position of greatest limitation
		Outer field is displaced close to
		   inner field in the position of
		   greatest limited movement

Forced duction test	Full passive movement	Limited passive movement

Intraocular pressure	Same in all positions of gaze	Increases when looking away
		   from the position of
		   limitation

Head tilt

The tilt is generally towards the hypotropic eye and may be adopted to utilise the torsional movements of the eyes.

Face turn

This moves the eyes away from the field of action of the paresed muscle for vertically acting muscles as well as horizontal. It also enables the eyes to fix centrally where there is gross limitation of movement.

Chin elevation or depression

This may be adopted to place the eyes away from the field of action of the affected muscle or to utilise other muscles having the same action. It can also be used for comfort in some mechanical limitations where movement is painful.

Assessment of head posture

The following factors should be considered.

(1) Ensure sitting upright or standing.
(2) Observe head posture from directly in front of the patient.
(3) Note facial symmetry/asymmetry.
(4) Straighten head and allow patient to assume usual position.
(5) Assess near and distance.
(6) May be intermittent, therefore observe throughout.
(7) Examine old photographs in suspected long-standing cases.
(8) Scoliosis of spine may be seen in congenital or early onset tilt.
(9) Compare which ear is more visible.
(10) Check whether eyes are level.
(11) Observe for chin position from side if not obvious.

Uses of the assessment of head posture

Diagnostic
(1) Diagnosis of the affected muscle in palsies.
(2) Differential diagnosis of congenital and acquired palsies by:
   — awareness of presence of a head posture
   — degree of head posture in relation to amount of limitation of movement
   — examination of old photographs.
(3) Presence of normal binocular functions in paralytic squint. An abnormal head posture without binocular single vision may indicate pre-existing binocular single vision.
(4) Use of the Bielchowsky head tilt test to differentiate the affected muscle.

Therapeutic
A marked abnormal head posture may be an indication for surgery in:

- ocular palsies
- musculofacial anomalies
- ptosis
- nystagmus.

Reasons for abnormal head postures

Non-ocular
(1) Non-ocular torticollis (contracture of the sternomastoid muscle)
(2) Deafness
(3) Arthritic and rheumatoid conditions
(4) Habit
(5) Shyness
(6) Mental development delay

Ocular
(1) To enable the development of binocular single vision in cases of congenital paralytic strabismus and musculofacial anomalies.
(2) To maintain binocular single vision in cases of acquired paralytic strabismus, mechanical limitations and A or V patterns.
(3) To overcome symptoms other than diplopia such as avoiding painful ocular movements or in cases of physiological V pattern.
(4) To gain foveal fixation in cases of marked infantile esotropia, bilateral lateral recti paralysis and in myogenic conditions with grossly limited movement.
(5) To improve visual acuity in cases of bilateral ptosis, nystagmus, under- or overcorrected spherical refractive errors, wrongly corrected astigmatism and visual field defects.
(6) To separate diplopia in paralytic strabismus by moving the images further apart so that the second image can be ignored.
(7) In DVD, there may be a tilt or turn towards the fixating eye.
(8) To protect the eyes.

Differential diagnosis between ocular and non-ocular torticollis

	Ocular	Non-ocular
Aetiology	Vertical extraocular muscle palsies	Contracture of sternomastoid muscle
Effect of straightened head	Vertical deviation decreases and may decompensate	Shoulder raises
Ocular movements	Over- and underactions of vertically acting muscles in the same direction as the face turn	Full or unrelated to head posture
Ocular deviation	Vertical and may have a horizontal and torsional component	None or not related to head posture
Type of head posture	Depends on affected muscle	Tilt to affected side Turn to opposite side
Head tilt	Of varying degree	Usually marked
Effect of occlusion	Head tilt reduced or is abolished with one eye occluded	Head tilt persists when one eye is occluded or with both eyes closed
Treatment	Surgery on the vertically acting muscles may succeed in abolishing or reducing the head posture	Treatment of the neck defects Physiotherapy

Conditions in which abnormal head postures are present

(1)   Bilateral ptosis: to achieve binocular single vision and better visual acuity.
(2)   Incomitant squint:
— neurogenic: to achieve binocular single vision or separate diplopic images where there has been a traumatic loss of fusion. A marked face turn makes use of the nose as an occluder
— mechanical: to avoid pain, achieve binocular single vision or separate the diplopic images.
(3)   Nystagmus: to make use of a null point. Face turn adopted.
(4)   Physiological V: alteration in chin position.
(5)   A and V patterns.
(6)   Heterophoria: a large heterophoria in the primary position may decrease on elevation or depression.
(7)   Manifest deviation: a small angle deviation may be controlled on elevation or depression.
(8)   Tripartite field: abnormal head posture to cross-fixate.
(9)   Monocular blindness, occlusion, field defects: abnormal head posture to centralise the field of vision.
(10) Uncorrected refractive errors: abnormal head posture to achieve better vision.
(11) Ill fitting spectacles/incorrect cylinder: head tilt.

FURTHER READING

Fells P. (1974) Management of paralytic strabismus. *British Journal of Ophthalmology*, 58: 255

Helveston EM. (1971) Muscle transposition procedures. *Survey of Ophthalmology*, 16: 92

Iacobucci I & Beyst-Martonyi J. (1978) The use of press-on prisms in the preoperative evaluation of adults with strabismus. *American Orthoptic Journal*, 28: 68

Jones ST. (1977) Treatment of hypertropia by vertical displacement of horizontal recti. *American Orthoptic Journal*, 27: 107

Knapp P. (1975) The use of membrane prisms. *Transactions of the American Academy of Ophthalmology and Otolaryngology*, 79: 718

Stephens KF & Reinecke RD. (1967) Quantitative forced duction. *Transactions of the American Academy of Ophthalmology and Otolaryngology*, 71: 324

Chapter 11
A and V patterns

A and V patterns are patterns of horizontal incomitance in which a significant increase or decrease in angle of a horizontal deviation is noted between an elevated and depressed position of gaze.

Classification

- **A pattern** (Fig. 11.1): this is a condition in which there is relative convergence on upgaze and relative divergence on downgaze. There must be a minimum of 10 prism dioptres difference between upgaze and downgaze.
- **V pattern** (Fig. 11.2): this is a condition in which there is relative divergence on upgaze and relative convergence on downgaze. There must be a minimum of 15 prism dioptres difference between upgaze and downgaze. This allows for a slight physiological V pattern.

Variants of A and V patterns include:

- **X pattern**: there is relative divergence on both up- and downgaze.
- **Y pattern**: there is relative divergence on upgaze with no significant difference between the primary position and downgaze.
- **λ pattern**: there is relative divergence on downgaze with no significant difference between the primary position and upgaze.
- **◊ pattern**: there is relative convergence on both up- and downgaze.

Aetiology

There are various theories relating to the aetiology of A and V patterns (Folk 1997). These may involve imbalance or abnormal insertions of horizontally acting extraocular muscles, imbalance of vertically acting extraocular muscles, sagittalisation or structural anomalies. Horizontal innervational muscle theories are based on the concept of physiological V pattern in which medial recti have greater power on downgaze and lateral recti have greater power on upgaze. Many have reported anomalies in the insertions of the horizontal recti muscles; thus, if the muscle insertions are higher or lower than the normal position, abduction or adduction is subsequently increased on upgaze or downgaze. Reports have appeared of insertion of the medial rectus at the time of surgery in patients with elevation on adduction and anomalies of the rectus muscle insertions, particularly in patients with A and V patterns with additional anomalies of the lid fissures (von Noorden 1995). Kushner (1985) reported that if muscles are displaced, they take on additional actions.

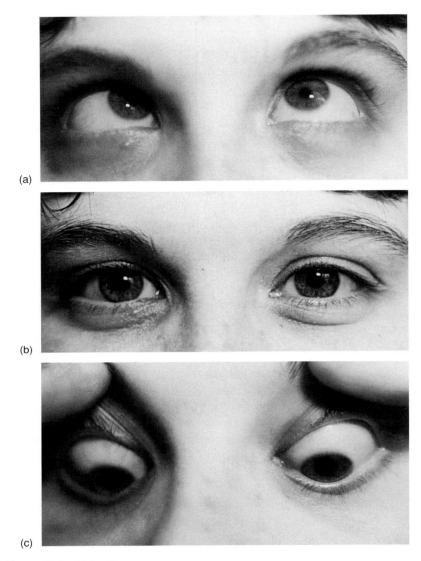

(a)

(b)

(c)

Figure 11.1   'A' pattern.

Brown (1953) reported A and V patterns caused by primary anomalies in function of vertical muscles. Urist (1958) stated that A and V patterns may be caused by anomalies of cyclovertical muscle actions. Fink (1959) found anomalies in the muscle planes of the superior oblique tendon and the inferior oblique muscle during anatomical dissection of the orbits.

Normally the planes of both the superior and inferior obliques are identical and form an angle of 51 degrees with the anterior-posterior

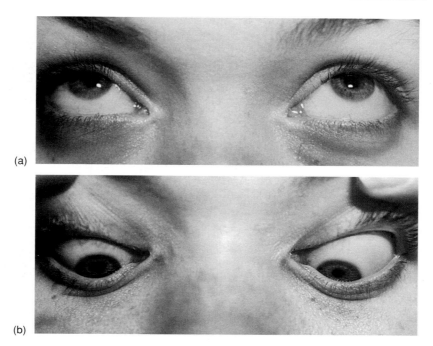

(a)

(b)

Figure 11.2   'V' pattern.

axis of the globe. If one insertion is more posterior than normal, the muscle axis will lie in a more sagittal plane, i.e. it is closer to the anterior-posterior axis of the globe. The effect of this 'sagittalisation' is to reduce the muscle's torsional action and there is muscle overaction to compensate (Gobin 1968).

Urrets-Zavalia *et al.* (1961) believed that anomalies in action of the cyclovertical muscles, which may cause variations of the horizontal deviations in up- and downgaze, are very different in patients with mongoloid and antimongoloid features.

Aetiology may also be related to muscle pulleys (Clark *et al.* 1998). Apparently overacting inferior obliques or superior obliques have shown difference in positions of lateral rectus muscle pulleys. The heterotopia alters the vertical position of the pulleys, thus changing the course and the action of the lateral rectus muscle which in turn produces elevation or depression in adduction of the fellow eye, depending on whether the pulley is displaced inferiorly or superiorly.

A eso pattern

(1)   Lateral rectus underaction results in less abduction on elevation.

(2)   Low medial rectus insertions result in more adduction on elevation due to different muscle position and increased muscle tension.

(3)   Inferior oblique underaction results in less abduction on elevation. The superior oblique will overact, resulting in more abduction on depression.

(4)   Superior oblique sagittalisation results in superior oblique overaction.

(5)   Mongoloid facial features.

A exo pattern

(1)   Medial rectus underaction results in less adduction on depression.

(2)   High lateral rectus insertions result in more abduction on depression.

(3)   Inferior rectus underaction results in less adduction on depression. The superior rectus will overact, resulting in more adduction on elevation.

(4)   Superior oblique sagittalisation results in superior oblique overaction.

(5)   Antimongoloid facial features.

V eso pattern

(1)   Lateral rectus overaction results in more abduction on elevation.

(2)   High medial rectus insertions result in more adduction on depression.

(3)   Superior oblique underaction results in less abduction on depression. The inferior oblique will overact, resulting in more abduction on elevation.

(4)   Inferior oblique sagittalisation results in inferior oblique overaction.

(5)   Antimongoloid facial features.

V exo pattern

(1)   Medial rectus overaction results in more adduction on depression.

(2)   Low lateral rectus insertions result in more abduction on elevation.

(3)   Superior rectus underaction results in less adduction on elevation. The inferior rectus will overact, resulting in more adduction on depression.

(4)   Inferior oblique sagittalisation results in inferior oblique overaction.

(5)   Mongoloid facial features.

Incidence/prevalence

There is a varied incidence of A and V patterns reported in the literature. However, it is accepted that the incidence is around 20%. The relative frequency of various types of patterns is not clearly established but is thought to be, in order of greatest to least frequent, V eso, A eso, V exo, A exo.

A and V patterns are especially prevalent in certain conditions.

- Infantile esotropia. High incidence of both A and V patterns along with DVD and inferior oblique overactions.
- Duane's retraction syndrome. V pattern with upshoots and A pattern with downshoots.
- Brown's syndrome. Most have V pattern explained by increased abduction occurring when mechanically inhibited inferior oblique receives increased innervation to elevate the eye.
- Acquired IV nerve palsy (particularly bilateral). V pattern esotropia.
- Thyroid eye disease. A pattern exotropia may result from overrecession of the inferior recti muscles or from orbital decompression.

Investigation

Aims

(1) Detect and measure A/V patterns.
(2) Assess ocular movements associated with A/V patterns.
(3) Assess significance of A/V patterns for prognosis and management.

Criteria for diagnosis

This is based on the amount of difference in measurement of the horizontal angle of deviation.

- V pattern: minimum difference of 15 prism dioptres from upgaze to downgaze.
- A pattern: minimum difference of 10 prism dioptres from upgaze to downgaze (Knapp 1959).

There is a physiological tendency to relatively diverge in upgaze and thus the minimum standards required for a V pattern are larger than for an A pattern.

Significance of A/V patterns

(1) Diagnosis of incomitance: the pattern may be the first sign of incomitance and not just a horizontal squint.
(2) Diagnosis of paretic element: strabismus may not have been noticed but A/V pattern indicates the presence of early onset squint.
(3) Indication of possible vertical element in apparent horizontal deviation.
(4) Suggestion of bilateral ocular muscle imbalance.
(5) Binocular single vision may be present in the position of minimal deviation even if it is not present in the primary position. Therefore test in that position.
(6) Cosmesis is more significant in certain positions such as primary gaze and elevation but less so for downgaze as the lids cover the eye position.

Case history	An abnormal head posture may be noted. Strabismus and abnormal eye movements may have been observed and patients may present with symptoms of decompensation.
Abnormal head posture	Chin elevation is seen with A eso and V exo patterns and chin depression with A exo and V eso patterns. In addition, a face turn and head tilt may be present due to associated extraocular muscle paresis.
Cover test	This should be performed with and without the abnormal head posture to assess the state of compensation or decompensation of the deviation. Perform in primary position, upgaze and downgaze for both near and distance.

Control accommodation by using an accommodative target for fixation and ensuring it is seen clearly, and by testing with glasses worn, particularly if hypermetropic. Repeat without glasses as frames may restrict fixation on up- and downgaze.

Failure to wear appropriate correction or use an accommodative target may result in true patterns being concealed (Knapp 1959; von Noorden & Olsen 1965).

Ocular motility	A and V patterns are common in some motility syndromes as detailed above. One should check for asymmetry of bilaterality in ocular movements. Where overacting extraocular muscles are noted, the corresponding underacting muscles should be assessed. If the patient is hypermetropic, use an accommodative target to assess in up- and downgaze.
Binocular function	A good level of binocular function may be maintained with an abnormal head posture. If negative in the primary position, test in the position of minimal deviation.

If no free space binocularity can be demonstrated, test on the synoptophore. If negative in the primary position, move tubes into the position of minimum deviation.

Angle of deviation	Measurements should be made in up- and downgaze to confirm presence and assess if it is diagnostically significant. There must be a difference of 15 prism dioptres between measurements on elevation and depression in cases of V patterns. This allows for a physiological V pattern. There must be a difference of 10 prism dioptres in cases of A patterns to confirm the diagnosis. Accommodation must be controlled when measuring the nine positions of gaze as a pseudo A or V pattern may result or a pattern can be masked if accommodation is exerted or not (Knapp 1959; von Noorden & Olsen 1965). Measurements are therefore preferable at distance fixation to prevent the influence of accommodation.

Measurements may be made using the synoptophore and moving the tubes or with the prism cover test by moving the head or the target. The synoptophore is a repeatable test but does not always reveal the full difference in the angle of deviation.

Knapp (1959) questioned whether errors in measurement were incurred by measuring the deviation with the head tilted backward and forward to obtain depression and elevation of the eyes or with the head fixed whilst the patient fixates above and below the horizontal plane. However, there has generally been little difference found whether the target or head is moved (Magee 1960; Scott 1968).

Breinin (1961) stated that the eyes should not be rotated in extreme positions since the mechanical effects of the check ligaments and musculofacial system may alter the deviation.

Hess chart and field of binocular single vision   Confirm A/V patterns and associated over- and underactions. A and V patterns are revealed by sloping sides to the two fields.

Management

It is important to determine whether the strabismus is functional, to differentiate between compensated and decompensated and the extent of the head posture, and to consider the cosmetic aspect. Give the refractive correction as appropriate.

Functional cases

Management consists of monitoring the patient to ensure that comfortable symptom-free binocular single vision is maintained without an excessive head posture. If a significant degree of abnormal head posture is present, surgery must be considered to eliminate this. Surgery may also be undertaken for upshots.

It is important to ensure that there are no factors which may contribute to decompensation such as a reduced near point of convergence.

Prisms are indicated where there are signs of decompensation with intermittent diplopia and loss of control. Prisms may be used diagnostically provided the incomitance is not excessive.

Cosmetic cases

Surgery is considered only for large deviations, marked abnormal head postures and upshoots. An increase in angle of deviation on depression is masked by the upper eyelids. Obvious strabismus on elevation may be cosmetically poor in children but is likely to be less obvious in adult life. In such cases the height of family members should be considered.

Aims of surgery

- Correct horizontal angle in primary position.
- Reduce incomitance in vertical gaze.
- Eliminate any noticeable upshoot on lateroversion.

General principles of surgery

- Bilateral symmetrical procedures.
- May require more than one operation.

- If no vertical extraocular muscle abnormality is present, operate on horizontal recti. If vertical extraocular muscle abnormalities are documented then surgery on the vertical muscles should be considered.

Surgery on horizontal recti

This is recommended when there is no evidence of vertical extraocular muscle dysfunction or minor vertical muscle incomitance is present only in extreme positions of elevation or depression.

- **Transpositions**. Vertical transposition of horizontal rectus muscles may be combined with a recession and less commonly with a resection. This is based on the principle that with the eyes in elevation or depression, the muscle plane, determined by the centre of rotation of the globe and centres of origin and insertion, changes. Extraocular muscles are usually displaced a distance which is equivalent to a muscle width or half a muscle width.
- **Boyd's technique**. Recessions are further enhanced by recessing the upper or lower margin of the horizontal rectus more than the opposite margin.

Surgery on vertically acting muscles

- Weakening procedures: recession or myectomy, tenotomy or tenectomy (Urist 1951; Villaseca 1961).
- Strengthening procedures: plication (tuck) or resection, Harado–Ito (Harado & Ito 1964).
- Anteropositioning.
- Transplant vertical recti: nasal or temporal muscle displacement (Miller 1960; von Noorden 1963).

A eso pattern

- Bilateral medial rectus recessions, moving the insertions up (Goldstein 1967; Urist 1968).
- Sloping medial rectus recessions with maximum recession on the upper border of muscles (Boyd et al. 1971).
- Weaken the superior oblique by tenotomy or tenectomy (Shin et al. 1996).
- Superior oblique anteropositioning.
- Transpositioning of the superior rectus temporally (Miller 1960).

A exo pattern

- Bilateral lateral rectus recessions, moving the insertions down (Urist 1968; Scott et al. 1989).
- Sloping lateral rectus recessions with maximum recession on the lower border of muscles (Boyd et al. 1971).

- Weaken the superior oblique by tenotomy or tenectomy (Shuey *et al.* 1992).
- Superior oblique anteropositioning (Caldeira 1975; Buckley & Flynn 1983; Romano & Roholt 1983; Souza-Dias & Uesugui 1986).
- Transpositioning of the inferior rectus medially.

V eso pattern

- Bilateral medial rectus recessions, moving the insertions down (Urist 1951; Goldstein 1967).
- Sloping medial rectus recessions with maximum recession on the lower border of muscles (Boyd *et al.* 1971).
- Weaken the inferior oblique (Billet & Freedman 1969).
- Strengthen the superior oblique with a tuck procedure (Hiles *et al.* 1985)
- Inferior oblique anteropositioning (Gobin 1964).
- Tranpositioning of the inferior rectus temporally (Miller 1960; von Noorden 1963).

V exo pattern

- Bilateral lateral rectus recessions, moving the insertions up (Urist 1968).
- Sloping lateral rectus recessions with maximum recession on the upper border of muscles (Boyd *et al.* 1971).
- Weaken the inferior oblique.
- Inferior oblique anteropositioning.
- Transpositioning of the superior rectus medially (Miller 1960).

REFERENCES

Billet E & Freedman M. (1969) Surgery of the inferior oblique muscles in V pattern exotropia. *Archives of Ophthalmology*, 82: 21

Boyd TAS, Leitch GT & Budd GE. (1971) A new treatment for 'A' and 'V' patterns in strabismus by slanting muscle insertions: a preliminary report. *Canadian Journal of Ophthalmology*, 6: 170

Breinin GM. (1961) Vertically incomitant horizontal strabismus. The A-V syndromes. *New York State Journal of Medicine*, 61: 2243

Brown HW. (1953) Vertical deviations. *Transactions of the American Academy of Ophthalmology and Otolaryngology*, 57: 157

Buckley EG & Flynn JT. (1983) Superior oblique recession versus tenotomy: a comparison of surgical results. *Journal of Pediatric Ophthalmology and Strabismus*, 20: 112

Caldeira JA. (1975) Graduated recession of the superior oblique muscle. *British Journal of Ophthalmology*, 59: 553

Clark RA, Miller JM, Rosenbaum AL & Demer JL. (1998) Heterotopic muscle pulleys or oblique muscle dysfunction? *Journal of the American Association of Pediatric Ophthalmology and Strabismus*, 2: 17

Fink WH. (1959) The A and V syndrome. *American Orthoptic Journal*, 9: 105

Folk ER. (1997) Costenbader lecture. A and V syndrome. A historical perspective. *Journal of Pediatric Ophthalmology and Strabismus*, 34: 154

Gobin MH. (1964) Anteroposition of the inferior oblique muscle in V-esotropia. *Ophthalmologica*, 148: 325

Gobin MH. (1968) Sagittalisation of the oblique muscles as a possible cause for the A, V and X phenomena. *British Journal of Ophthalmology*, 52: 13

Goldstein JH. (1967) Monocular vertical displacement of the horizontal rectus muscles in the A and V patterns. *American Journal of Ophthalmology*, 64: 265

Harado M & Ito Y. (1964) Surgical correction of cyclotropia. *Japanese Journal of Ophthalmology*, 8: 88

Hiles DA, Baker JD & Biglan AW. (1985) Six muscle surgery for V pattern esotropia. *Binocular Vision*, 1: 27

Knapp P. (1959) Vertically incomitant horizontal strabismus; the so-called A and V syndrome. *Transactions of the American Optical Society*, 57: 666

Kushner BJ. (1985) The role of ocular torsion on the etiology of A and V patterns. *Journal of Pediatric Ophthalmology and Strabismus*, 22: 171

Magee AJ. (1960) Minimal values for the A and V syndromes. *American Journal of Ophthalmology*, 50: 753

Miller JE. (1960) Vertical recti transplantation in the A and V syndromes. *Archives of Ophthalmology*, 64: 175

Romano P & Roholt P. (1983) Measured graduated recession of the superior oblique muscle. *Journal of Pediatric Ophthalmology and Strabismus*, 20: 134

Scott AB. (1968) A and V patterns in exotropia. An electromyography study of horizontal rectus muscles. *American Journal of Ophthalmology*, 65: 12

Scott WE, Drummond GT & Keech RV. (1989) Vertical offsets of horizontal recti muscles in the management of A and V pattern strabismus. *Australian and New Zealand Journal of Ophthalmology*, 17: 281

Shin GS, Elliott RL & Rosenbaum AL. (1996) Posterior superior oblique tenectomy at the scleral insertion for collapse of A pattern strabismus. *Journal of Pediatric Ophthalmology and Strabismus*, 33: 211

Shuey TF, Parks MM & Friendly DS. (1992) Results of combined surgery on the superior oblique and horizontal rectus muscles for A pattern horizontal strabismus. *Journal of Pediatric Ophthalmology and Strabismus*, 29: 199

Souza-Dias C & Uesugui CF. (1986) Efficacy of different techniques of superior oblique weakening in the correction of A anisotropia. *Journal of Pediatric Ophthalmology and Strabismus*, 23: 82

Urist MJ. (1951) Horizontal squint with secondary vertical deviations. *Archives of Ophthalmology*, 46: 245

Urist MJ. (1958) The etiology of the so-called A and V syndromes. *American Journal of Ophthalmology*, 46: 835

Urist MJ. (1968) Recession and upward displacement of the medial rectus muscles in A-pattern esotropia. *American Journal of Ophthalmology*, 65: 769

Urrets-Zavalia A, Solares-Zamora J & Olmos HR. (1961) Anthropological studies on the nature of cyclo-vertical squint. *British Journal of Ophthalmology*, 45: 578

Villaseca A. (1961) The A and V syndromes. *American Journal of Ophthalmology*, 52: 172

von Noorden GK. (1963) Temporal transplantation of the inferior rectus muscle in V-esotropia. *American Journal of Ophthalmology*, 56: 919

von Noorden GK & Olsen CL. (1965) Diagnosis and surgical management of vertically incomitant horizontal strabismus. *American Journal of Ophthalmology*, 60: 434

von Noorden GK. (1995) *Binocular Vision and Ocular Motility. Theory and Management of Strabismus*, 5th edn. Mosby, St Louis

FURTHER READING

Apt L & Call NB. (1978) Inferior oblique muscle recession. *American Journal of Ophthalmology*, 85: 95

Caldeira JA. (1978) Bilateral recession of the superior oblique in 'A' pattern tropias. *Journal of Pediatric Ophthalmology and Strabismus*, 15: 306

Cheng H, Burdon MA, Shun-Shin GA & Czypionka S. (1993) Dissociated eye movements in craniosynostosis: a hypothesis revived. *British Journal of Ophthalmology*, 77: 563

Costenbader FD. (1964) Introduction to symposium: the A and V patterns in strabismus. *Transactions of the American Academy of Ophthalmology and Otolaryngology*, 68: 354

Diamond S. (1964) Conjugate and oblique prism correction for noncomitant ocular deviations. *American Journal of Ophthalmology*, 58: 89

Drummond GT, Pearce WG & Astle WF. (1990) Recession of the superior oblique tendon in A pattern strabismus. *Canadian Journal of Ophthalmology*, 25: 301

Fells P. (1975) The superior oblique, its actions and anomalies. *British Orthoptic Journal*, 32: 43

Fells P. (1987) Orbital decompression for severe dysthyroid eye disease. *British Journal of Ophthalmology*, 71: 101

Guyton DL & Weingarten PE. (1994) Sensory torsion as the cause of primary oblique muscle overaction/underaction and A- and V- pattern strabismus. *Binocular Vision and Eye Muscle Surgery*, 9 (suppl): 209

Harley RD & Manley DR. (1969) Bilateral superior oblique tenectomy in A-pattern exotropia. *Transactions of the American Ophthalmology Society*, 67: 324

Helveston EM & Cofield DD. (1970) Indications for marginal myotomy and technique. *American Journal of Ophthalmology*, 70: 574

Jampolsky A. (1965) Oblique muscle surgery of the A and V pattern. *Journal of Pediatric Ophthalmology*, 2: 31

Jampolsky A. (1984) Unusual eye movements in alert humans with attached and detached eye muscles. In: Ravault AP, Lenk M (eds) *Transactions of the Fifth International Orthoptic Congress*. LIPS, Lyon, p. 201

Lang J. (1968) Squint dating from birth or with early onset. In: *Transactions of the First International Orthoptic Congress*. Kimpton, London, p. 231

Mein J. (1968) Clinical features of the retraction syndrome. *Transactions of the First International Orthoptic Congress*. Kimpton, London, p. 165

Mein J & Johnson F. (1981) Dissociated vertical divergence and its association with nystagmus. In: Mein J, Moore S (eds) *Orthoptics, Research and Practice. Transactions of the Fourth International Orthoptic Congress*. Kimpton, London, p. 14

Miller M & Folk E. (1975) Strabismus associated with craniofacial anomalies. *American Orthoptic Journal*, 25: 27

Parks MM. (1974) The overacting inferior oblique muscle. *American Journal of Ophthalmology*, 77: 787

Parks MM. (1977) The superior oblique tendon. *Transactions of the Ophthalmological Society of the United Kingdom*, 97: 288

Robb RM & Boger WP. (1983) Vertical strabismus associated with plagiocephaly. *Journal of Pediatric Ophthalmology and Strabismus*, 20: 58

Roper-Hall G & Burde RM. (1987) Management of A pattern exotropia as a complication of thyroid ophthalmopathy. In: Lenk-Schafer M, Calcutt C, Doyle M & Moore S (eds) *Transactions of the Sixth International Orthoptic Congress*. BOS, London, p. 361

Scott AB & Stella SL. (1968) Measurement of A and V syndromes. *Journal of Pediatric Ophthalmology*, 5: 181

Chapter 12
Accommodation and convergence disorders

Accommodation is the ability to increase the convexity of the intraocular lens in order to obtain a clear image of a near object. It is associated with convergence and pupil constriction. Circular muscles of the ciliary body contract and this brings about accommodation. The ciliary body is supplied by the III nerve and parasympathetic nerve supply. Brucke's muscles are meridional muscles which contract when looking into the distance and are supplied by sympathetic nerves.

Accommodative disorders

A defect of the focusing mechanism may result in:

- deficient accommodation
  — presbyopia (physiological, premature)
  — accommodative weakness (insufficiency, fatigue)
  — accommodative paralysis
- excessive accommodation
  — accommodative spasm
- failure to alter accommodation
  — accommodative inertia.

PRESBYOPIA – PHYSIOLOGICAL

Aetiology

Normal ageing changes of the crystalline lens.

Investigation

Refraction   A near addition is often required.

Case history   Blurred vision is experienced for reading print, especially in poor light. Asthenopic symptoms are common. Symptoms depend on age, refractive error (earlier in hypermetropia), the individual's normal reading position and requirements for close work.

Cover test   Often exophoric. This increases in angle when wearing the reading correction and may decompensate or become an intermittent near exotropia.

Binocular function   The control of the deviation must be assessed at near fixation.

Management

The minimum convex lenses are given to get rid of symptoms, taking into account the reading and near working position.

PRESBYOPIA – PREMATURE (NON-PHYSIOLOGICAL)

Aetiology

Lens changes, glaucoma, poor general health, drugs. This may be permanent or temporary depending on the cause.

Investigation

Refraction   A near addition is often required.
Case history   Blurred vision is noted for reading print with asthenopic symptoms.
Cover test   Often exophoric. This increases in angle when wearing the reading correction and may decompensate or become an intermittent near exotropia.
Binocular   The control of the deviation must be assessed at near fixation.
function

Management

A permanent spectacle correction is only given if the cause cannot be treated. However, it may be necessary to give a temporary correction while the cause is being treated.

ACCOMMODATIVE INSUFFICIENCY

This is a deficiency in the ability to obtain the amount of accommodation which would be expected from the patient's refractive state and age.

Aetiology

Drugs (high oestrogen contraceptive pill, tranquillisers, valium, antihypertensive drugs, atropine based drugs), poor general health, history of prolonged fever, vitamin deficiencies, virus infection, trauma (Mazow & France 1989).

Investigation

Case history   Blurred vision is noted for near vision with general asthenopia and micropsia if there is marked insufficiency.
Visual acuity   Distance vision is normal with poor near vision.
Cover test   An exophoria is demonstrated for near fixation with good recovery, becoming esophoria on extreme effort to accommodate.
Convergence   Overconvergence is possible which improves with convex lenses.
                     Pupils should be carefully assessed to ensure normal reaction.
Accommodation   This is assessed uniocularly and binocularly and also retested with concave lenses. The condition normally affects both eyes but if one eye is affected, a local cause should be suspected, such as:

- cyclitis
- glaucoma, lens change
- trauma.

Management

Elicit the cause and treat this where possible. The refractive error is corrected by giving the minimum convex lenses on a temporary or permanent basis. Miotics may be of use to increase the depth of focus. By reducing the pupil size, less accommodative effort is required which helps to alleviate symptoms. Orthoptic exercises may be of benefit with mild insufficiency and where associated with convergence insufficiency.

ACCOMMODATIVE FATIGUE

There is a deficiency in the ability to maintain the amount of accommodation which would be expected from the patient's refractive state and age. Accommodation is sufficient but tires easily and therefore differs from accommodation insufficiency which is a more constant condition.

Aetiology

Prolonged close work, poor general health, general fatigue, drugs, hysterical reaction, uncorrected refractive error.

Investigation

Visual acuity   Distance vision is normal but near vision deteriorates with time.
Cover test   Esophoria for near fixation is demonstrated.
Convergence   Poor.
Accommodation   The range is poor for the patient's age, deteriorating on repeated testing.
Binocular function A poor fusion range is demonstrable, particularly the convergent range.

Management

This is a temporary condition which improves with rest and restoration of good general health. The refractive error should be corrected. Temporary convex lenses may be used to alleviate symptoms. Orthoptic exercises to improve the fusional range may be necessary.

ACCOMMODATIVE PARALYSIS

There is a total inability to accommodate due to ciliary paralysis.

Aetiology

Drugs (anticholinergic, cycloplegic), toxins (botulism), trauma (direct injury to the eye, head trauma, whiplash), congenital (e.g. III nerve palsy), neurogenic (III nerve palsy, late feature of diphtheria, progressive midbrain disorder, pineal tumour).

Investigation

Case history   The severity of the symptoms depends on the refractive error.

An emmetrope will see clearly in the distance but not for near fixation. Hypermetropes see little at any distance and myopes have mild symptoms.

Visual acuity   Near vision is defective.

Cover test   Exotropia is seen at near fixation or exophoria, dependent on the state of convergence.

Convergence   There may be an associated convergence paralysis.

Accommodation   Complete loss of accommodation with fixed dilated pupil is demonstrable. It usually affects both eyes and, if uniocular, indicates a III nerve palsy.

Binocular function   Reduced binocularity is noted at near fixation, particularly stereopsis.

Management

Treat the cause if possible. The refractive error is corrected and convex lenses and base-in prisms are given for close work. The minimum strength prism should be given.

Miotics are useful for a partial palsy to increase the depth of focus.

ACCOMMODATIVE SPASM

A condition in which the ciliary muscle is contracted and cannot be relaxed. As a result accommodation is continuously exerted.

Aetiology

Functional cases may have an underlying emotional cause, uncorrected moderate degree of hypermetropia, effort to control intermittent divergent strabismus, overwork and fatigue or temporary spasm from miotics. Organic cases are due to irritative lesions of the brainstem, trigeminal neuralgia, drugs (morphine, vitamin B), trauma and cyclic oculomotor spasm (Dagi *et al.* 1987; Goldstein & Schneekloth 1996).

Investigation

Case history   Mild symptoms involve difficulty in relaxing accommodation, leading to blurred vision (pseudomyopia). Marked symptoms include pseudomyopia, pain and tenderness of the globe, macropsia, headaches and an inability to concentrate.

Visual acuity   Mild cases note that vision is better without a hypermetropic correction. Marked cases note severe loss of distance vision and near vision can also be affected. Vision improves with a pinhole or concave lenses.

Cover test Mild cases are usually esophoric at distance. Marked cases have an esotropia at distance with diplopia and spasmodic miosis.

Ocular motility Jerky movements are often noted with defective abduction.

Convergence There is usually an associated convergence spasm.

Accommodation Excessive accommodation is detected and this is usually a bilateral condition.

Management

Treat the underlying cause where possible. Correct the refractive error but initially undercorrect hypermetropes and then gradually increase. Marked spasms are treated with atropine for several weeks and the atropine is then gradually reduced. Where atropine is not tolerated, alternative mydriatics may be tried, such as cyclopentolate. However, these are less effective and generally not well tolerated either.

It is possible to give orthoptic exercises to increase negative relative convergence once the spasm has relaxed and this may help to prevent recurrence. Mild spasms may respond to orthoptic exercises, especially improving negative relative convergence.

Where there is an associated convergence spasm, botulinum toxin may be used.

ACCOMMODATIVE INERTIA

This is a condition in which there is difficulty in changing the accommodative state from one fixation distance to another. Patients experience difficulty in changing focus quickly.

Aetiology

Poor general health, fatigue, unequal refractive errors. If unilateral, the likely diagnosis is Adie's syndrome.

Investigation

Case history The condition is more common over the age of 30 years. Intermittent blurring of vision is noted for near fixation and/or distance.

Visual acuity Initially blurred vision for near fixation is noted. This eventually clears and then becomes blurred for distance due to slow relaxation.

Cover test Patients may show signs of decompensation or an exophoria.

Accommodation The range is below normal for the patient's age.

Management

The refractive error is corrected and general health should be improved. The fusion range and convergence may be returned to normal levels with orthoptic exercises.

MICROPSIA

Objects appear smaller than their natural size. If excessive accommodative effort is exerted the brain will interpret the retinal image as being produced by an object close to the eye and therefore this will appear smaller than natural size, i.e. micropsia occurring in accommodative palsy.

MACROPSIA

Objects appear larger than their natural size. If reduced accommodative effort is required, the brain will interpret that the object producing the retinal image is further away and therefore this will appear larger than normal size, i.e. macropsia in accommodative spasm.

Convergence disorders

Convergence is the mechanism which keeps the visual axes directed towards the object.

A defect in the convergence mechanism may result in:

- convergence insufficiency
- convergence paralysis
- convergence spasm.

CONVERGENCE INSUFFICIENCY

This is the inability to obtain and/or maintain adequate binocular convergence without undue effort. Convergence insufficiency may be primary or secondary (Mazow & France 1989; Rowe *et al.* 2001).

Aetiology

Primary

Predisposing causes include a wide interpupillary distance, occupations using mainly distance vision, occupations using mainly uniocular vision.

Precipitating causes include illness, ocular fatigue from prolonged close work and poor lighting, exams, advancing age, drugs, pregnancy.

Secondary

Secondary or organic convergence insufficiency is due to a variety of factors. A number of reports associate convergence insufficiency with whiplash injuries following road traffic accidents (Anderson 1961; Greaves 1987) where the aetiology is presumed to be at brainstem level.

Other associated factors include refractive error such as uncorrected myopia or correction of presbyopia, iatrogenic (weakened medial rectus), poor general health, neurological impairment due to multiple sclerosis or space occupying lesions, heterophoria (convergence weakness exophoria), vertical deviation, accommodative insufficiency and defective fusion (Lyle & Wybar 1970; Schwyzer 1978; Mills 1994; Wicks 1994; Rowe *et al.* 2001). Cases of convergence insufficiency have also been reported with superior oblique myokymia (Waddingham 1995).

Investigation

Case history   Symptoms are those of headache, difficulty in changing focus, blurring of print, intermittent diplopia, asthenopia. The patient may have had treatment before.

Visual acuity   Near vision may be reduced if accommodation is involved.

Cover test   An exophoria is usually present on cover testing and tends to be of the convergence weakness type.

Convergence   There is a reduced level of convergence which should be assessed with the RAF rule and fatigue noted.

Accommodation   There is a good level of monocular accommodation but when tested binocularly, the accommodative amplitude is reduced (von Noorden *et al.* 1973).

Binocular function   A reduced positive fusion range is elicited.

Management

Primary convergence insufficiency has been termed functional where conventional orthoptic exercises are usually successful in the treatment of the convergence weakness. Correct the refractive error and treat the cause if possible.

Orthoptic treatment. Recognition of pathological diplopia should be taught if not already appreciated. Binocular convergence is improved with pen convergence exercises. Recognition of physiological diplopia is then taught and the patient should continue to improve binocular convergence using jump pen convergence with appreciation of physiological diplopia. The range of positive fusional convergence is improved with base-out prisms, the synoptophore, dotcards and stereograms with near fixation. Good voluntary convergence is established where possible. Exercises are discontinued for one month and if then still asymptomatic, with adequate binocular convergence obtained and maintained with ease, the patient is discharged.

Base-in prisms. If the patient is unable to start orthoptic exercises due to very reduced convergence, a small prism (approximately half the measurement of the near angle of deviation) may be given to achieve binocularity at a closer distance. Orthoptic exercises may then be commenced and once convergence has begun to improve, the strength of prism may be decreased and eventually removed.

Many cases respond to conventional treatment by orthoptic exercises and tend to be primary in nature. Those that do not respond to treatment are often of secondary nature and may also have poorer levels of convergence and fusional amplitude or need additional treatment with prisms or surgery (Schwyzer 1978; Wicks 1994; Rowe *et al.* 2001).

Convergence insufficiency associated with accommodative insufficiency may be treated with plus lenses and base-in prisms.

Medial rectus resection with bifocals may be considered with larger angle deviations (von Noorden 1976).

CONVERGENCE PARALYSIS

This is a condition in which there is an absence of convergence.

Aetiology

There is usually a history of closed head injury. The condition may be secondary to various organic processes such as encephalitis, diphtheria, multiple sclerosis and occlusive vascular disease involving the rostral midbrain. It may also occur in isolation as a sequence of a viral illness.

Investigation

Case history   Diplopia is appreciated but often not for distance.
Cover test   Exotropia is noted for near fixation with crossed diplopia.
Accommodation This is often normal unless the intraocular muscles are involved, leading to mydriasis and absent accommodation.
Convergence   There is an absent near point of convergence.
Binocular function An absent base-out prism fusion range is detected.

Management

The cause of the condition is treated where possible.
Occlusion is often the best practical treatment.
Base-in prisms. Diplopia is not appreciated equally at all distances and as a result it is difficult to join with prisms.
Surgery. Unpredictable results are usual.

CONVERGENCE SPASM

This is a condition in which there is excessive convergence, most often associated with accommodation spasm, which has been discussed in the previous section on accommodative anomalies (pp. 200–201).

REFERENCES

Anderson M. (1961) Orthoptic treatment of loss of convergence and accommodation caused by road accidents (whiplash injury). *British Orthoptic Journal*, 18: 117

Dagi LR, Chronsos GA & Cogan DC. (1987) Spasm of the near reflex associated with organic disease. *American Journal of Ophthalmology*, 582: 103

Goldstein JH & Schneekloth BB. (1996) Spasm of the near reflex: a spectrum of anomalies. *Survey of Ophthalmology*, 40: 269

Greaves BPB. (1987) Role of the oblique muscles in convergence insufficiency. In: Lenk-Schafer M, Calcutt C, Doyle M & Moore S (eds) *Orthoptic Horizons. Transactions of the Sixth International Orthoptic Congress.* Harrogate, UK, p. 412

Lyle TK & Wybar KC. (1970) *Lyle and Jackson's Practical Orthoptics in the Treatment of Squint.* Lewis, London

Mazow ML & France TD. (1989) Acute accommodative and convergence insufficiency. *Transactions of the American Ophthalmology Society*, 87: 158

Mills A. (1994) The incidence of symptom producing near exophoria with or without a convergence deficit and associated neurological disease. *British Orthoptic Journal*, 51: 30

Rowe FJ, Swift J & Noonan CP. (2001) Convergence insufficiency with associated superior oblique weakness. *British Orthoptic Journal*, 58: 42

Schwyzer EB. (1978) Aspects of the treatment of convergence insufficiency. *British Orthoptic Journal*, 35: 28

von Noorden GK. (1976) Resection of both medial rectus muscles in organic convergence insufficiency. *American Journal of Ophthalmology*, 81: 223

von Noorden GK, Brown DJ & Parks MM. (1973) Associated convergence and accommodative insufficiency. *Documenta Ophthalmologica*, 34: 393

Waddingham PE. (1995) Convergence and accommodative insufficiency associated with superior oblique myokymia. *British Orthoptic Journal*, 52: 21

Wicks HR. (1994) A report of a clinical audit of the management of convergence insufficiency. *British Orthoptic Journal*, 51: 35

FURTHER READING

Bruce GM. (1935) Ocular divergence: its physiology and pathology. *Archives of Ophthalmology*, 13: 639

Burian HM & Brown AW. (1972) Unusual adverse effect of prismatic corrections in a child with divergence insufficiency. *American Journal of Ophthalmology*, 74: 336

Capobianca NM. (1952) The subjective measurement of the near point of convergence and its significance in the diagnosis of convergence insufficiency. *American Orthoptic Journal*, 2: 40

Dunphy EB. (1928) Paralysis of divergence. *American Journal of Ophthalmology*, 11: 298

Harrison RL. (1987) Loss of fusional vergence with partial loss of accommodative convergence and accommodation following head injury. *Binocular Vision*, 2: 93

Hermann JS. (1981) Surgical therapy for convergence insufficiency. In: Mein J & Moore S (eds) *Orthoptics, Research and Practice.* Kimpton, London, p. 179

Jacobsohn DM. (2000) Divergence insufficiency revisited: natural history of idiopathic cases and neurological associations. *Archives of Ophthalmology*, 118: 1237

Lyle DJ. (1954) Divergence insufficiency. *Archives of Ophthalmology*, 52: 858

Rutkowsky PC & Burian HM. (1972) Divergence paralysis following head trauma. *American Journal of Ophthalmology*, 73: 660

Trimble RB. (1977) Loss of accommodation and convergence. *Proceedings of the Royal Society of Medicine*, 70: 261

Chapter 13
Ptosis and pupil disorders

PTOSIS

The levator muscle is the primary elevator of the upper lid. Its failure to function properly produces a ptosis. Secondary elevators include Muller's muscle and the frontalis muscle.

Aetiology

Congenital

(1) Isolated simple ptosis. This may be due to weakness of the levator muscle alone or with ipsilateral superior rectus muscle paresis.
(2) Blepharophimosis. There are pronounced inverse epicanthic folds, thickening and ptosis of the lids, wide separation of the medial canthi and slit-like palpebral apertures.
(3) Congenital III nerve palsy (see Chapter 14).
(4) Double elevator palsy (see Chapter 14).
(5) Marcus Gunn jaw winking syndrome.
(6) Congenital misdirection syndrome/aberrant regeneration (see Chapter 14).
(7) Congenital fibrosis syndrome (see Chapter 15).
(8) Periodic ptosis as with cyclic oculomotor palsy (see Chapter 14).
(9) Transient neonatal myasthenia gravis (see Chapter 16).
(10) Congenital Horner's syndrome.

Acquired

Myogenic (see also Chapter 16)
(1) Myasthenia gravis
(2) Muscular dystrophy
(3) Myotonic dystrophy
(4) Chronic progressive external ophthalmoplegia
(5) Myositis
(6) Senile

Neurogenic (see also Chapter 14)
(1) III nerve palsy
(2) Aberrant regeneration
(3) Horner's syndrome

Mechanical (see also Chapter 15)
(1)   Space occupying lesions involving the lid
(2)   Trauma
(3)   Scar tissue

Differential diagnosis

Ptosis must be differentially diagnosed from pseudoptosis, some causes for which include:

- ipsilateral hypotropia
- ipsilateral enophthalmos
- ipsilateral microphthalmos
- ipsilateral pthisis bulbi
- contralateral proptosis
- contralateral lid retraction

Investigation

Case history   Signs of ptosis are often first observed while taking a case history. One should also look for the presence of strabismus, abnormal head posture and pupil abnormalities. The patient is asymptomatic if congenital but with acquired ptosis it may appear worse in the evenings or with fatigue (myasthenia gravis). The patient may appreciate diplopia with associated strabismus and may have blurred vision if mydriasis is present.

Refraction   There is an increased frequency of myopia in congenital ptosis (Gusek-Schneider & Martus 2001).

Visual acuity   Unilateral ptosis causes stimulus deprivation amblyopia depending on the degree of ptosis and age of patient and can occasionally cause anisometropic amblyopia (Anderson & Baumgartner 1980; Dray & Leibovitch 2002). There is a high risk for amblyopia and the need for head posturing indicates that the visual axis is at least partially obscured (Fiergang *et al.* 1999).

With III nerve palsy, there may be blurred vision due to mydriasis.

Cover test   There may be an associated strabismus.

Ocular motility   It is necessary to observe superior rectus function and changes in degree of ptosis in different positions of gaze and with jaw movement. The pupils are examined for signs of miosis or mydriasis. Assessment of lid position and levator function is important and both eyes must always be assessed for comparison. Patients often use frontalis muscle over-action to compensate for ptosis and it is important that this is abolished when assessing the lids. The patient closes the eyes and the examiner presses the brow against the frontal bone to prevent use of the frontalis muscle. The patient then opens the eyes.

The presence or absence and the height of the skin crease must be noted. The lid crease tends to be higher than the other eye in cases of congenital ptosis and lower in cases of senile ptosis. When assessing the patient to ensure that the ptosis is truly unilateral and not masked bilateral due to frontalis overaction, frontalis muscle action should be abolished in the apparent ptotic eye and the lid position of the other eye reassessed.

It is important to measure the palpebral aperture of either eye for evaluation of the extent of ptosis. This can be measured with the patient fixing in the primary position and a measurement taken using a rule held against the patient's eyes.

Levator function is assessed by comparing the degree of levator action between up- and downgaze. The patient looks down and the upper lid position is measured on a rule held against the face/eye. The patient looks up and the lid position is again measured on the rule (without the rule being moved). The difference is noted and the normal measurement is in the region of 15 mm.

The presence of Bell's phenomenon should be assessed and any associated pupil abnormalities or synkinetic movements documented.

Abnormal head posture   Chin elevation is often seen.

Accommodation   Defective accommodation is frequent with III nerve palsy and Horner's syndrome.

Non-orthoptic tests   Ophthalmic, photographs, neurological, radiological, muscle biopsy, general medical.

Management

Orthoptic management

Aims of management are to improve visual acuity and eliminate symptoms. Correct the refractive error and treat amblyopia if present. If unable to assess acuity in young children with obscuration of the visual axis by ptosis, prophylactic part time occlusion should be considered until acuity can be reliably assessed (Fiergang *et al.* 1999).

- **Observation**: Marcus Gunn syndrome often improves. It is important to monitor the vision of children with unilateral ptosis and monitor the progress of the condition and ptosis for signs of deterioration or recovery.
- Eliminate or join associated diplopia with **prisms** or **occlusion.**
- Treat the cause of acquired conditions and await any recovery.

Surgical management

Surgery is considered according to the degree of ptosis, the type and cosmesis. Ptosis procedures include brow suspension, levator resection or reinsertion and Fasanella servat.

For a small degree with good levator function, a levator resection or Fasanella servat procedure may be considered. For a moderate degree with good levator function, a levator resection may be considered. For a moderate degree with fair levator function, a large levator resection, tuck or advancement are options. For a severe degree with poor levator function, a frontalis sling or brow suspension is considered.

Non-surgical management
- Drugs
- Ptosis props
- Magnets

Post-operative complications
These may include:

- corneal exposure
- eye lid too high or too low post-operatively
- lash eversion and ectropion
- defective skin crease
- conjunctival prolapse

Marcus Gunn jaw winking syndrome

Aetiology

Congenital

The condition is due to abnormal innervation between III and Vc nerves.

Acquired

The acquired form of the condition is rare and often secondary to space occupying lesions or syphilis where aberrant regeneration has occurred.

Investigation

Refraction	Patients are often anisometropic and astigmatic.
Case history	The condition is usually detected early as it is noticed when the baby is being fed. It is reported as becoming less obvious with time. Familial occurrence is rare although dominant inheritance can occur.
Visual acuity	There is a high incidence of amblyopia.
Cover test	Strabismus is frequently detected and is commonly unilateral.
Ocular motility	Unilateral, partial ptosis is present on the affected side. The ptosis is variable and may be bilateral. Retraction of the affected upper lid occurs on movement of the lower jaw, particularly when sucking, chewing or speaking. This occurs when the jaw is moved to the opposite side. Retraction and ptosis phases alternate rapidly, producing the winking effect. Associated extraocular muscle paresis may occur.
Binocular function	This may be absent or there may be abnormal retinal correspondence dependent on the type of manifest deviation. If latent, there is usually good binocular function.

Management

Correct the refractive error if present and treat amblyopia if indicated.

Surgery may be considered for strabismus if a functional result is expected and for cosmetic appearance. Surgery for ptosis is required if marked. Generally ptosis surgery is delayed as much as possible as many cases appear to improve with age. However, if ptosis is marked and covering the pupil, intervention is advisable earlier to prevent amblyopia. Bilateral surgery involving brow suspensions should be considered to achieve a symmetrical result.

Lid retraction

Lid retraction may be noted in a number of conditions.

- Thyroid eye disease.
- Inferior rectus tethering.
- Ptosis of the contralateral eye.
- Midbrain disease.
- Post-operatively due to overliberal ptosis surgery or surgery involving the superior rectus or inferior rectus.

PUPILS

The sphincter pupillae receives parasympathetic nerve supply and constricts the pupil (miosis). This pupillary light reflex is a four neuron arc. The first order neuron passes from the retina to the pretectal nucleus. The second neuron passes from the pretectal nucleus to the Edinger–Westphal nucleus and the third neuron passes from there to the ciliary ganglion via the III cranial nerve. The fourth order neuron passes from the ciliary ganglion to the sphincter pupillae via the short ciliary nerves.

The dilator pupillae receives sympathetic nerve supply and dilates the pupil (mydriasis). This is a three neuron pathway. The first order neuron passes from the posterior hypothalamus to the ciliospinal centre of Budge, situated from C8 to T2 in the spinal cord. The second order neuron (pre-ganglionic pathway) passes from the spinal cord to the superior cervical ganglion via the vertebral sympathetic chain. The third order neuron (post-ganglionic pathway) passes from the superior cervical ganglion via the internal carotid artery, through the cavernous sinus to the short posterior ciliary nerves and on to the dilator pupillae.

The near reflex is a triad of miosis, accommodation and convergence. The final pathway of the near reflex is the same as the light reflex. The centre is thought to be in the midbrain in a more ventral position than the light reflex pretectal nucleus.

Factors affecting pupil size

- Intensity of retinal illumination
- Near effort reflex
- State of retinal light adaptation
- Supranuclear influences; frontal and occipital cortex
- Reticular formation of brainstem
- Age
- Constant state of movement = hippus

Pupil functions

The functions of the pupils are to:

- regulate the amount of light reaching the retina
- reduce chromatic and spherical aberrations produced by peripheral imperfections of cornea and lens
- increase depth of focus/field.

Classification of pupil anomalies

Unilateral

(1) Amaurotic pupil
(2) Anisocoria
(3) Drugs: cycloplegics such as cyclopentolate and atropine will cause mydriasis. Miosis occurs with drugs such as pilocarpine and phospholine iodide.
(4) Holmes-Adie pupil
(5) Horner's syndrome
(6) Internal ophthalmoplegia
(7) Relative afferent pupil defect
(8) III nerve palsy: mydriasis if pupil involvement

Bilateral

(1) Accommodative convergence spasm
(2) Argyll Robertson pupil
(3) Drugs: as above

Investigation

Case history   Pupil abnormalities may be noted while taking a case history. Other signs may include ptosis, strabismus and heterochromia.

Visual acuity   This may be blurred with mydriasis. An increased depth of focus may be noticed with miosis.

Cover test   Associated strabismus may be seen in cases involving III nerve palsy. Esotropia is frequently seen with accommodative convergence spasm.

Ocular motility   Extraocular muscle pareses will be noted with associated III nerve palsy. Vertical gaze palsies are commonly noted with dorsal midbrain (Parinaud's) syndrome.

Accommodation Response to a near target should be noted as normal miosis in response to accommodation and an absent reaction to light stimulus is indicative of light–near dissociation. Accommodation may be defective where mydriasis is noted and an increased depth of focus may be noted with miosis.

Pupil size and reaction The normal pupils are round and of equal size in either eye. Both react equally to light and accommodation.

Pupil size may be irregular due to posterior synechiae from trauma or ocular inflammation. Difference in pupil size (anisocoria) will be noted as either mydriasis of one eye or miosis of the other eye. The pupillary response to a light stimulus should be noted in either eye and any difference between either eye noted, such as an absent or sluggish reaction to light.

When examining the pupils, use a distant fixation to prevent accommodation miosis. General observations should note the speed, quality and symmetry of responses.

Swinging flashlight test The patient fixates on a distant object which prevents accommodative miosis. A bright light is shone onto the pupil of one eye, which should immediately constrict, followed by a slow dilation to an intermediate point. This is repeated for the other eye with the light being rapidly transferred from one eye to the other and back several times. A comparison of the pupil reactions will identify the presence of an afferent or efferent pupil defect. The direct reflex occurs in the eye stimulated by the light whereas the consensual (indirect) reflex occurs in the other eye.

Amaurotic pupil

Defective pupil reflexes are due to damage to the optic nerve and blindness. Both pupils are seen to react with stimulation of the normal eye. No reaction is seen with stimulation of the affected eye. The near reflex response is normal.

Holmes-Adie pupil

This is a myotonic pupil with absent or diminished tendon reflexes. A dilated pupil is noted with poor reaction to light. There is accommodative paresis and vermiform movements of the iris may be seen on slit-lamp examination. The diagnosis is confirmed with instillation of either pilocarpine 0.1% or mecholyl 2.5% which will constrict the affected pupil but not the normal pupil.

Horner's syndrome

There is total or partial interruption of the sympathetic chain to the dilator pupillae with resulting ipsilateral pupil miosis, ptosis, apparent enophthalmos and heterochromia. An increased amplitude of accommodation may be present. If the lesion is pre-ganglionic, there will also be an associated anhydrosis of the ipsilateral side of the face. The diagnosis is confirmed with instillation of cocaine 4% in both eyes which will dilate the normal eye but not the affected pupil. For differential diagnosis of pre- and post-ganglionic lesions, hydroxyamphetamine 1% (paredrine) is instilled which dilates the affected pupil if there is a pre-ganglionic lesion but not if it is post-ganglionic.

Internal ophthalmoplegia

This is due to a lesion in the efferent parasympathetic pupillary pathway which causes loss of direct and consensual light reflexes and loss of miosis to a near stimulus on the affected side.

Relative afferent pupillary defect

This is caused by an optic nerve lesion which is not severe enough to cause an absence of light perception. The affected pupil does not constrict to direct light stimulation but does react on consensual testing. The pupil of the affected eye will be seen to dilate as the light is transferred to it on the swinging flashlight test.

Argyll Robertson pupil

A lesion in the rostral midbrain affects the light reflex fibres to the Edinger–Westphal nucleus. This results in miotic irregular pupils and light–near dissociation. Both pupils are involved but often to an asymmetrical degree. Causes of the condition include neurosyphilis, diabetes and multiple sclerosis.

REFERENCES

Anderson RL & Baumgartner SA. (1980) Amblyopia in ptosis. *Archives of Ophthalmology*, 98: 1068
Dray J-P & Leibovitch I. (2002) Congenital ptosis and amblyopia; a retrospective study of 130 cases. *Journal of Pediatric Ophthalmology and Strabismus*, 39: 222
Fiergang DL, Wright KW & Foster JA. (1999) Unilateral or asymmetric congenital ptosis, head posturing and amblyopia. *Journal of Pediatric Ophthalmology and Strabismus*, 36: 74
Gusek-Schneider G-C & Martus P. (2001) Stimulus deprivation myopia in human congenital ptosis; a study of 95 patients. *Journal of Pediatric Ophthalmology and Strabismus*, 38: 340

FURTHER READING

Collin JRO. (1984) *A Manual of Systematic Eyelid Surgery*. Churchill Livingstone, Edinburgh
Ficker LA, Collin JRO & Lee JP. (1986) Management of ipsilateral ptosis with hypotropia. *British Journal of Ophthalmology*, 70: 732

Harrad RA, Graham CM & Collin JR. (1988) Amblyopia and strabismus in congenital ptosis. *Eye,* 2: 625

Lyness RW, Collin JR, Alexander RA & Garner A. (1988) Histological appearances of the levator palpebrae superioris in the Marcus Gunn phenomenon. *British Journal of Ophthalmology,* 72: 104

Trobe JD. (1988) Third nerve palsy and the pupil (editorial). *Archives of Ophthalmology,* 106: 601

von Noorden GK & Middleditch PR. (1975) Histology of the monkey lateral geniculate nucleus after unilateral lid closure and strabismus: further observations. *Investigative Ophthalmology,* 14: 674

Chapter 14
Neurogenic disorders

This chapter discusses the neurogenic disorders, including cranial nerve palsies, isolated extraocular muscle pareses and the ophthalmoplegic syndromes. A palsy indicates loss of nerve function. This may be complete (no function) or partial (some residual function). The term paresis also applies to a partial palsy.

III (THIRD) CRANIAL NERVE

The III nerve divides into two branches. The superior branch supplies the levator palpebrae superioris muscle and the superior rectus. The inferior branch supplies the medial rectus, inferior rectus and inferior oblique muscles. A complete lesion of the III nerve involving both branches will result in a deficit of elevation, adduction and depression in abduction. There will be an accompanying ptosis and pupil dilation.

Alternatively, there may be a lesion affecting one or other of the branches only and these lesions may be partial or complete.

Aetiology

Localisation of lesion

- **Nuclear**: a nuclear lesion may result in:
    - unilateral III with bilateral ptosis
    - bilateral III with spared levator function.
- **Internuclear**
    - INO
    - Weber's syndrome: III and contralateral hemiplegia due to lesion of corticospinal tract
    - Benedikt's syndrome: III and contralateral ataxia and intension tremor.
- **Infranuclear**: this is due to a lesion along the nerve pathway.

III nerve palsy may be central, sparing the pupil, or peripheral with pupil involvement. If the pupil is spared the cause is most likely vascular. When the pupil is involved the cause is likely to be an aneurysm (Goldstein & Cogan 1960). The two most common causes are:

- *aneurysms* in the circle of Willis. Those involving the posterior communicating artery are particularly associated. There is often pupil involvement resulting in dilation

- *diabetes*: III nerve lesions associated with underlying vascular disorders are often pupil sparing.

Trauma and space occupying solid lesions are other major factors which may result in III nerve palsies.

Typical III nerve palsy

Investigation

Visual acuity It is necessary to lift the ptotic lid to evaluate visual acuity. This may be reduced due to mydriasis.

Cover test An exo- and hypodeviation is present.

Ocular motility There will be limited elevation, depression and adduction (Fig. 14.1). The examiner should always check for the presence of IV nerve function by asking the patient to attempt to look down and outwards and observe for the presence of incyclotorsion during this movement.

There is likely to be a ptosis present in which case the upper lid will have to be raised by the examiner (or an assistant) in order to perform the ocular motility assessment. The pupil may be dilated depending on the underlying pathology.

Convergence This will be absent if the medial rectus muscle is paralysed.

Binocular function This is usually absent unless the III nerve paresis is mild and partial.

Accommodation If the underlying cause of the lesion has resulted in pupillary dilation, then fibres to the ciliary body are also likely to be involved so that accommodation will be defective.

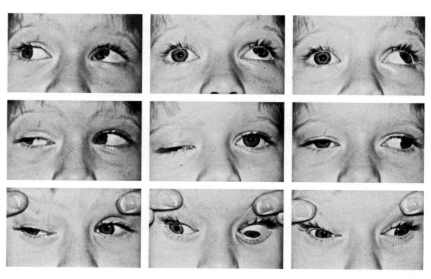

Figure 14.1   Right III nerve palsy.

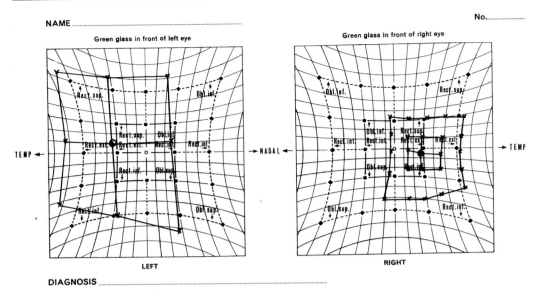

NAME ....   No. ....

Green glass in front of left eye   Green glass In front of right eye

LEFT   RIGHT

DIAGNOSIS ....

Figure 14.2   Hess chart of right III nerve palsy.

Hess chart	(Fig. 14.2) The affected eye will show a markedly constricted field whereas the other eye demonstrates overaction of its muscles.
Diplopia	There will be constant diplopia unless complete ptosis is present and blocks the vision of the affected eye.

Aberrant regeneration

This is a change in the actions of muscles supplied by the III nerve due to regrowth of damaged nerve fibres following complete or severe III nerve palsy (Shuttleworth *et al.* 1998). It is liable to occur when either trauma or an aneurysm has caused the lesion (Cox *et al.* 1979). Aberrant regeneration may occur from weeks to months after the onset of the III nerve paresis. The factors underlying aberrant regeneration are unclear but may involve either a central or peripheral response. In the former, there is a mass response of the damaged nerve resulting in growth to the wrong muscle. In the latter, abnormal growth of damaged axons may occur locally.

Investigation

Ocular motility	Abnormal movements often involve the eye lids and pupils.
Ptosis	The lid may rise on attempted depression, adduction and occasionally abduction (pseudo Graefe phenomenon).
Pupil	This may constrict on attempted adduction, elevation and depression (pseudo Argyll Robertson pupil).
Convergence	This may occur on attempted elevation.

Cyclic oculomotor palsy

This rare condition is usually congenital and unilateral in origin (Burian & van Allen 1963). It is often associated with a partial III nerve palsy with some degree of ptosis. The condition is described as having cyclical fluctuation in two phases:

(1) **Paralytic phase**. There is a partial III nerve palsy.
(2) **Miotic phase**. There is convergence, lid retraction, accommodation and pupil constriction.

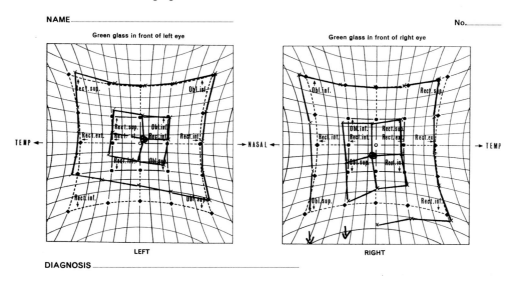

Figure 14.3   Hess chart of left inferior rectus palsy.

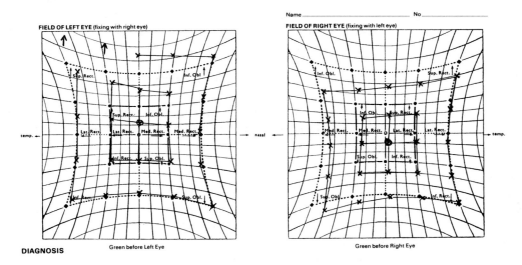

Figure 14.4   Hess chart of right inferior oblique palsy.

Single muscle palsy

The following isolated muscle palsies are all recognised.

(1) **Medial rectus**. This produces an exodeviation which is greater for near.
(2) **Inferior rectus**. This produces hyper- and exodeviation (Fig. 14.3).
(3) **Superior rectus**. This is often bilateral and may present with a V exo pattern.
(4) **Inferior oblique**. This is a feature of an A eso pattern (Fig. 14.4).

Differential diagnosis of single muscle palsies

The following conditions should be considered.

Palsy	Differential diagnosis
Medial rectus	Atypical Duane's retraction syndrome
	Unilateral/bilateral internuclear ophthalmoplegia
Inferior rectus	Myogenic (myasthenia gravis)
	Mechanical limitation (thyroid eye disease)
	Trauma (blow-out fracture)
Inferior oblique	Brown's syndrome
Superior rectus	Trauma (blow-out fracture)
	Mechanical limitation (thyroid eye disease)

Double elevator palsy

This often has a congenital origin and is presumed to be caused by a supranuclear defect. The superior rectus and inferior oblique muscles of the same eye are affected (Jampel & Fells 1968).

Investigation

Cover test
There is a hypodeviation in the primary position which may be manifest or latent.

Ocular motility
There is limited elevation of one eye in both adduction and abduction. Ptosis and/or pseudoptosis may be present. Bell's phenomenon is usually present.

Abnormal head posture
The chin is elevated to compensate for the palsy.

Binocular function
If there is only a small angle of deviation in the primary position, this may be controlled with or without an abnormal head posture, resulting in a latent hypodeviation. In these circumstances, binocular single vision is present.

Forced duction test
There will be full passive movement (negative result).

Differential diagnosis of double elevator palsy

The following conditions should be differentiated from double elevator palsy as they will have a positive forced duction test:

- blow-out fracture
- thyroid eye disease
- Brown's syndrome
- congenital fibrosis of the inferior rectus muscle
- general fibrosis syndrome.

Conditions with a negative forced duction test which should be included in the differential diagnosis are anomalous superior or inferior rectus muscle insertions.

Management of III nerve palsy

In children, any associated amblyopia should be treated. Any underlying cause for the lesion should be investigated and treated. As with most conditions affecting the extraocular muscles, it is important to allow a period for recovery of any muscle function and then wait until stability of this has been demonstrated.

Surgery is indicated to correct the strabismus and any associated ptosis. Squints are treated initially as the ptosis acts as a mechanical barrier to diplopia. However, if the action of raising the lid has an effect on the strabismus this must be accounted for in the surgery undertaken.

In the case of a complete palsy, the aim of surgery is to improve cosmesis and if possible to achieve some field of binocular single vision. Any ptosis is subsequently corrected. It should be noted that an adequate Bell's phenomenon is needed before ptosis can be repaired.

Strabismus surgery for complete palsies is usually performed in stages. The level of function of each involved muscle must be carefully evaluated and the presence of secondary ipsilateral lateral rectus contracture identified. All patients require evaluation for possible disruption of central fusion. If serious neurological disease is found, treatment may need to be modified in light of the patient's general condition.

Total III nerve palsy

A very large lateral rectus recession to totally abolish abduction is undertaken. Superior oblique tendon resection and transposition to the area between the medial rectus and superior rectus insertions may create a chronic adducting force that will ensure long term stability (Peter 1934; Metz & Yee 1973; Saunders & Rogers 1982: Maruo *et al.* 1996; Villasenor *et al.* 2000; Young *et al.* 2000).

Partial III nerve paresis

Where there is isolated muscle involvement the paretic muscle with residual function is resected and the antagonist is recessed, preferably with adjustable sutures. Where there is multiple muscle involvement, resection of the paretic muscles with recession of the lateral rectus is advised. The insertions may be transposed down with absent inferior rectus function to provide a downward force (Metz 1988, 1993). Recession or Faden to the contralateral inferior rectus to match a deficient field can be considered. A Knapp procedure for inferior division III nerve palsy is a useful option.

Botulinum toxin to the lateral rectus may aid horizontal alignment. The patient may then adopt a vertical abnormal head posture to attain fusion (Metz 1988).

In cases of double elevator palsy, a Knapp's procedure may be indicated (Knapp 1969; Burke *et al.* 1992). In this operation, the lateral and medial recti are transposed to the superior rectus insertion. If the inferior rectus muscle in the affected eye is limited, then this muscle may be recessed. Ptosis surgery may or may not be required.

IV (FOURTH) CRANIAL NERVE

The IV cranial nerve supplies the superior oblique muscle only. Any lesion affecting the nerve may result in difficulties of depression, intorsion and abduction of the eye.

Aetiology

The condition may be congenital or acquired. The latter group may be caused by the following:

- trauma: particularly bilateral cases, as the IV cranial nerve is the only nerve to arise from the dorsal surface of the midbrain and therefore follows a long, winding route which renders it susceptible to injury
- vascular causes: e.g. hypertension
- diabetes
- space occupying lesions.

In congenital superior oblique palsy the tendon is usually lax and abnormally long (Plager 1990, 1992).

Investigation

Case history   In congenital cases the patients are often affected bilaterally. They may present with any of the following:

- manifest strabismus without binocular function
- binocular function but there may be an abnormal head posture, depending on the extent of paresis

- symptoms of decompensation. These occur when the patient has been binocular, possibly with an abnormal head posture, but it has become too difficult to control the deviation. The patient may suffer from symptoms of diplopia, headaches and asthenopia.

These effects are experienced particularly by older patients and it is therefore necessary to establish the underlying congenital nature of the disorder from an acquired cause.

There is often facial asymmetry in congenital superior oblique palsy, consisting of shallowing of the midfacial region between the lateral canthus and the edge of the mouth (Parks 1958). This is found in three-quarters of patients with congenital palsy (Wilson & Hoxie 1993; Paysee *et al.* 1995).

In acquired cases, the paresis may be unilateral or bilateral. The latter is often associated with major closed head trauma. Symptoms of cyclovertical diplopia are experienced, which worsen on downgaze. The presence of an abnormal head posture tends to indicate more long-standing deviations.

Abnormal head posture
In unilateral IV nerve paresis, the patient may present with chin depression with face turn and head tilt away from the affected side. Bilateral cases demonstrate chin depression but there may be no face turn or head tilt unless one side is affected more than the other.

Cover test
The test is performed with and without the abnormal head posture for comparison. A latent deviation exists if a compensatory abnormal head posture is adopted. When the test is repeated with the head straight, the deviation will increase and may become manifest.

The affected eye shows a hyperdeviation and an associated esodeviation. (However, an exodeviation may be seen if this was present before the onset of the palsy.) It is useful to note that the vertical deviation is commonly greater on near testing than for distance. In bilateral cases, the main deviation usually tends to be a small angle horizontal deviation.

Ocular motility
The primary underaction of the affected superior oblique muscle results in a number of sequelae. There is overaction of the contralateral inferior rectus and ipsilateral inferior oblique muscles (Fig. 14.5). The contralateral superior rectus shows secondary underaction. The combination of these muscle effects is variable and often depends on whether or not the deviation is of long standing.

In bilateral cases, a V pattern is often present. In the presence of this, one should always suspect a bilateral case, especially where there is an excyclotorsion of greater than 7 degrees and a tendency towards reversal of any hyperdeviation or diplopic images on lateral gaze (Hermann 1981).

Convergence
This may be reduced, due to either convergence insufficiency or the vertical deviation. Differentiation is achieved by correcting the deviation and seeing if convergence improves.

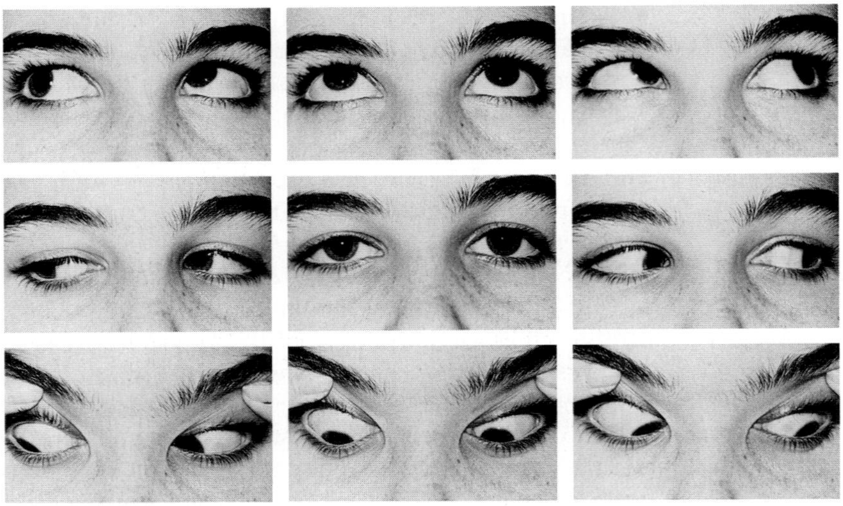

Figure 14.5   Left IV nerve palsy.

Binocular function	Assessment of binocular function is carried out with and without the abnormal head posture if one is present. Binocular single vision cannot be maintained if there is a significant degree of torsion and therefore is often not present in acquired bilateral palsies.
	Patients who maintain binocularity tend to have a small angle of deviation associated with a congenital palsy. Some patients with long-standing acquired palsies can maintain binocularity if there is a good fusional control with an extended vertical fusion range.
Hess chart	The Hess chart provides a useful record for the notes and demonstrates the effects of the paresis on the other extraocular muscles (Fig. 14.6).
Field of binocular single vision	The area in which binocular single vision is retained is displaced upwards to the affected side (Fig. 14.7).
Diplopia	The patient experiences a greater degree of diplopia on near testing when looking down. The diplopia is vertical and usually uncrossed. If, however, an exodeviation is present, the horizontal element of diplopia will be crossed.
Bielchowsky head tilt test	A cover test in the primary position with the head straight will show a hyperdeviation in the affected eye. If there is a positive Bielchowsky test, on tilting the head towards the affected side, this vertical deviation increases. Tilting towards the unaffected side will show a decrease which is indicative of a IV nerve palsy.
Torsion	Excyclotorsion is frequently present in acquired bilateral cases.
Diagnostic prisms	Fresnel prisms may be used temporarily to correct the angle of deviation. If the prism alleviates the need for an abnormal head posture,

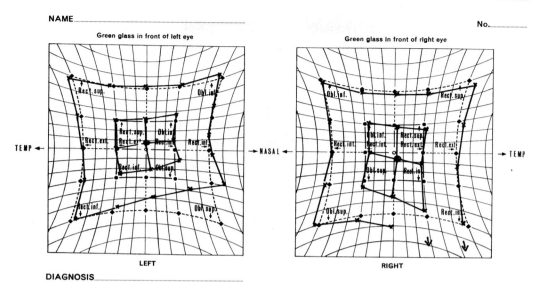

Figure 14.6 Hess chart of left IV nerve palsy.

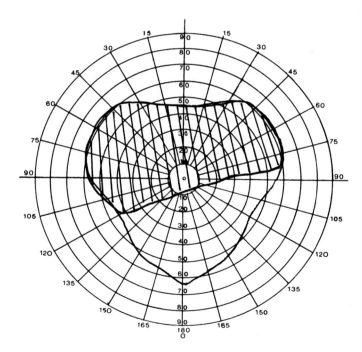

Figure 14.7 Field of binocular single vision of left IV nerve palsy.

this indicates that the IV nerve was responsible for the abnormal head posture rather than a non-ocular cause.

Differential diagnosis with skew deviation is by the presence of torsion. Typically excyclotorsion is seen in IV nerve palsy and incyclotorsion is seen in skew deviation.

The following table indicates the differences to be found on examination between a superior oblique palsy and a contralateral superior rectus palsy in long-standing cases.

Investigation	Superior oblique	Superior rectus
Cover test	Hyperdeviation if fixing with unaffected eye	Hypodeviation if fixing with unaffected eye
	Deviation greater for near	Deviation greater for distance
Abnormal head posture	Chin depression	Chin elevation
Ocular motility	Increase in angle on depression	Increase in angle on elevation
Hess chart	Greatest negative displacement on depression	Greatest negative displacement on elevation
Extorsion	Very common	Rare
Bielchowsky head tilt test	Often positive	Usually negative

Unilateral and bilateral cases of superior oblique palsy show the following set of different examination results.

Investigation	Unilateral	Bilateral
Cover test	Hyperdeviation in primary position reflects extent of palsy	Often only slight hyperdeviation in primary position
Ocular motility	No reversal of hypertropia or diplopia on lateral versions	Reversal of hyperdeviation and diplopia on lateral versions
	Slight V pattern may be noted	Large V pattern
Abnormal head posture	Chin depression, head tilt and head turn	Chin depression
Torsion	Slight extorsion	Extorsion > 10 degrees
Bielchowsky head tilt test	Positive with head tilt to affected side	Positive with head tilt to either shoulder

Management

Congenital

Correct any refractive error present and treat amblyopia if indicated. Surgery may be required for any of the following:

- strabismus
- marked abnormal head posture
- decompensating cases which show moderate/large angle deviations.

Abnormal superior oblique tendons are found in many cases of congenital IV nerve palsy and these cases may respond to a superior oblique tuck procedure (Helveston *et al.* 1981, 1992). Further procedures include weakening of overacting muscles, including the inferior oblique and inferior rectus.

Acquired

Treat the underlying cause of the IV nerve palsy, e.g. hypertension. Many cases recover within 3–6 months of onset.

Prisms. These can be used for small angles of deviation. Prisms of up to 10 prism dioptre strength can be incorporated in each lens, depending on the patient's spectacle prescription. Prism incorporation occurs at the stage where the condition is considered to be stable, usually with static reports for a minimum of six months.

Occlusion. This eliminates diplopia whilst waiting for static reports prior to further treatment.

Surgery. Once the degree of recovery is considered to be stable and static (usually a period of six months minimum is required for this), surgery may be undertaken. Knapp (1974; Knapp & Moore 1976) emphasised the importance of the relative magnitude of hyperdeviation in the various fields of gaze. The fields of greatest deviation should be matched to the muscles that exert their strongest action in those fields. For example, if the inferior oblique muscle overacts, this should be recessed. If the inferior oblique does not overact and the ipsilateral superior rectus is restricted, the superior rectus should be recessed. If the superior oblique is lax, it should be tucked.

Where the deviation measures more than 15 prism dioptres, surgery on two or more muscles is required: ipsilateral inferior oblique recession plus ipsilateral superior rectus recession if restricted or ipsilateral superior oblique tuck if lax or contralateral inferior rectus recession or a combination as necessary.

Generally, for large angle deviations with/without torsion, surgical procedures include the following.

- Weaken the overacting muscles:
  - ipsilateral inferior oblique recession
  - contralateral inferior rectus recession.
  Adjustable sutures may be used.

- For torsion, a Harado–Ito procedure (Fell's modification) can be performed (Harado & Ito 1964). In this procedure, the anterior portion of the affected superior oblique tendon is placed further anteriorly and laterally. This increases the sagittal axis on the globe and leads to a greater amount of incyclotorsion compared to depression as the muscle functions.
- In bilateral cases, Harado–Ito procedures may be carried out on both sides where there is torsion. If there is no torsion, bilateral inferior oblique recessions may suffice.

  Sometimes, a combination of these two procedures is required.

Superior oblique myokymia

This very rare, benign, self-limiting disorder is found unilaterally and may follow an acquired superior oblique palsy.

The condition is characterised by the following features.

- The patient suffers recurrent episodes of involuntary rapid eye movements which may be vertical or torsional. These movements are clearly visible when observed through a slit-lamp or direct ophthalmoscope.
- These movements are experienced by the patient with the production of intermittent oscillopsia.
- The patient may also experience torsional monocular diplopia.

The cause is usually unknown but it has been suggested that it occurs following an alteration in membrane threshold of the IV nerve nucleus. An occasional association has been made with the presence of multiple sclerosis. The patient's symptoms sometimes reduce with time and episodes are often brief, occurring at irregular intervals. There may be long periods of remission which may last for several years (Kommerell & Schaubele 1980).

Management

Carbamazepine (Tegretol) has been used with some success (Brazis *et al.* 1994). The therapeutic effect is probably related to an elevation of the neural threshold of the IV nerve to repeated stimulation. The patients need to be followed up at regular intervals with full blood counts and liver function tests due to possible unwanted effects of bone marrow suppression, aplastic anaemia and hepatic toxicity. Surgery may be considered in severe cases but is rarely associated with a complete cure. The procedure involves a superior oblique intrasheath tenotomy combined with an ipsilateral inferior oblique recession.

VI (SIXTH) CRANIAL NERVE

The VI cranial nerve supplies the lateral rectus muscle only. A lesion affecting the nerve will result in defective abduction of the eye.

Aetiology

The commonly recognised causes of VI nerve palsy include space occupying lesions, trauma, vascular insults and inflammation. VI nerve palsy secondary to raised intracranial pressure is also commonly regarded as a typical false localising sign. Other causes have included pseudo-tumor cerebri (idiopathic intracranial hypertension), post-operative complications, viral infection, multiple sclerosis and otitis.

Congenital

- Following birth trauma
- Hereditary
- Infection (maternal)
- Failure of lateral rectus development

Acquired

This differs according to age.

- *Children* (Afifi *et al.* 1992):
  — space occupying lesions
  — infections, bacterial or viral*
  — trauma
  — raised intracranial pressure.
- *Young adults*:
  — trauma
  — space occupying lesions
  — post-viral inflammation
  — multiple sclerosis
  — diabetes
- *Older adults*:
  — vascular
  — diabetes
  — space occupying lesions.

* Gradinego's syndrome is the association of a VI nerve palsy with middle ear infection which has spread to the VI nerve at the petrous-temporal bone.

Investigation

Case history

There may be a significant medical history, as indicated above. Birth history may also be significant. The patient may complain of horizontal

Visual acuity   diplopia and relatives or friends may notice the presence of squint (esodeviation) or an abnormal head posture.

This may be reduced if the affected eye fails to fixate properly due to the presence of a marked deviation. Amblyopia will develop in children with unilateral strabismus.

Abnormal head posture   The face is turned towards the affected side.

Cover test   An esodeviation is present which is often greater on distance testing. The test should be carried out with and without an abnormal head posture, if one is present. The deviation increases without the head posture but does not necessarily become manifest.

Ocular motility   The primary underaction of the affected lateral rectus results in limited abduction (Fig. 14.8) and is followed by a number of sequelae. There is overaction of both the contralateral and ipsilateral medial recti. There is also secondary underaction of the contralateral lateral rectus.

Binocular function   This is often retained in the presence of an abnormal head posture. As the angle of deviation is often smaller for near fixation, binocular function is usually present on near fixation. In cases of head trauma, fusion may have been lost.

Hess chart   This provides a record for the notes and illustrates the associated muscle sequelae (Fig. 14.9).

Field of binocular single vision   The field of binocular single vision is displaced away from the affected side (Fig. 14.10).

Diplopia   This is uncrossed and becomes worse for distance fixation.

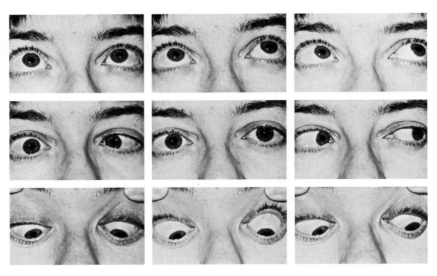

Figure 14.8   Right VI nerve palsy.

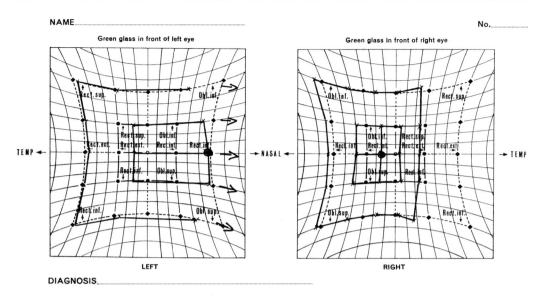

Figure 14.9   Hess chart of right VI nerve palsy.

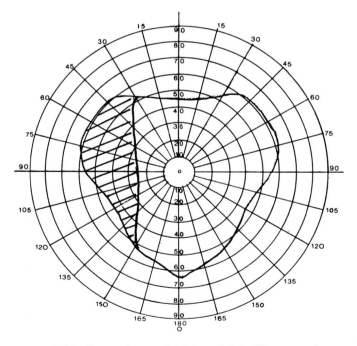

Figure 14.10   Field of binocular single vision of right VI nerve palsy.

Differential diagnosis

Differential diagnosis should be made with the following conditions: Duane's retraction syndrome, infantile esotropia, nystagmus block syndrome.

Management

Recovery of VI nerve palsy can be expected in at least 50% of cases although a higher percentage of recovery is likely in those cases due to vascular insults, trauma and inflammation. Good recovery of cranial nerve palsies following raised intracranial pressure is also expected. However, poor recovery is more likely with an aetiology of space occupying lesions where the nerve is involved in the mass lesion with compression or stretching of the nerve, resulting in shearing injuries or contusion.

Congenital

Treat amblyopia if indicated. Surgery may be required for cosmesis (see below). In young children treatment is aimed at preventing amblyopia and preserving binocular function (Rosenbaum 1991; Aroichane & Repka 1995).

Children often suppress, leading to amblyopia. Therefore occlusion is required. If they adopt an abnormal head posture this should not be discouraged.

Acquired

Treat the underlying cause of the VI nerve palsy if possible. In adult cases allow for recovery, but during this period, **prisms** or **occlusion** can be used to join or eliminate diplopia. Where small angle deviations are present, it may be possible to incorporate prisms into a spectacle correction once the deviation is static, to provide long term management. Fresnel prisms are useful for small deviations. However, vision may be blurred by the prisms in proportion to the amount of prism applied.

Surgery may be employed once the condition is static, with a minimum of six months of stable measurements. Depending on the size of the angle of deviation, unilateral or bilateral medial recti recessions may be required. The lateral rectus may be resected in addition (Rosenbaum *et al.* 1989).

If the palsy is complete, a medial rectus recession can be combined with muscle transposition of the superior and inferior recti to the affected lateral rectus (Berens & Girard 1950; Parks 1974; Metz 1976; Wybar 1981; Ciancia *et al.* 1984). Three muscle surgery increases the risk of anterior segment ischaemia.

Where there is residual lateral incomitance, a recession or Faden on the contralateral medial rectus may be considered.

Botulinum toxin A may be injected into the medial rectus muscle in recent onset palsies. This helps prevent contracture and allows the eyes to adopt a straighter position in order to obtain binocular single vision. It may help to restore binocular function in the long term (Scott *et al.* 1989, 1990). The use of botulinum toxin A may be combined with surgery when performing a transposition procedure (Fitzsimmons *et al.* 1988, 1989).

Prospective randomised clinical trials have shown no evidence of any difference between the treated and untreated groups in terms of ultimate outcome. However, patients treated with botulinum reported subjective improvement (Lee *et al.* 1994).

MULTIPLE SCLEROSIS

Aetiology

Multiple sclerosis is due to demyelination. If there is inflammation there are also biochemical changes. Improvement occurs because inflammation settles, there is a degree of remyelination and reorganisation of cell functions such as an increase in sodium channels. There is also plasticity of the nervous system with rerouting of impulses.

Investigation

The orthoptic investigation is dependent on the type of ocular motility defect that has occurred. Generally there are isolated muscle palsies, internuclear ophthalmoplegia and nystagmus.

The prognosis for patients with normal baseline brain scans is very good, with few developing multiple sclerosis. Most cases with abnormal scans at baseline assessment develop multiple sclerosis. The more lesions at baseline, the more severe and disabling in the long term the condition will be.

Management

For an isolated episode, steroids will settle the condition faster. These are given intravenously for three days if the patient has shown little recovery after 7–10 days. Interferon over 18–24 months at a low dose may delay conversion to the chronic disease.

Counselling should address issues such as the risk of developing multiple sclerosis, patient access to medical information and financial/insurance issues.

Relapse management includes the use of steroids, multidisciplinary involvement of nurses, occupational therapists, physiotherapists and the orthoptist. Symptoms must be actively managed while waiting for recovery.

Mitoxantrone may be effective for switching off aggressive relapsing multiple sclerosis but cannot be used long term due to its toxicity. However, it stabilises patients and further treatment can be instigated at that point.

ACQUIRED MOTOR FUSION DEFICIENCY

Aetiology

This occurs after closed head trauma, after cerebrovascular accidents, as a result of intracranial tumours and after brain surgery (Avilla & von Noorden 1984). There is an assumed midbrain lesion.

Investigation

Case history   Patients complain of severe asthenopia, intractable diplopia and inability to maintain single vision for any length of time. Diplopia may be crossed, then uncrossed, then vertical.

Accommodation This may be associated with a reduced range of accommodation (Wade 1965; Pratt-Johnson 1973; Pratt-Johnson & Tillson 1979; Harrison 1987).

Binocular
function   There is no motor fusion. Sensory fusion and stereopsis are intermittently demonstrable (Avilla & von Noorden 1984).

Management

There is no effective treatment. Prisms are not useful due to variable diplopia and patients cannot use motor fusion once aligned. There is no suppression area to move the image into.

The condition can spontaneously improve but this is uncommon (Hart 1969; MacLellan 1974; McLean & Lee 1998).

Filters and occlusion are required (McIntyre & Fells 1996).

OPHTHALMOPLEGIA

This is a group of conditions which have a variety of causative factors, where there is a paresis of two or more extraocular muscles.

Cavernous sinus syndrome

There is a lesion in the cavernous sinus causing paresis of the ocular motor nerves and the first two divisions of the V nerve (Hunt *et al.* 1961).

Aetiology

- Tumour affecting both cavernous sinuses
- Cavernous sinus thrombosis
- Cavernous sinus fistula

Investigation

Case history   Diplopia is due to ophthalmoplegia and reduced visual acuity. There is often a marked conjunctival injection. An ocular bruit may be present which is audible with the use of a stethoscope.

Cover test	Proptosis is often present which may be pulsatile.
Intraocular pressure	Raised intraocular pressure is due to the proptosis.
Ocular motility	Pupillary reaction is often spared. Ophthalmoplegia is due to involvement of the III, IV and VI nerves. Ptosis may be evident.

Sphenoidal fissure syndrome

Aetiology

A lesion in the region of the superior orbital fissure may affect any structure passing through.

Investigation

| *Case history* | Diplopia is due to III, IV and VI cranial nerve involvement. Symptoms are variable depending on the extent and combination of nerve involvement. Pain and anaesthesia are due to involvement of the V cranial nerve. |
| *Ocular motility* | There is progressive involvement of the III (sometimes only the superior branch), IV and VI cranial nerves. Proptosis is noted. |

Orbital apex syndrome

Aetiology

A lesion in the posterior part of the orbit near its apex is responsible for this condition. Orbital pseudotumour may produce this although visual loss is infrequent. Orbital cellulitis may also produce this syndrome.

Investigation

Case history	V nerve involvement will give symptoms of severe pain. Diplopia is due to defective ocular motility.
Visual acuity	Reduced visual acuity is due to compression of the optic nerve.
Ocular motility	Limited ocular movement is seen with III, IV and VI nerve involvement according to the muscles involved. There is often marked swelling and redness of the eye lids with chemosis of the conjunctiva. Proptosis and raised intraocular pressure are also documented.

Guillain–Barré syndrome (Fisher's syndrome)

Aetiology

This syndrome is thought to be the result of an allergic response of the peripheral nervous system to an antigen, possibly of viral origin. Fisher's syndrome is a variant with less severe clinical features.

Investigation

Ocular motility   Facial nerve paralysis may be noted. There is mild to complete ophthalmoplegia and ptosis, anisocoria and nystagmus may be noted.

Visual acuity   Optic neuritis may occur with papilloedema evident on fundus examination.

Associated paralysis   There may be variable paralysis of motor nerves beginning in the lower extremities with absent tendon reflexes. There may also be involvement of the respiratory muscles.

Recovery is a slow and gradual process but in general the prognosis is favourable.

Fisher's syndrome is characterised by total external ophthalmoplegia, ataxia and hyporeflexia. Ophthalmoplegia involves symmetrical impairment of conjugate upward and lateral gaze progressing frequently to complete ophthalmoplegia. There is absence of limb weakness and patients usually recover spontaneously within 7–12 weeks.

Ophthalmoplegia migraine

This condition involves migraine and usually an associated III nerve palsy without pupil sparing. Other oculomotor nerves may also be affected leading to corresponding muscle paresis.

Aetiology

It is postulated that the III nerve is compressed in the cavernous sinus by a dilated or oedematous carotid artery but this is not a consistent finding. Alternatively, vasospasm may affect the small vessels supplying the nerve itself.

Investigation

A typical episode consists of pain in and around the involved eye. There may be associated nausea and vomiting. With the onset of ophthalmoplegia, the head pain often resolves. The paresis usually completely resolves within one month but there may be permanent full or partial disability. The onset is usually in childhood and there is often a positive family history of migraine.

Tolosa–Hunt syndrome

This is an acute inflammatory condition that involves the superior orbital fissure or the anterior cavernous sinus resulting in a painful ophthalmoplegia.

Aetiology

There may be non-specific granulation tissue in the cavernous sinus or pachymeningitis of the superior orbital fissure.

Investigation

Case history   The patient may complain of a steady, boring pain in or around the eye. Diplopia may be appreciated. Hypoaesthesia or anaesthesia in the distribution of the ophthalmic division of the V nerve may be experienced.

Visual acuity   Occasionally there is a reduction in visual acuity.

Ocular motility   Ophthalmoplegia with complete or partial palsy of extraocular muscles may be documented and the pupil may or may not be affected.

The condition occurs acutely or subacutely and usually responds to high doses of corticosteroids. Spontaneous remission may occur with complete or partial recovery.

Ocular neuromyotonia

This is a rare condition resulting in transient, aperiodic ocular misalignment.

Aetiology

There is spontaneous firing of ocular motor nerves resulting in impairment of muscle relaxation. The spontaneous firing is thought to occur in injured axons or with radiation plexopathy and peripheral trauma neuropathy. Many patients have had prior radiation therapy to the sellar and parasellar regions. The condition is particularly noted following pituitary fossa surgery and irradiation. Experimental evidence has implicated extracellular potassium concentration in causing the spontaneous firing of axons.

Investigation

Case history   There is episodic diplopia which occurs either spontaneously or after sustained eccentric gaze.

Ocular motility   There is often a cranial nerve palsy and a III nerve palsy is most commonly noted with aberrant regeneration. Attacks can be provoked by overaction of the muscles supplied by the cranial nerve involved and therefore may be elicited by sustained gaze in that direction (Spiritus *et al.* 1995; Ezra *et al.* 1996).

Management

Treatment with anticonvulsants is extremely effective. Carbamazepine is most frequently employed.

REFERENCES

Afifi AK, Bell WE & Menezes AH. (1992) Etiology of lateral rectus palsy in infancy and childhood. *Journal of Child Neurology*, 7: 295

Aroichane M & Repka MX. (1995) Outcome of sixth nerve palsy or paresis in young children. *Journal of Pediatric Ophthalmology and Strabismus*, 32: 152

Avilla CW & von Noorden GK. (1984) Post-traumatic fusion deficiency. In: Ravault AP & Lenk M (eds) *Transactions of the Fifth International Orthoptic Conference*. LIPS, Lyon, p. 143

Berens C & Girard L. (1950) Transplantation of the superior and inferior rectus muscles for paralysis of the lateral rectus muscle. *American Journal of Ophthalmology*, 33: 1041

Brazis PW, Miller NR, Henderer JD & Lee AG. (1994) The natural history and results of treatment of superior oblique myokymia. *Archives of Ophthalmology*, 112: 1063

Burian HM & van Allen MW. (1963) Cyclic oculomotor paralysis. *American Journal of Ophthalmology*, 55: 529

Burke JP, Ruben JB & Scott WE. (1992) Vertical transposition of the horizontal recti (Knapp procedure) for the treatment of double elevator palsy: effectiveness and long-term stability. *British Journal of Ophthalmology*, 76: 734

Ciancia AO, Garcia HA & Lavin R. (1984) Treatment of the lateral rectus palsy. *Documenta Ophthalmologica*, 58: 57

Cox TA, Wurster JB & Godfrey WA. (1979) Primary aberrant oculomotor regeneration due to intracranial aneurysm. *Archives of Neurology*, 36: 570

Ezra E, Spalton D, Sanders MD, Graham EM & Plant GT. (1996) Ocular neuromyotonia. *British Journal of Ophthalmology*, 80: 350

Fitzsimmons R, Lee JP & Elston J. (1988) Treatment of sixth nerve palsy in adults with combined botulinum toxin chemodenervation and surgery. *Ophthalmology*, 95: 1535

Fitzsimmons R, Lee JP & Elston J. (1989) The role of botulinum in the management of sixth nerve palsy. *Eye*, 3: 391

Harado M & Ito Y. (1964) Surgical correction of cyclotropia. *Japanese Journal of Ophthalmology*, 8: 88

Harrison RL. (1987) Loss of fusional vergence with partial loss of accommodative convergence and accommodation following head injury. *Binocular Vision and Strabismus Quarterly*, 2: 93

Hart CT. (1969) Disturbances of fusion following head injury. *Proceedings of the Royal Society of Medicine*, 62: 704

Helveston EM, Giangiacomo JD & Ellis FD. (1981) Congenital absence of the superior oblique tendon. *Transactions of the American Ophthalmological Society*, 79: 124

Helveston EM, Krach D, Plager DA & Ellis FD. (1992) A new class of superior oblique palsy based on congenital variations in the tendon. *Ophthalmology*, 99: 1609

Hermann JS. (1981) Masked bilateral superior oblique paresis. *Journal of Pediatric Ophthalmology and Strabismus*, 18: 43

Hunt WE, Meagher JN, Lefever HE & Zeman W. (1961) Painful ophthalmoplegia: its relationship to indolent inflammation of the cavernous sinus. *Neurology*, 11: 56

Jampel RS & Fells P. (1968) Monocular elevation paresis caused by a central nervous system lesion. *Archives of Ophthalmology*, 80: 45

Knapp P. (1969) The surgical treatment of double-elevator paralysis. *Transactions of the American Ophthalmological Society*, 67: 304

Knapp P. (1974) Classification and treatment of superior oblique palsy. *American Orthoptic Journal*, 24: 18

Knapp P & Moore S. (1976) Diagnosis and surgical options in superior oblique surgery. *International Ophthalmic Clinics*, 16: 137

Kommerell G & Schaubele G. (1980) Superior oblique myokymia: an electromyographical analysis. *Transactions of the Ophthalmological Society of the United Kingdom,* 100: 504

Lee J, Harris S, Cohen J, Cooper K, MacEwen C & Jones S. (1994) Results of a prospective randomised trial of botulinum toxin therapy in acute unilateral sixth nerve palsy. *Journal of Pediatric Ophthalmology and Strabismus,* 31: 283

MacLellan AV. (1974) A case of recovery from traumatic loss of fusion. *British Orthoptic Journal,* 31: 102

Maruo T, Iwashiga H, Kubota N, Sakaue T, Ishida T, Honda M, Nemoto Y & Usui C. (1996) Results of surgery for paralytic exotropia due to oculomotor palsy. *Ophthalmologica,* 210: 163

McIntyre A & Fells P. (1996) Bangerter foils: a new approach to the management of pathological intractable diplopia. *British Orthoptic Journal,* 53: 43

McLean CJ & Lee JP. (1998) Acquired central fusion disruption with spontaneous recovery. *Strabismus,* 6: 175

Metz HS. (1976) The diagnosis and treatment of abduction deficiencies. *Annals of Ophthalmology,* 8: 683

Metz HS. (1988) The use of vertical offsets with horizontal strabismus surgery. *Ophthalmology,* 95: 1094

Metz HS. (1993) 20th Annual Frank Costenbader Lecture – muscle transposition surgery. *Journal of Pediatric Ophthalmology and Strabismus,* 30: 346

Metz HS & Yee D. (1973) Third nerve palsy: superior oblique transposition surgery. *Annals of Ophthalmology,* 5: 215

Parks MM. (1958) Isolated cyclovertical muscle palsy. *Archives of Ophthalmology,* 60: 1027

Parks MM. (1974) The overacting inferior oblique muscle. *American Journal of Ophthalmology,* 77: 787

Paysee EA, Coats DK & Plager DA. (1995) Facial asymmetry and tendon laxity in superior oblique palsy. *Journal of Pediatric Ophthalmology and Strabismus,* 32: 158

Peter LC. (1934) The use of the superior oblique as an internal rotator in third-nerve paralysis. *American Journal of Ophthalmology,* 17: 297

Plager DA. (1990) Traction testing in superior oblique palsy. *Journal of Pediatric Ophthalmology and Strabismus,* 27: 136

Plager DA. (1992) Tendon laxity in superior oblique palsy. *Ophthalmology,* 99: 1032

Pratt-Johnson JA. (1973) Central disruption of fusional amplitude. *British Journal of Ophthalmology,* 57: 347

Pratt-Johnson JA & Tillson G. (1979) Acquired central disruption of fusional amplitude. *Ophthalmology,* 86: 2140

Rosenbaum AL. (1991) The clinical use of botulinum toxin in acute and chronic sixth nerve palsy. *Current Opinion in Ophthalmology,* 2: 69

Rosenbaum AL, Kushner BJ & Kirschen D. (1989) Vertical rectus muscle transposition and botulinum toxin (Oculinum) to medial rectus for abducens palsy. *Archives of Ophthalmology,* 107: 820

Saunders RA & Rogers GL. (1982) Superior oblique transposition for third nerve palsy. *Ophthalmology,* 89: 310

Scott AB, Magoon EH, McNeer KW & Stager DR. (1989) Botulinum toxin for strabismus in children. *Transactions of the American Ophthalmology Society,* 87: 174

Scott AB, Magoon EH, McNeer KW & Stager DR. (1990) Botulinum toxin of childhood strabismus. *Ophthalmology,* 97: 1434

Shuttleworth GN, Steel DHW, Silverman BW & Harrad RA. (1998) Patterns of third nerve synkinesis. *Strabismus*, 6: 181

Spiritus M, Boschi A & Bergmans J. (1995) Ocular neuromyotonia: report of two clinical cases. In: Louly M, Doyle M, Hirai T & Tomlinson E (eds) *Transactions of the Eighth International Orthoptic Congress*. Japan, p. 77

Villasenor Solares J, Riemann BI, Romanelli Zuazo AC & Riemann CD. (2000) Ocular fixation to nasal periosteum with a superior oblique tendon in patients with third nerve palsy. *Journal of Pediatric Ophthalmology and Strabismus*, 37: 260

Wade SL. (1965) Loss of fusion following brain damage. *British Orthoptic Journal*, 22: 81

Wilson ME & Hoxie J. (1993) Facial asymmetry in superior oblique muscle palsy. *Journal of Pediatric Ophthalmology and Strabismus*, 30: 315

Wybar KC. (1981) Management of sixth nerve palsy and Duane's retraction syndrome. *Transactions of the Ophthalmic Society of the United Kingdom*, 101: 276

Young TL, Conahan BM, Summers CG & Egbert JE. (2000) Anterior transposition of the superior oblique tendon in the treatment of oculomotor nerve palsy and its influence on postoperative hypertropia. *Journal of Pediatric Ophthalmology and Strabismus*, 37: 149

FURTHER READING

Baker RS & Steed MM. (1990) Restoration of function in paralytic strabismus: alternative methods of therapy. *Binocular Vision*, 5: 203

Bechac G, Bec P & Delfour N. (1984) Bilateral fourth nerve palsy. Excyclovergence, as a warning of peri-aqueduct stenosis. In: Ravault A & Lenk M (eds) *Transactions of the Fifth International Orthoptic Congress*. LIPS, Lyon, p. 135

Berlit P. (1991) Isolated and combined pareses of cranial nerves III, IV and VI. A retrospective study of 412 patients. *Journal of Neurological Science*, 103: 10

Bixenman WW & von Noorden GK. (1981) Benign recurrent sixth nerve palsy in childhood. *Journal of Pediatric Ophthalmology and Strabismus*, 18: 29

Brown WB. (1957) Isolated inferior oblique paralysis. *Transactions of the American Ophthalmological Society*, 55: 415

Buckley EG & Meekins BB. (1988) Fadenoperation for the management of complicated incomitant vertical strabismus. *American Journal of Ophthalmology*, 105: 304

Burian HM & Cahill JE. (1952) Congenital paralysis of medial rectus muscle with unusual synergism of the horizontal muscles. *Transactions of the American Ophthalmological Society*, 50: 87

Carlson MR & Jampolsky A. (1979) An adjustable transposition procedure for abduction deficiencies. *American Journal of Ophthalmology*, 78: 382

Cobbs WH, Schatz HJ & Savino PJ. (1980) Nontraumatic bilateral fourth nerve palsies. A dorsal midbrain sign. *Annals of Neurology*, 8: 107

de Decker W. (1981) The fadenoperation. When and how to do it. *Transactions of the Ophthalmology Society of the United Kingdom*, 101: 264

Fells P. (1974) Management of paralytic strabismus. *British Journal of Ophthalmology*, 58: 255

Fells P. (1976) Surgical management of extorsion. *International Ophthalmology Clinics*, 16: 161

Fells P & Collin JRO. (1979) Cyclic oculomotor palsy. *Transactions of the Ophthalmology Society of the United Kingdom*, 99: 192

Ficker LA, Collin JRO & Lee JP. (1986) Management of ipsilateral ptosis with hypotropia. *British Journal of Ophthalmology*, 70: 732

Freedman HL, Waltman DD & Patterson JH. (1992) Preservation of anterior ciliary vessels during strabismus surgery: a nonmicroscopic technique. *Journal of Pediatric Ophthalmology and Strabismus*, 29: 38

Frueh BR & Henderson JW. (1971) Rectus muscle union in sixth nerve paralysis. *Archives of Ophthalmology*, 85: 191

Goldstein JE & Cogan DG. (1960) Diabetic ophthalmoplegia with special reference to the pupil. *Archives of Ophthalmology*, 64: 592

Gottlob I, Catalano RA & Reinecke RD. (1991) Surgical management of oculomotor nerve palsy. *American Journal of Ophthalmology*, 111: 71

Green WR, Hackett ER & Schlezinger NS. (1964) Neuro-ophthalmic evaluation of oculo motor nerve paralysis. *Archives of Ophthalmology*, 72: 154

Hamed LM & Silbiger J. (1992) Periodic alternating esotropia. *Journal of Pediatric Ophthalmology and Strabismus*, 29: 240

Harcourt B, Almond S & Freedman H. (1981) The efficacy of inferior oblique myectomy operations. In: Mein J & Moore S (eds) *Orthoptics, Research and Practice*. Kimpton, London, p. 20

Harley RD. (1980) Paralytic strabismus in children. Etiologic incidence and management of the third, fourth and sixth nerve palsies. *Ophthalmology*, 87: 24

Helveston EM. (1971) Muscle transposition procedures. *Survey of Ophthalmology*, 16: 92

Holmes JM, Beck RW, Kip KE, Droste PJ & Leske DA. (2001) Predictors of nonrecovery in acute traumatic sixth nerve palsy and paresis. *Ophthalmology*, 108: 1457

Hoyt WF & Keane JR. (1970) Superior oblique myokymia. Report and discussion on five cases of benign intermittent uniocular microtremor. *Archives of Ophthalmology*, 84: 461

Iacobucci I & Beyst-Martonyi J. (1978) The use of press-on prisms in the preoperative evaluation of adults with strabismus. *American Orthoptic Journal*, 28: 68

Jensen CDF. (1964) Rectus muscle union: a new operation for paralysis of the rectus muscle. *Transactions of the Pacific Coast Ophthalmological Society*, 45: 359

Jones ST. (1977) Treatment of hypertropia by vertical displacement of horizontal recti. *American Orthoptic Journal*, 27: 107

Keech RV, Morris RJ, Ruben JB & Scott WE. (1990) Anterior segment ischemia following vertical muscle transposition and botulinum toxin injection. *Archives of Ophthalmology*, 108: 176

Khawam E, Scott A & Jampolsky A. (1967) Acquired superior oblique palsy. Diagnosis and management. *Archives of Ophthalmology*, 77: 761

Knapp P. (1971) Diagnosis and surgical treatment of hypertropia. *American Orthoptic Journal*, 21: 29

Knapp P. (1978) Paretic squints. In: Allen JH (ed) *Symposium on Strabismus. Transactions of the New Orleans Academy of Ophthalmology*. Mosby, St Louis, p. 350

Kodsi SR & Younge BR. (1992) Acquired oculomotor, trochlear and abducent cranial nerve palsies in pediatric patients. *American Journal of Ophthalmology*, 114: 568

Kraft SP, O'Reilly C, Quigley PL, Allan K & Eustis HS. (1993) Cyclotorsion in unilateral and bilateral superior oblique paresis. *Journal of Pediatric Ophthalmology and Strabismus*, 30: 361

Kraft SP & Scott WE. (1986) Masked bilateral superior oblique palsy. Clinical features and diagnosis. *Journal of Pediatric Ophthalmology and Strabismus*, 23: 264

Kushner BJ. (1992) A surgical procedure to minimize lower eyelid retraction with inferior rectus recession. *Archives of Ophthalmology*, 110: 1011

Lee JP. (1984) Superior oblique myokymia. A possible etiologic factor. *Archives of Ophthalmology*, 102: 1178

Lee JP. (1992) Modern management of sixth nerve palsy. *Australian and New Zealand Journal of Ophthalmology*, 20: 41

Lessel S. (1975) Supranuclear paralysis of monocular elevation. *Neurology*, 25: 1134

Loewenfeld IE & Thompson HS. (1975) Oculomotor paresis with cyclic spasms. A critical review of the literature and a new case. *Survey of Ophthalmology*, 20: 81

Lustbader JM & Miller NR. (1988) Painless, pupil sparing but otherwise complete oculomotor nerve paresis caused by basilar artery aneurysm. *Archives of Ophthalmology*, 106: 583

McDonald WI, Compston A, Edan G, Goodkin D, Hartung HP, Lublin FD, McFarland HF, Paty DW, Polman CH, Reingold SC, Sandberg-Wollheim M, Sibley W, Thompson A, van den Noort S, Weinshenker BY & Wolinsky JS. (2001) Recommended diagnostic criteria for multiple sclerosis: guidelines from the International Panel on the diagnosis of multiple sclerosis. *Annals of Neurology*, 50: 121

Manners RM, O'Flynn E & Morris RJ. (1994) Superior oblique lengthening for acquired superior oblique overaction. *British Journal of Ophthalmology*, 78: 280

Metz HS & Dickey CF. (1991) Treatment of unilateral acute sixth nerve palsy with botulinum toxin. *American Journal of Ophthalmology*, 112: 381

Metz HS & Mazow M. (1988) Botulinum toxin treatment of acute sixth and third nerve palsy. *Graefe's Archives of Clinical and Experimental Ophthalmology*, 226: 141

Miller NR. (1977) Solitary oculomotor nerve palsy in childhood. *American Journal of Ophthalmology*, 83: 106

Mitchell PR & Parks MM. (1982) Surgery for bilateral superior oblique palsy. *Ophthalmology*, 89: 484

Mulvihill A, Murphy M & Lee JP. (2000) Disinsertion of the inferior oblique muscle for treatment of superior oblique paresis. *Journal of Pediatric Ophthalmology and Strabismus*, 37: 279

Murray AD. (1991) Early botulinum toxin treatment of acute sixth nerve palsy. *Eye*, 5: 45

Ohtsuki H, Hasebe S, Hanabusa K, Fujimoto Y & Furuse T. (1994) Intraoperative adjustable suture surgery for bilateral superior oblique palsy. *Ophthalmology*, 101: 188

Pacheco EM, Guyton DL & Repka MX. (1992) Changes in eyelid position accompanying vertical rectus muscle surgery and prevention of lower lid retraction with adjustable surgery. *Journal of Pediatric Ophthalmology and Strabismus*, 29: 265

Palmer EA & Shults WT. (1984) Superior oblique myokymia: preliminary results of surgical treatment. *Journal of Pediatric Ophthalmology and Strabismus*, 21: 96

Parks MM. (1974) Management of acquired esotropia. *British Journal of Ophthalmology*, 58: 240

Richards BW, Jones FR & Younge BR. (1992) Causes and prognosis in 4278 cases of paralysis of the oculomotor, trochlear and abducens cranial nerves. *American Journal of Ophthalmology*, 113: 489

Roper-Hall G & Burde RM. (1978) Superior oblique myokymia. *American Orthoptic Journal*, 28: 58

Rosenberg ML & Glaser JS. (1983) Superior oblique myokymia. *Annals of Neurology*, 13: 667

Rowe FJ. (2000) Acquired ocular motility disorders in idiopathic intracranial hypertension. *Neuro-ophthalmology*, 24: 445

Rucker CW. (1958) Paralysis of the third, fourth and sixth cranial nerves. *American Journal of Ophthalmology*, 46: 787

Rucker CW. (1966) The causes of paralysis of the third, fourth and sixth cranial nerves. *American Journal of Ophthalmology*, 61: 1293

Rush JA & Younge BR. (1981) Paralysis of cranial nerves III, IV and VI: causes and prognosis in 1,000 cases. *Archives of Ophthalmology*, 99: 76

Schatz NJ, Savino PJ & Corbett JJ. (1977) Primary aberrant oculomotor regeneration: a sign on intracavernous meningioma. *Archives of Neurology*, 34: 29

Schmal B, Verlohr D & Schulz E. (1999) Benign VIth nerve palsies in childhood. In: Pritchard C, Kohler M, Verlohr D (eds) *Transactions of the Ninth International Orthoptic Congress: Orthoptics in Focus*. Stockholm, p. 219

Scott AB & Kraft SP. (1985) Botulinum toxin injection in the management of lateral rectus paresis. *Ophthalmology*, 92: 676

Scott WE & Kraft SP. (1986) Classification and surgical management of superior oblique palsies: 1 Unilateral superior oblique palsies. In: Allen JH (ed) *Pediatric Ophthalmology and Strabismus: Transactions of the New Orleans Academy of Ophthalmology*. Raven Press, New York, p. 15

Strachan IM & Innes JR. (1987) Congenital paralysis of vertical gaze. In: Lenk-Schafer M, Calcutt C, Doyle M & Moore S (eds) *Transactions of the Sixth International Orthoptic Congress*. British Orthoptic Society, London, p. 140

Tiffin PAC, MacEwen CJ, Craig EA & Clayton G. (1996) Acquired palsy of the oculomotor, trochlear and abducens nerves. *Eye*, 10: 377

Trimble RB. (1977) Loss of accommodation and convergence. *Proceedings of the Royal Society* of *Medicine*, 70: 261

Tolosa EJ. (1954) Peri-arteritic lesions of the carotid siphon with clinical features of carotid infra-clinoid aneurysms. *Journal of Neurology, Neurosurgery and Psychiatry*, 17: 300

Trobe JD. (1988) Third nerve palsy and the pupil (editorial). *Archives of Ophthalmology*, 106: 601

Tsuzuki K & Awaya S. (1992) Long-term follow up of Jensen's procedure in cases of sixth nerve palsy. *Folia Ophthalmologica Japonica*, 43: 866

von Noorden GK, Awaya S & Romano PE. (1971) Past-pointing in paralytic strabismus. *American Journal of Ophthalmology*, 71: 27

von Noorden GK & Hansell R. (1991) Clinical characteristics and treatment of isolated inferior rectus paralysis. *Ophthalmology*, 98: 253

Werner DB, Savino PJ & Schatz NJ. (1983) Benign recurrent sixth nerve palsies in childhood. *Archives of Ophthalmology*, 101: 607

Wolff E. (1928) A bend in the 6th cranial nerve – and its probable significance. *British Journal of Ophthalmology*, 12: 22

Chapter 15
Mechanical disorders

Mechanical strabismus is paralytic strabismus which is caused by factors which interfere with muscle contraction or relaxation, or prevent free movement of the globe. There may be a physical restraint which interferes with normal function and is sometimes referred to as a leash. This may be:

- **direct** for example tight muscles. This limits movement in the position of gaze opposite to the leash
- **indirect** for example, posteriorly inserted muscle. This limits movement in the position towards the leash.

Classification

Congenital

- Duane's retraction syndrome
- Strabismus fixus syndrome
- Moebius' syndrome
- General fibrosis syndrome
- Brown's syndrome
- Adherence syndrome

Acquired

- Brown's syndrome
- Adherence syndrome
- Thyroid eye disease
- Orbital injuries } causing muscle fibrosis and development
- Orbital inflammation } of fibrotic tethers
- Conjunctival shortening syndrome
- Retinal detachment
- Space occupying lesions
- Iatrogenic

Characteristics

- The deviation in the primary position and the abnormal head posture are generally small.
- Ocular motility:
  — ductions and versions are equally limited
  — movement in the opposite direction of gaze is often limited

— muscle sequelae are often limited to overaction of the contralateral synergist
— abnormal patterns of movement may be present, such as upshoots
— normal saccadic velocity is present up to the point of limitation
— pain on movement may be experienced.
- Forced duction test shows limitation of passive movement.
- Globe retraction is diagnostic of mechanical restrictions.

Management

The primary aim of management is to ensure that the patient is symptom free and the deviation is cosmetically satisfactory.

Treatment is indicated where the condition produces symptoms and there is poor cosmesis.

Aims of surgical treatment

- Centralise and enlarge the field of binocular single vision and therefore reduce the abnormal head posture.
- Obtain good cosmesis.
- Reduce corneal exposure due to absence of Bell's phenomenon.
- Reduce or eliminate any obvious abnormal pattern of movement.

Principles

- Reduction of the mechanical restriction.
- Weaken the overacting contralateral synergist to induce relative concomitance.
- Decrease abnormal movement by stabilising the positions of other muscles.

DUANE'S RETRACTION SYNDROME

This is a congenital condition although it has been described as an acquired condition in rare cases. The condition may be bilateral (Rowe *et al.* 1991) or unilateral, the left eye is more commonly affected and the incidence is higher in females.

Classification

Brown and Lyle

The condition was classified separately by Brown and Lyle in 1950, according to the clinical findings.

- **Type A**. Typical convergent deviation with limited abduction and limited adduction to a lesser degree.
- **Type B**. Typical convergent deviation with limited abduction and normal adduction.

- **Type C**. Atypical divergent deviation with limited adduction and limited abduction to a lesser degree.

Huber (1974)

The condition is classified on the basis of EMG recordings and the co-contraction theory where the lateral rectus receives co-innervation from the III and VI nerves.

- **Type I**. There is limited abduction and limited adduction to a lesser degree. The lateral rectus has little or no innervation on abduction but has some innervation on adduction.
- **Type II**. There is limited adduction. The lateral rectus has innervation on abduction and adduction. It can therefore abduct, and on adduction it counteracts the medial rectus, producing limited adduction and globe retraction.
- **Type III**. There is limited abduction and adduction. The lateral rectus has little or no innervation to abduct, but is innervated on adduction and therefore counteracts the medial rectus.

Aetiology

Mechanical

- Thin, elastic muscles.
- Muscles bound to the orbital wall.
- Posterior insertion of the medial rectus.
- Abnormal attachments from the medial rectus to the orbital apex resulting in a tight medial rectus unable to relax or contract.
- Inelastic, fibrotic lateral rectus with abnormal attachments.

Innervational

- Absent VI nucleus. The lateral rectus shows atrophy and fibrosis (Hotchkiss *et al.* 1980; Parsa *et al.* 1998)
- Partially formed VI nerve.
- Co-contraction theory. The lateral rectus is partially innervated by the III nerve with or without VI nerve innervation. This produces co-contraction of the medial and lateral recti on adduction and limited adduction with retraction of the globe.

Investigation

Case history   Children present because parents have noted abnormal eye movements, head posture and/or strabismus. Adults may present with symptoms of decompensation. Diplopia is rarely noticed.

Visual acuity   Amblyopia may be present if there is associated manifest strabismus or anisometropia.

Abnormal head posture   A face turn to the affected side is most often seen.

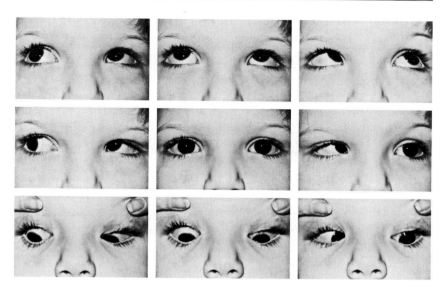

Figure 15.1 Duane's retraction syndrome.

Cover test	This is performed with and without the abnormal head posture. A typical condition has a convergent deviation and the atypical condition has a divergent deviation.
Ocular motility	Limited abduction occurs to a variable degree and limited adduction occurs often to a lesser degree (Fig. 15.1). Retraction of the globe on adduction with narrowing of the palpebral fissure is often noted. Widening of the palpebral fissure may be seen on attempted abduction. Up- or downshoots of the affected eye may occur on adduction with depression or elevation of the affected eye on abduction and bulging of orbital fat through the orbital septum may occur as the eye is adducted. An A or V pattern may be documented. Vertical retraction syndrome is a rare variant where there is limited elevation with lid retraction and limited depression with narrowing of the palpebral fissure.
	Upshoots are more common than downshoots and occur because of globe slippage between the tight horizontal recti (Bridal effect) or because of slippage of the tight horizontal recti over the globe.
Convergence	This is poor if there is limited adduction.
Binocular function	There is usually a good level of binocular function present which is maintained with an abnormal head posture. A mixture of binocular and suppression responses are recorded on clinical testing.
Angle of deviation	Primary and secondary angles differ, indicating incomitance.
Hess chart	Retention of incomitance is documented (Fig. 15.2).
Field of binocular single vision	The area of binocular single vision is positioned away from the position of maximum limitation (Fig. 15.3).

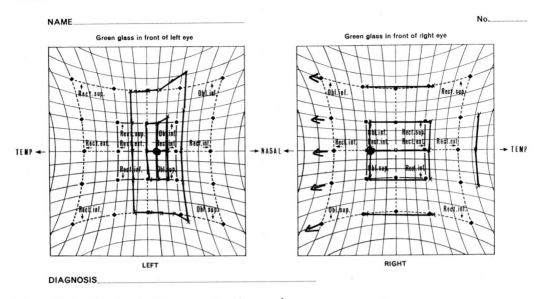

Figure 15.2   Hess chart of Duane's retraction syndrome.

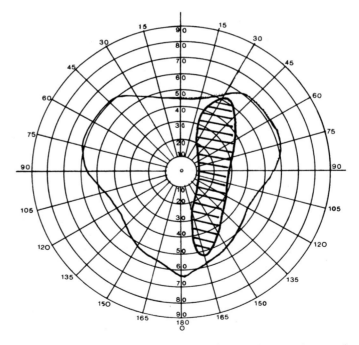

Figure 15.3   Field of binocular single vision of Duane's retraction syndrome.

Differential diagnosis	It is necessary to ensure the deviation is not due to a VI nerve palsy, medial wall fracture, localised inflammation, Moebius syndrome or iatrogenic cause such as a liberal lateral rectus recession.
Associated eye signs	Associated eye signs include lens opacities, heterochromia iridies, fundal defects, microphthalmos and crocodile tears (Ramsey & Taylor 1980).
Associated general signs	Two associated general conditions are those of Klippel-Feil and Goldenhar.

- **Klippel-Feil**. The patient has a short, immobile, rigid neck with a low posterior hairline.
- **Goldenhar**. The patient has ocular, auditory and vertebral anomalies with a poor mental performance (Pieroni 1970).
- **Kirkham's triad**. The triad is composed of Duane's retraction syndrome, Klippel-Feil and perceptive deafness. This is inherited as a single gene defect (Kirkham 1969).

Management

Correct the refractive error if present and treat any amblyopia. There is usually no further treatment as the majority of patients are comfortable and remain compensated, often with only a slight abnormal head posture. Symptoms are uncommon.

Indications for treatment

- Decompensation resulting in strabismus in children and symptoms in adults.
- Cosmetically poor abnormal head posture.
- Cosmetically poor strabismus.

Aims of treatment

- Place the field of binocular single vision more centrally and enlarge the field where possible.
- Reduce or eliminate the abnormal head posture.
- Achieve a good cosmesis.

Prisms

Prisms may be used first in cases of decompensation to assess if correction of the deviation helps or if the abnormal head posture is helped. They are given as an alternative method of treatment if possible.

Surgery

The purpose of surgery is not to obtain an improvement of ocular movement and it is unlikely that any significant increase in abduction or adduction will occur post-operatively.

The forced duction test will give a positive result due to the presence of fibrotic muscles. It is important never to resect the lateral rectus in either eye as this would result in further restriction of ocular motility.

Typical (esodeviation)

Ipsilateral or bilateral medial rectus recessions are advocated depending on the degree of the deviation. For large angle esodeviations and retraction, bilateral medial recti and ipsilateral lateral rectus recessions are useful.

Fells has used temporal transfer of superior and inferior recti to the lateral rectus combined with ipsilateral medial rectus recession < 3.5 mm. This procedure increases abduction and reduces esodeviation and abnormal head posture.

Atypical (exodeviation)

Ipsilateral or bilateral lateral rectus recessions are performed depending on the degree of the deviation.

Up/downshoots and globe retraction

In the Faden procedure, prevent globe slippage by adding a fixation suture to medial rectus and lateral rectus. This prevents the globe from slipping as it is tethered to the horizontal muscles.

Globe retraction and up- or downshoots are dealt with effectively with ipsilateral medial and lateral recti recessions (von Noorden 1992).

Up- and downshoots may also be innervational in origin and may be reduced with superior and inferior rectus recessions (Mohan & Saroha 2002).

Vertical retraction syndrome (Malbran 1963)

This is a rare syndrome where there is absence or impairment of elevation with lid retraction. To a lesser degree there may be limitation of depression with narrowing of the palpebral fissure.

STRABISMUS FIXUS SYNDROME

This is a rare condition, usually congenital, where one or both eyes are anchored in a position of extreme adduction or abduction (the former is more commonly found) (Villaseca 1959).

Aetiology

Extraocular muscle fibrosis occurs where normal elastic muscle fibres are replaced by fibrous tissue.

Investigation

Visual acuity   Amblyopia will be present where there is unilateral strabismus.

Cover test   A marked unilateral or bilateral esotropia is commonly noted. The deviation may, however, be exotropic or a vertical angle. There is no movement on testing to fix with the affected eye.

Abnormal head posture   With bilateral deviations, there is a marked head posture which is often a face turn to fix with one eye.

Ocular motility   Marked limitations of lateral gaze are demonstrated.

Forced duction test   Positive.

Management

Correct the refractive error if present and treat amblyopia. Surgery is required for a cosmetic result for the existing esotropia. Surgery may involve liberal medial rectus recessions, medial rectus tonotomy, medial rectus recession on loops or use of stay sutures to anchor the eye in abduction post-operatively.

MOEBIUS' SYNDROME

Aetiology

This congenital condition may be due to a primary developmental defect of the central nervous system with aphasia of the motor nuclei of the VI and VII nerves and denervation atrophy of facial and extraocular muscles. This is often associated with infranuclear defects (Lengyel *et al.* 2000; Cronemberger *et al.* 2001). There may be a primary mesodermal defect causing abnormal musculature with a secondary supranuclear brainstem disorder.

Investigation

Visual acuity   There are often defects in vision in one or both eyes.

Cover test   Strabismus is present in most cases and is usually esotropic. Where there is an associated III nerve palsy, the deviation may be exotropic.

Ocular motility   There is an absence of abduction of either eye. An occasional weakness of adduction is sometimes noted and may resemble that in internuclear ophthalmoplegia. It is postulated that this is due to an interruption of pathways in the medial longitudinal fasciculus. A disturbance of vestibular nystagmus may be demonstrated and ptosis may be noted where there is an associated III nerve palsy. Bilateral facial weakness is present with defective lid closure and a reduction of corneal sensitivity. Bell's phenomenon is retained.

Associated clinical signs   The associated signs may include tongue deformities, facial diplegia, deafness, dental defects, hand deformities (webbed fingers, asymmetrical fingers), feet deformities (webbed toes, clubbed feet), intellectual difficulties (variable), hypotonia and pectoral muscle hypoplasia.

Management

Correct the refractive error if present and treat amblyopia. Surgery may be required for strabismus and lateral tarsorrhaphy may be indicated for cosmesis and protection of an exposed cornea. Results of strabismus surgery are disappointing.

Where there is a negative forced duction test bilateral transpositions to the lateral rectus may be considered (Molarte & Rosenbaum 1990). This may be followed by graded medial rectus recessions or botulinum toxin for residual esotropia. Botulinum toxin is useful in young children before development of medial rectus contracture.

Where there is a positive forced duction test transposition surgery and medial recti recessions are required. Maximum medial recti recessions are undertaken and stay sutures may be employed to improve alignment.

GENERAL FIBROSIS SYNDROME

This is a hereditary form of musculofascial anomaly, involving most or all of the extraocular muscles. It is present from birth and is non-progressive (Sugawara *et al.* 1982).

Aetiology

The condition is due to fibrotic or degenerative changes in the extra-ocular muscles. There is autosomal dominant inheritance.

Investigation

Case history   There is a positive family history. Signs are present from birth and are almost always bilateral.

Cover test   The eyes are fixed in a depressed position with no elevation beyond the midline.

Abnormal head posture   Chin elevation is adopted.

Ocular motility   Severely limited movements are demonstrated, particularly on upgaze as the inferior muscles are affected first. There is often a spasm of convergence on elevation, producing a shallow A pattern. The condition may be unilateral but is more commonly bilateral. Bilateral ptosis is symmetrical or asymmetrical and Bell's phenomenon is absent.

The patient may have some nystagmus on attempted elevation.

Management

Treat amblyopia where indicated. Surgery may be required for strabismus or ptosis. The aim is to remove obstacles to the visual axes in primary gaze, alleviate abnormal head posture and align the eyes in primary gaze. A forced duction test is required pre-operatively and during surgery.

Strabismic surgery, however, tends to have disappointing results. The procedure usually involves an inferior rectus recession and/or superior rectus resection and the use of stay sutures may be considered. Large recessions and hangback sutures are used as necessary with careful extensive posterior dissection of the rectus muscles from the intermuscular septal attachments. Conjunctival recession may also be undertaken.

Ptosis surgery if undertaken should only partially correct the ptosis as where there is an absent Bell's phenomenon, full correction of the ptosis may result in corneal exposure. A conservative fascia lata frontalis sling procedure is advised.

BROWN'S SYNDROME

The natural history of Brown's syndrome shows there is clear evidence for spontaneous improvement in some cases (Adler 1959; Dyer 1970; Scott & Knapp 1972). The syndrome may be unilateral or bilateral.

Aetiology

Congenital

- Short anterior superior oblique tendon sheath.
- Tight, inelastic superior oblique tendon. Sometimes the musculo-fascial anomaly is posterior to the globe and is not found on surgical exploration.
- A swelling or nodule on the superior oblique tendon will prevent free movement of the muscle through the trochlea. The click syndrome occurs because the nodule is forced through the trochlea. Such a swelling may be found on surgical exploration of the trochlear area (Maggi & Maggi 2002).
- Anomalous innervation to the superior and inferior oblique muscles of the affected eye.

Acquired

- Injury to the trochlea leading to scar tissue formation. This may be from a penetrating injury to the trochlear area or a fracture in this area.
- Rheumatoid conditions which have developed in later life (Killian *et al.* 1977).
- Swelling on tendon.
- Inflammation spreading from ethmoid.

Investigation

Case history   Children present as parents notice abnormal eye movement, head posture and strabismus. Adults present as they appreciate diplopia, pain, discomfort, tugging around the trochlear area, palpable or audible clicks. Associated conditions may include rheumatism or trigger-finger syndrome. There may be a history of inflammatory conditions, trauma or previous surgery (involving a superior oblique tuck procedure) (Roper-Hall & Roper-Hall 1972).

Visual acuity   Amblyopia may be present if manifest strabismus is present.

Abnormal head posture   The patient may have a slight chin elevation, head tilt to the affected side and face turn away from the affected side. The head posture is rarely marked.

Cover test   A small primary position hypodeviation of the affected eye is demonstrated which is commonly latent.

Ocular motility   There is limitation of the affected eye on elevation in adduction and often the eye cannot elevate beyond the midline (Fig. 15.4). There is generally slight limitation on direct elevation. A downshoot of the affected eye occurs on adduction. Muscle sequelae are limited to overaction of the contralateral synergist. A V pattern phenomenon is likely where the eyes diverge on elevation due to the abducting action of the inferior oblique muscle as it attempts to elevate the eye. Sometimes the movement of the affected eye increases on repeated testing and may show improvement of the defective elevation. There may be a click and the eye may remain in an elevated position if the muscle has managed to pass through the trochlea.

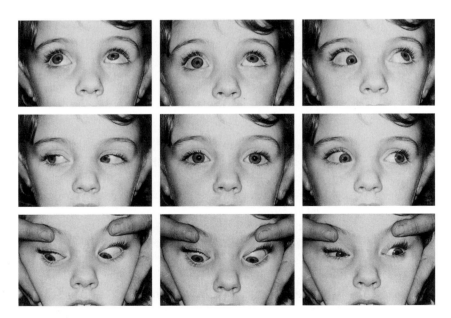

Figure 15.4   Right Brown's syndrome.

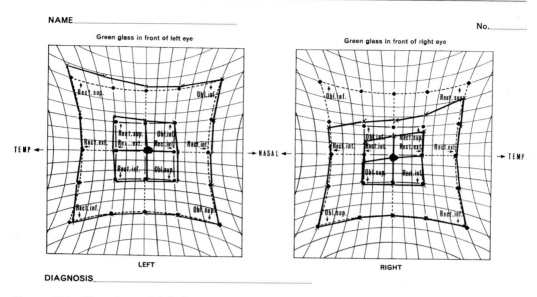

Figure 15.5   Hess chart of right Brown's syndrome.

Binocular function	Binocular single vision is usually present in the primary position and in the lower field.
Hess chart	Retention of incomitance is documented. This shows inferior oblique underaction and overaction of the contralateral superior rectus only (Fig. 15.5).
Field of binocular single vision	Diplopia is limited to elevated positions of gaze (Fig. 15.6).
Forced duction test	Positive.

Differential diagnosis

Investigation	Inferior oblique underaction	Brown's syndrome
Abnormal head posture	Marked head tilt	Slight head posture
Angle in primary position	Moderate	Slight
Muscle sequelae	Develops full sequelae	Limited to overaction of contralateral synergist
A/V pattern	A pattern	V pattern
Forced duction test	Negative	Positive

Management

It is advisable not to intervene with invasive treatment unless there is noticeable chin elevation or vertical squint in primary position. Spontaneous improvement begins around seven years of age and most

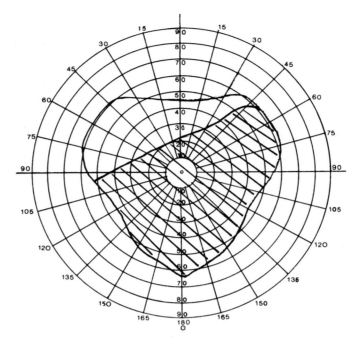

Figure 15.6   Field of binocular single vision of right Brown's syndrome.

cases show virtually full improvement by 12–15 years old. The 'click' syndrome may be a phase in this natural improvement. Correct the refractive error if present and treat amblyopia where indicated.

Local steroids may be useful in acquired cases with inflammation (Saunders *et al.* 1990). These may be oral or injected corticosteroids (Hermann 1978; Beck & Hickling 1980).

Prisms compensate for the deviation in the primary position but may be used with small angle deviations only.

Surgery is rarely indicated and tends to be a last resort (Adler 1959). It rarely improves the ocular rotations significantly (Sprunger *et al.* 1991). The choice of surgery is governed by the result of the forced duction test and the findings at operation which may establish the aetiology.

Indications for surgery

(1)   Diplopia in the primary position.
(2)   Marked abnormal head posture.
(3)   Decompensating deviation.
(4)   Allows development of binocular single vision.

Contraindications

(1) Spontaneous recovery may occur.
(2) Presence of normal comfortable binocularity in the primary position.
(3) Only a slight abnormal head posture present.

Procedures

(1) Division and stripping of the superior oblique tendon sheath. This has been found to be insufficient on its own.
(2) Superior oblique tendon elongation (Stolovitch *et al*. 2002).
(3) Free any adhesions around the trochlear area. This may be combined with a complete superior oblique tenectomy. If a superior oblique paresis occurs, a contralateral inferior rectus recession may be performed as a second procedure.
(4) Contralateral superior rectus recession.

Surgery does not usually produce immediate improvement in motility and can cause additional fibrosis and, as a result, results may be disappointing.

ADHERENCE SYNDROME

This syndrome results from a fusion of the fascial sheaths, giving rise to various adherence syndromes.

Aetiology

Congenital

The syndrome is due to defective cleavage of the mesoderm where extraocular muscles are not differentiated from each other.

Acquired

The condition is due to trauma, inflammation or surgery. Where the cause is iatrogenic, there may be adherence of the muscle belly and globe, the muscle and conjunctiva or sclera and conjunctiva. This results from excessive bleeding, excessive cautery, multiple procedures, excessive tissue reaction, suture reaction, operative or post-operative infection.

Investigation

Ocular motility The type of defective ocular motility depends on the muscles or tendons which have adhered to each other (Johnson 1950).

The lateral rectus and inferior oblique adhering where they cross produce a pseudolateral rectus palsy.

Superior rectus and superior oblique adherence may produce a pseudosuperior rectus palsy.

Superior rectus and superior oblique adhering near the superior oblique insertion produce a pseudosuperior oblique palsy with torsion.

Adherence of superior oblique tendon sheath and superior rectus produces a pseudo Brown's syndrome.

Adherence syndrome of Parks occurs after weakening of the inferior oblique, most frequently after myectomy. In this situation the inferior oblique adheres to Tenon's capsule and produces hypotropia of the involved eye.

Management

Management usually requires surgery where there is division of adhesions while the muscles are temporarily detached from the globe. Use of Supramidextra implants in sleeve or sheet form after division of adhesions may prevent redevelopment of adhesions.

THYROID EYE DISEASE

Thyroid dysfunction is due to disturbance of the immune system. The condition may be termed active, when thyroid stimulating immuno-globulin (TSIgG) activity is most evident, or inactive, which follows active thyroid eye disease and occurs when normal thyropituitary homeostasis has returned. The inflammatory wet phase of the thyroid condition is a myogenic disorder and the following fibrotic dry phase is a mechanical disorder. The active state (congestive, inflammatory signs of eye and orbit, conjunctival injection, chemosis, lid oedema, proptosis) is followed by the fibrotic state (restricted extraocular muscles and infiltration of mucopolysaccharide ground substance through the orbit). Pathologically the extraocular muscle bellies are the primary site of the disease. Inflammation of the muscle stimulates fibroblasts to produce mucopolysaccharides and collagen, resulting in muscle degeneration and fibrosis.

Lymphocytosis and mucopolysaccharide infiltration crowds the orbital spaces, affecting orbital muscle tissue pressure and resilience.

The confined orbit rapidly shows any increase in volume by forward movement of the globe (proptosis).

Investigation

Case history

There is often an insidious onset of diplopia. The condition is a bilateral process but motility can be unilaterally or asymmetrically impaired. Signs include upper lid retraction, lid lag, reduced frequency of blinking, weak convergence, inability to hold fixation on extreme lateral gaze, staring appearance, resistance to retrodisplacement of the eye, oedema and injection of conjunctiva and tremor on gentle lid closure.

General signs include an enlarged thyroid gland, weight loss despite a good appetite, raised body temperature resulting in sweating and heat intolerance, raised blood pressure which may lead to tachycardia, nervous agitation and tremors, irritability and emotional lability (moodiness).

Symptoms include diplopia associated with some degree of external ophthalmoplegia which is often worse in the morning, pain on eye movement due to fibrosed muscles, epiphora, grittiness of eyes and general discomfort, photophobia and visual loss.

Visual acuity Visual loss in extreme cases may be due to an increase in orbital pressure with II nerve compression or corneal exposure from marked proptosis with exposure keratitis.

Abnormal head posture Presence of an abnormal head posture varies in each case. Where there is bilateral limitation of upgaze, there is chin elevation and face turns are adopted with limited lateral gaze.

Cover test The presence of lid retraction should be noted. Central fixation may not be possible with the affected eye if a marked deviation is present. Observe recovery of large vertical heterophorias as this can indicate extended fusional reserves if good recovery exists.

Ocular motility Extraocular muscles are thickened markedly due to cellular infiltration. This interferes with relaxation and contraction and slows movement. Limited movement occurs with restriction in the field of action of the affected muscle due to inadequate muscle contracture and restriction in the field opposite to the affected muscle because of inadequate relaxation (main limitation).

The most commonly affected muscle is the inferior rectus followed by the medial rectus, superior rectus and lateral rectus. Limited elevation is most common (Fig. 15.7) followed by limited abduction, depression

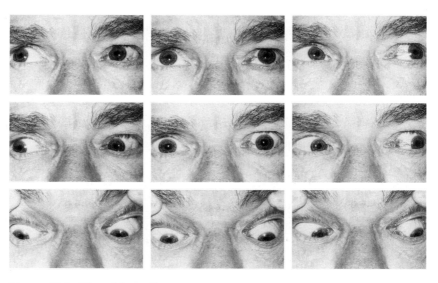

Figure 15.7   Thyroid eye disease.

and adduction. The oblique muscles are also involved but to a much lesser extent. There may be retraction of the globe on downgaze.

Thyroid eye disease may be associated occasionally with myasthenia gravis and a 5% association is cited.

Lid lag (von Graefe's sign) and lid retraction may be observed. Lid lag is noted where the upper lid does not follow the eye fully when changing fixation from up- to downgaze. An area of white sclera will be exposed. Lid retraction is a raised upper lid due to overaction of Muller's muscle.

There may be raised intraocular pressure on attempted elevation (Spierer & Eisenstein 1991).

The degree of ocular involvement can be graded according to the severity of the condition (Werner 1969, 1977).

1   N   No signs or symptoms
2   O   Only symptoms
3   S   Soft tissue involvement
4   P   Proptosis > 21 mm
5   E   Extraocular muscle involvement
6   C   Corneal exposure
7   S   Sight loss due to optic nerve involvement

Convergence   This is reduced (Moebius' sign) where the medial rectus is involved.
Binocular   Normal binocular function is often maintained with an abnormal head
function   posture. Where there is a long-standing vertical deviation, it is not uncommon to have an extended vertical fusion range which can maintain control of large angle vertical deviations.

Hess chart   It is important to plot the outer fields. It is necessary to ensure that the patient maintains foveal fixation of each point without moving the head. This is particularly important in cases of severe limitation of movement when documenting an accurate record of the range of ocular motility (Figs 15.8, 15.9).

Field of   This is frequently much larger than the extent of limitation seen on the
binocular   Hess chart (Fig. 15.10).
single vision

Field of   This is plotted if the limitation is too severe for a Hess chart to be
uniocular   completed.
fixation

Ophthalmic   ● Measure intraocular pressure
tests   ● Exophthalmometry
    ● Fundus and media
    ● Note any corneal exposure
    ● Forced duction test to prove tethering
    ● Visual fields may be reduced if signs of optic nerve compression present

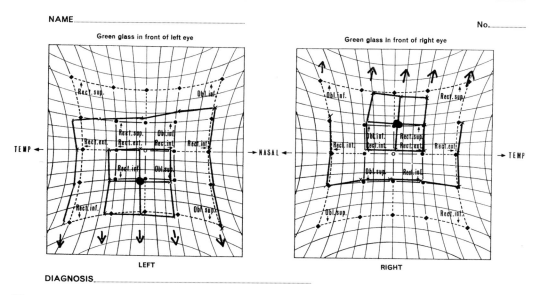

Figure 15.8 Hess chart of thyroid eye disease.

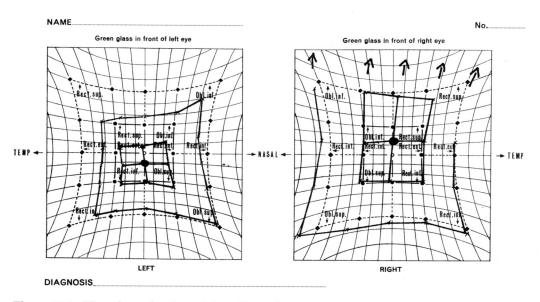

Figure 15.9 Hess chart of unilateral thyroid eye disease.

- Refraction – high intraocular pressure can cause secondary hypermetropia
- CT/MRI scan confirms thyroid eye disease by showing up thickened extrinsic muscles. A STIR sequence highlights current activity within the extraocular muscles.

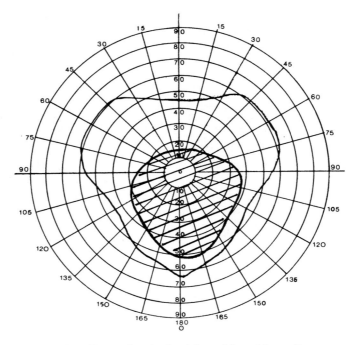

Figure 15.10 Field of binocular single vision of thyroid eye disease.

Management

Long term observation of the ocular condition is required while the medical condition is treated.

Aims of treatment

- Preserve visual acuity
- Relief of symptoms
- Improve cosmesis

Visual acuity

Where visual acuity is compromised, an orbital decompression is indicated. This may take the form of medical decompression, surgical decompression or radiotherapy. Medical decompression involves the oral or intravenous pulse administration of high dose steroids. Immuno-suppressants such as cyclosporin A and azathioprine are also used. Surgical decompression involves the removal of orbital walls, often the orbital floor and the medial orbital wall. Displacement of inferior and medial recti paths may occur after decompression surgery, resulting in patterns of ocular motility restriction (Abramoff et al. 2002).

Radiotherapy to the orbital apex area reduces inflammation but its effect is not seen until approximately six weeks post radiotherapy and therefore it is not useful where immediate decompression is required.

Prisms

Success with prisms depends on the size of deviation, the amount of incomitance and variability of the deviation and, as such, frequent changes may be necessary.

If a small deviation is present, the whole vertical deviation may need to be corrected to make the patient comfortable with prisms. With a large deviation it may be possible to manage with a considerably lower power prism because of the gradual increase in deviation and the consequent increased vertical fusion range.

Strabismus

When the ocular condition has been stable for at least 12 months and the general condition is euthyroid, **surgery** may be considered to correct the strabismic angle.

The tethered muscles are recessed on adjustable sutures, principally the inferior and medial recti. With bilateral tethered muscles, the more tethered muscle is put on adjustable suture. When recessing the inferior rectus, it is important to ensure that lower lid retraction does not occur (Kushner 1992).

Botulinum toxin A may be of use with recent thyroid cases where there is some cellular infiltration, particularly with the inferior rectus and medial rectus. Early injection may prevent development of fibrotic contracture and as a result may delay tethering.

General symptoms

Lid retraction may be improved by antithyroid drugs (propranolol and guanethidine) or surgery. Henderson's operation (a disinsertion of the smooth muscle component of the levator from the upper border of the tarsal plate) gives a good correction of established lid retraction and never produces an overaction.

Lid swelling is a cosmetic problem. Diuretics can be used and will also reduce epiphora. Small doses of systemic steroids may also be considered.

For grittiness and general discomfort, palliative drops and artificial tears give temporary relief. If there is a conjunctival or corneal infection, antibiotic drops are needed. Tinted glasses are useful if the patient is photophobic.

Lateral tarsorrhaphy may be undertaken in severe cases. This is useful in protecting the lateral conjunctiva from irritation due to dryness caused by chronic exposure associated with proptosis.

ORBITAL INJURIES

Orbital injuries may encompass the following:

- blow-out fracture
- soft tissue injury
- supraorbital fracture
- naso-orbital fracture
- zygoma fracture.

Blow-out fracture

A blow-out fracture occurs when a smooth contoured object of diameter larger than the orbit hits the orbit with sufficient force to force the soft contents backwards without rupturing the globe. The subsequent rise in intraocular pressure fractures one of the orbital walls, most commonly the orbital floor. Fractures are either pure or impure.

(1) **Pure**
   — Trap door
   — Linear
   — Hanging
   — Hinged bone crack
   — Depressed
   — Or a combination of fractures
(2) **Impure**. The orbital rim is also involved.

Mechanism

The limitation of ocular motility results occasionally from direct entrapment and damage to an extraocular muscle (commonly the inferior rectus). However, predominantly the limitation of ocular motility results from entrapment of orbital fascia, the septum, connective tissue and muscle pulleys which subsequently impair extraocular muscle action (Koornneef 1979a,b; Demer *et al.* 1995).

Investigation

Case history   Signs include periorbital ecchymosis, surgical emphysema, enophthalmos, depression of the globe, traumatic mydriasis, subconjunctival haemorrhage, hyphaema and facial asymmetry. Symptoms include diplopia (usually vertical), infraorbital anaesthesia and pain on eye movements.

Visual acuity   Visual acuity is expected to be reduced where hyphaema or perforation of the globe has occurred.

Abnormal head posture   An abnormal head posture is used to maintain binocular single vision and avoid painful areas of ocular movement. There is usually some chin elevation/depression with orbital floor fractures. There may be a face turn with medial wall fractures.

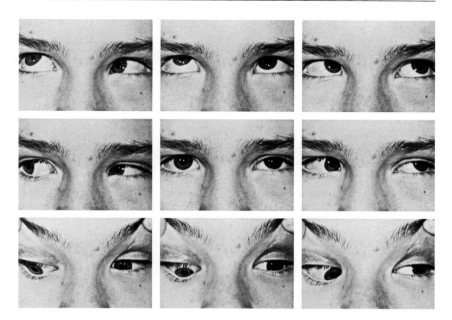

Figure 15.11   Left orbital floor fracture.

Cover test   The cover test should be performed with and without any abnormal head posture and there is often a small deviation in the primary position which is controlled to a latent deviation.

A hypotropia is noted where there is entrapment of tissue anterior to the equator with associated limitation of elevation. Hypertropia is noted with entrapment of tissue posterior to the equator with associated limitation of depression.

Ocular motility   Enophthalmos may be apparent from initial observation. There is limited elevation and depression with orbital floor fractures (Fig. 15.11) and limited abduction and adduction with medial wall fractures. Retraction of the globe may be noted in the position of maximum limitation.

Diplopia may alter depending on position of gaze, due to limitations in elevation and depression. Infraorbital anaesthesia is seen with damage/bruising to the infraorbital nerve, leading to numbing of distribution of this nerve, i.e. cheek, upper lips and side of nose.

Diplopia   This reverses with limitations in opposite positions of gaze.

Binocular function   There is usually a good level of binocular function maintained in the primary position with an abnormal head posture.

Hess chart   This demonstrates limitations in opposite positions of gaze. It is important to plot the outer fields as slight limitations may not be demonstrable on the inner fields alone (Figs 15.12, 15.13).

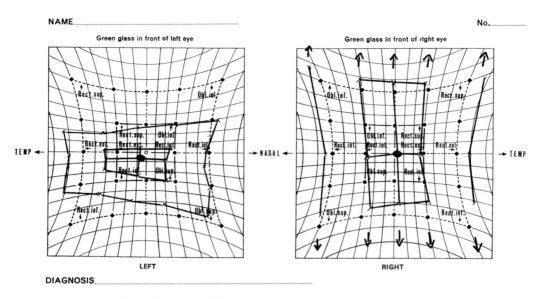

Figure 15.12   Hess chart of left orbital floor fracture.

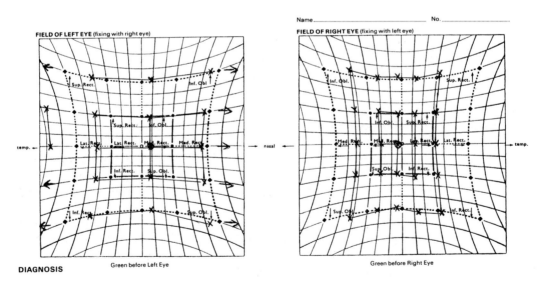

Figure 15.13   Hess chart of right medial wall fracture.

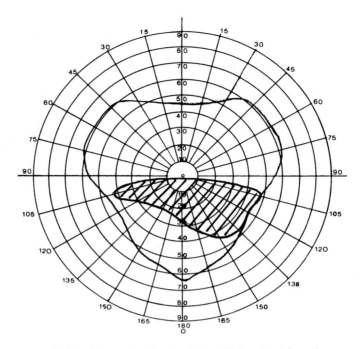

Figure 15.14   Field of binocular single vision of left orbital floor fracture.

Field of binocular single vision Ophthalmic tests

The field is spread out across or along the centre portion (Fig. 15.14).

- Examination of fundus and media to check if the globe has been damaged.
- Radiological examination (X-rays, CT) to pinpoint the location of the fracture.
- Measurement of intraocular pressure particularly if hyphaema is present. Measure in primary position and in position of greatest limitation.
- Forced duction test to assess if limitation is mechanical/neurogenic.
- Measurement of enophthalmos assessed with exophthalmometer.
- Measurement of saccadic velocity.

Management

It is usual to wait for recovery in ocular motility and a wait of approximately 14 days is advisable. It was first suggested by Waddell *et al.* (1982) that patients under the age of 20 years responded less well to treatment than older patients. This was confirmed in a later study

(McCarry *et al.* 1984) where it was suggested that the poorer outcome might be due to the faster formation of fibrous scar tissue in the younger age group. Further conflicting studies of childhood orbital fractures have found poor outcomes in children in contrast to the resolution of symptoms in adults (Cope *et al.* 1999) or little difference in post-operative residual diplopia whether adults or children (Leitch *et al.* 1990).

Many cases resolve symptomatically despite residual limitations of ocular motility. However, patients with fractures involving a significant proportion of the orbital floor should be operated on early as enophthalmos is more common in such patients and its repair is more successful if performed early. Oral antibiotics and prednisolone aid the reduction of infection and inflammation respectively. Treatment options for orbital injuries include observation, conventional treatment (prisms, exercises and occlusion) and surgical intervention.

Early versus later surgical repair of orbital fractures has been debated. Bleeker (1967) reported that early intervention yielded better results whereas old cases were hard to deal with and responded poorly. Putterman *et al.* (1974), however, advocated non-surgical management and suggested a period of 4–6 months' wait after injury before surgery could be undertaken. At that stage conventional extraocular muscle surgery on the unaffected eye was performed to relieve residual diplopia. Dulley & Fells (1974) stated that late orbital repair had a high complication rate of both limited ocular motility and enophthalmos. They examined the optimum time for orbital repair and found it to be within 10–14 days post injury and specified criteria for surgical intervention in this time period (see below). Catone *et al.* (1988) recommended surgical intervention in patients who demonstrate residual diplopia in primary gaze and restricted ocular motility that persists after 10–14 days, the presence of enophthalmos greater than 2 mm and gross disruption of the orbital floor as confirmed by CT or X-ray. Patients with severe limitation of ductions and pain, nausea and vomiting often have direct entrapment of muscle in the fracture site and early surgical repair within one week of injury has been shown to result in a more rapid improvement than surgery performed later (Egbert *et al.* 2000). Urgent surgery has also been advocated for patients with the 'missing muscle syndrome' where there is severe entrapment of the inferior rectus muscle and an absence of the inferior rectus muscle on CT study (Wachler & Holds 1998).

Prisms may be required to join diplopia in the primary position.

Indications for surgery (Dulley & Fells 1974)

(1) Diplopia not resolving
(2) Enophthalmos >3 mm
(3) Large fracture

(4)   Incarceration of tissue with globe retraction

(5)   Intraocular pressure increased on upgaze

Aims of surgery

(1)   Free the trapped tissue and repair the fracture site.

(2)   Correct the strabismus.

Procedures

The fracture site may be approached along the floor of the orbit or inferiorly via the maxilla sinus. Trapped tissue is freed and a Silastic plate placed over the fracture site to prevent further entrapment of tissue in the fracture site.

Where surgery is indicated for strabismus, the overacting muscles of the unaffected eye may be weakened. With limited movements, recessions on adjustable sutures in the affected eye will free movement (inferior rectus if floor fracture). Where there is an associated extraocular muscle palsy, the affected muscle may be resected if a partial palsy or, if complete, weaken the overacting antagonist, consider a Faden suture on the contralateral eye to match the deficit of ocular movement or perform horizontal recti transpositions (Knapp procedure).

Soft tissue injury

This injury is due to trauma to the orbital area not causing a fracture of any bone, but resulting in damage to the orbital area and/or its contents. Orbital injuries include:

- muscle damage
- lacerations
- damage to the nerve supply to the extraocular muscles
- retrobulbar haemorrhage causing limitation of movement and proptosis.

Lid injuries include:

- lid lacerations
- injuries involving the lacrimal canal
- swelling and pseudoptosis
- levator damage with traumatic ptosis.

Ocular signs may include any or a combination of the following:

- subconjunctival haemorrhage
- corneal abrasions/lacerations
- lens dislocation
- damage to iris sphincter with traumatic mydriasis

- hyphaema
- retinal detachment/haemorrhage
- optic nerve damage
- choroidal ruptures.

Differential diagnosis between blow-out fracture and soft tissue injury

	Fracture with tissue entrapment	Fracture without tissue entrapment	Soft tissue injury
X-ray	Fracture	Fracture	No fracture
CT scan	Tissue entrapment	No entrapment	No entrapment
Forced duction test	Positive	Negative	Negative
Intraocular pressure	Increased on gaze opposite to fracture	No increase	No increase
Exophthalmometry	Enophthalmos	No enophthalmos	No enophthalmos
V nerve function	Infraorbital anaesthesia	Infraorbital anaesthesia	No infraorbital anaesthesia
Diplopia	Persistent	Usually resolving	Usually resolving
Ocular motility	Limitation opposite fracture site	Limitation opposite fracture site	Less marked limitation
Globe retraction	Present	Absent	Absent

Supraorbital fracture

This fracture of the orbit is caused by sharp objects going through the orbital roof.

Characteristics

(1) Superior periorbital swelling and haemorrhage
(2) Lid oedema
(3) Supraorbital anaesthesia
(4) Damage to the levator muscle and/or its nerve supply
(5) Diplopia due to muscle or nerve damage or damage to the trochlea
(6) Retrobulbar haemorrhage
(7) Depression of the supraorbital rim causing globe retraction
(8) Cerebrospinal fluid discharge if severe

Naso-orbital fracture

This fracture is produced by direct trauma to the naso-orbital region. It usually results from road traffic accidents.

Characteristics

(1)   Dish-face appearance
(2)   Traumatic telecanthus
(3)   Oedema and bruising
(4)   Epistaxis
(5)   Nasal obstruction
(6)   Surgical emphysema
(7)   Damage to the tear duct and lacrimal sac

Zygoma fracture

Direct trauma to the zygoma may cause fracture and displacement of the zygoma. The bone may be displaced outwards, resulting in traumatic enophthalmos, which is most noticeable after the swelling has subsided. The bone may be displaced inwards, resulting in traumatic proptosis which is most noticeable initially.

Characteristics

(1)   Muscle or nerve damage
(2)   Oedema which may impair ocular movement
(3)   Infraorbital anaesthesia
(4)   There is a tendency to recover fairly quickly
(5)   Any severe head trauma could cause extraocular muscle palsies

CONJUNCTIVAL SHORTENING SYNDROME

There is limited ocular movement caused by contracture of the conjunctiva.

Aetiology

A long-standing deviation with contracture of the conjunctiva in marked deviations may produce this syndrome. The condition may also occur post-operatively where limitations are due to the conjunctiva not being recessed at the same time as the muscle surgery.

Investigation

Case history   This syndrome is associated with long-standing conditions such as thyroid eye disease, III and VI nerve palsy and long-standing concomitant deviations.

Cover test   A marked deviation is noted.

Ocular motility   Limited movement is demonstrable.

Forced duction test   Positive.

Management

Surgery is usually required in the form of conjunctival recession performed at the same time as muscle surgery. The conjunctiva may be recessed and left to reattach. Alternatively, the conjunctiva may be resutured to the sclera in a new recessed position.

It is also possible to take a flap of conjunctiva from the fornix and graft it to the recessed conjunctiva.

RETINAL DETACHMENT

Retinal detachment is a separation of the main neuroretina from the pigment epithelium. The incidence of muscle restrictions, regardless of diplopia, can be high. This increases with the complexity and number of procedures (Portnoy et al. 1972; Sewell et al. 1974; Munoz & Rosenbaum 1987). In most cases, the muscle restriction is slight and often resolves with time (Kanski et al. 1973; Price & Pederzolli 1982; Waddell 1983; Peduzzi et al. 1984).

Causes of restrictions include:

- excessive or prolonged traction on a muscle(s) to position the eye for surgery
- the mechanical bulk of a plomb, bend or tyre under a muscle, which will limit its movement
- formation of scar tissue around a muscle(s)
- disinsertion of a muscle to gain access to a certain area and then reinsertion.

Investigation

Case history   Symptoms are caused by post-operative oedema, reduced vision, extraocular muscle swelling and haemorrhage.

Cover test   Patients may have had a pre-existing strabismus. Decompensation may be due to occlusion following surgery or reduced vision.

Ocular motility   Following disinsertion of a muscle, it may not be reattached correctly (Kanski et al. 1973; Metz 1983; Waddell 1983; Wolff 1983).

Encircling bands are associated with motility disturbances (Mets et al. 1985). Problems increase with posterior or obliquely placed buckles. Radial buckles predispose to problems (Wolff 1983; Fison & Chigwell 1987).

There may be development of adhesions and mass effect, direct muscle trauma, muscle ischaemia, muscle slippage, disinsertion, neural factors, oblique muscle inclusion or rotation, macular ectopia or gliosis.

Binocular function   Most patients adapt and use fusional vergences (Mets et al. 1985). There may be fusion breakdown and sensory deprivation, aniseikonia and anisometropia, and image distortion.

Management

Recovery is usually rapid but may take 3–6 months in some cases.

Patients may adopt an abnormal head posture. Prisms, filters and frosted lenses may alleviate diplopia in both the short and long term.

Surgery may be required in the long term. The forced duction test should be used pre-operatively and during surgery. It may be necessary to remove the buckle, dissect adhesions and undertake a conjunctival recession. Adjustable sutures are recommended. Consider recessing overacting muscles or using a Faden suture to match the limitation of ocular movement.

REFERENCES

Abramoff MD, Kalmann R, de Graaf MEL, Stilma JS & Mourits MP. (2002) Rectus extraocular muscle paths and decompression surgery for Grave's orbitopathy: mechanism of motility disturbances. *Investigative Ophthalmology and Visual Science*, 43: 300

Adler FH. (1959) Spontaneous recovery in a case of superior oblique tendon sheath syndrome of Brown. *Archives of Ophthalmology*, 61: 1006

Beck M & Hickling P. (1980) Treatment of bilateral superior oblique tendon sheath syndrome complicating rheumatoid arthritis. *British Journal of Ophthalmology*, 64: 358

Bleeker GM. (1967) *Blow Out Fractures of the Orbit. Transactions of the First International Orthoptic Congress*, Kimpton, London, p. 207

Catone GA, Morrissette MP & Carlson ER. (1988) A retrospective study of untreated orbital blow-out fractures. *Journal of Oral and Maxillofacial Surgery*, 46: 1033

Cope MR, Moos KF & Speculand B. (1999) Does diplopia persist after blow-out fractures of the orbital floor in children? *British Journal of Oral and Maxillofacial Surgery*, 37: 46

Cronemberger MF, Belmiro de Castro Moreira JB, Brunoni D, Mendonca TS, Alvarenga EH, Rizzo AM & Diogo SM. (2001) Ocular and clinical manifestations of Mobius syndrome. *Journal of Pediatric Ophthalmology and Strabismus*, 38: 156

Demer JL, Miller JM, Poukens V, Vinters HV & Glasgow BJ. (1995) Evidence for fibromuscular pulleys of the recti extraocular muscles. *Investigative Ophthalmology and Visual Science*, 36: 1125

Dulley B & Fells P. (1974) Orbital blow-out fractures. To operate or not to operate, that is the question. *British Orthoptic Journal*, 31: 47

Dyer JA. (1970) Superior oblique tendon sheath syndrome. *Annals of Ophthalmology*, 2: 790

Egbert JE, May K, Kersten RC & Kulwin DR. (2000) Pediatric orbital floor fracture: direct extraocular muscle involvement. *Ophthalmology*, 107: 1875

Fison PN & Chigwell AH. (1987) Diplopia after retinal detachment surgery. *British Journal of Ophthalmology*, 71: 521

Hermann JS. (1978) Acquired Brown's syndrome of inflammatory origin: response to locally injected steroids. *Archives of Ophthalmology*, 96: 1228

Hotchkiss MG, Miller NR, Clark AW & Green WM. (1980) Bilateral Duane's retraction syndrome. A clinical-pathologic case report. *Archives of Ophthalmology*, 98: 870

Huber A. (1974) Electrophysiology of the retraction syndrome. *British Journal of Ophthalmology*, 58: 293

Johnson LV. (1950) Adherence syndrome: pseudoparalysis of the lateral or superior rectus muscle. *Archives of Ophthalmology*, 44: 870

Kanski JJ, Elkington AR & Davies MS. (1973) Diplopia after retinal detachment surgery. *American Journal of Ophthalmology*, 76: 38

Killian PJ, McClain B & Lawless OJ. (1977) Brown's syndrome. An unusual manifestation of rheumatoid arthritis. *Arthritis and Rheumatism*, 20: 1080

Kirkham TH. (1969) Duane's syndrome and familial perceptive deafness. *British Journal of Ophthalmology*, 53: 335

Koornneef L. (1979a) *Sectional Anatomy of the Orbit*. Esculapius, Birmingham

Koornneef L. (1979b) Orbital septa; anatomy and function. *Ophthalmology*, 86: 876

Kushner BJ. (1992) A surgical procedure to minimize lower eyelid retraction with inferior rectus recession. *Archives of Ophthalmology*, 110: 1011

Leitch RJ, Burde JP & Strachan IM. (1990) Orbital blow-out fractures – the influence of age on surgical outcome. *Acta Ophthalmologica*, 68: 118

Lengyel D, Zaunbauer W, Keller E & Gottlob I. (2000) Mobius syndrome: MRI findings in three cases. *Journal of Pediatric Ophthalmology and Strabismus*, 37: 305

Malbran J. (1963) *Strabismes et Paralysies*. Heraly, Charleroi

McCarry B, Fells P & Waddell E. (1984) Difficulties in the management of orbital blow-out fractures in patients under 20 years old. In: Ravault AP & Lenk M (eds) *Transactions of the Fifth International Orthoptic Congress*. LIPS, Lyon, p. 283

Maggi R & Maggi C. (2002) Tendon surgery in Brown's syndrome. *Journal of Pediatric Ophthalmology and Strabismus*, 39: 33

Mets MB, Wendell ME & Gieser RG. (1985) Ocular deviation after retinal detachment surgery. *American Journal of Ophthalmology*, 99: 667

Metz HS. (1983) Restrictive factors in strabismus. *Survey of Ophthalmology*, 28: 71

Mohan K & Saroha V. (2002) Vertical rectus recession for the innervational upshoot and downshoot in Duane's retraction syndrome. *Journal of Pediatric Ophthalmology* and *Strabismus*, 39: 94

Molarte AB & Rosenbaum AL. (1990) Vertical rectus muscle transposition surgery for Duane's syndrome. *Journal of Pediatric Ophthalmology and Strabismus*, 27: 171

Munoz M & Rosenbaum AL. (1987) Long-term strabismus complications following retinal detachment surgery. *Journal of Pediatric Ophthalmology and Strabismus*, 24: 309

Parsa CF, Grant E, Dillon WP Jr, du Lac S & Hoyt WF. (1998) Absence of the abducens nerve in Duane syndrome verified by magnetic resonance imaging. *American Journal of Ophthalmology*, 125: 399

Peduzzi M, Campos EC & Guerrieri F. (1984) Disturbances of ocular motility after retinal detachment surgery. *Documenta Ophthalmologica*, 58: 115

Pieroni D. (1970) Goldenhar's syndrome associated with bilateral Duane's retraction syndrome. *American Journal of Ophthalmology*, 70: 945

Portnoy GL, Campbell LH & Casebeer JC. (1972) Acquired heterotropia following surgery for retinal detachment. *American Journal of Ophthalmology*, 73: 985

Price RL & Pederzolli A. (1982) Strabismus following retinal detachment surgery. *American Orthoptic Journal*, 32: 9

Putterman AM, Stevens T & Urist MJ. (1974) Nonsurgical management of blow-out fractures in the orbital floor. *American Journal of Ophthalmology*, 77: 232

Ramsey J & Taylor D. (1980) Congenital crocodile tears: a key to the aetiology of Duane's syndrome. *British Journal of Ophthalmology*, 64: 518

Roper-Hall MJ & Roper-Hall G. (1972) The superior oblique 'click' syndrome. In: Mein J, Bierlaagh JJM & Brummelkamp-Dons TEA (eds) *Transactions of the Second International Orthoptic Congress*. Excerpta Medica, Amsterdam, p. 360

Rowe FJ, Wong ML & MacEwen CJ. (1991) Duane's retraction syndrome – bilateral until proven otherwise. *British Orthoptic Journal*, 48: 36

Saunders RA, Stratas BA, Gordon RA & Holgate RC. (1990) Acute-onset Brown's syndrome associated with pansinusitis. *Archives of Ophthalmology*, 108: 58

Scott AB & Knapp P. (1972) Surgical treatment of the superior oblique tendon sheath syndrome. *Archives of Ophthalmology*, 88: 282

Sewell JJ, Knobloch WH & Eifrig DE. (1974) Extraocular muscle imbalance after surgical treatment for retinal detachment. *American Journal of Ophthalmology*, 78: 321

Spierer A & Eisenstein Z. (1991) The role of increased intraocular pressure on upgaze in the assessment of Graves' ophthalmopathy. *Ophthalmology*, 98: 1491

Sprunger DT, von Noorden GK & Helveston EM. (1991) Surgical results in Brown's syndrome. *Journal of Pediatric Ophthalmology and Strabismus*, 28: 164

Stolovitch C, Leibovitch I & Loewenstein A. (2002) Long-term results of superior oblique tendon elongation for Brown's syndrome. *Journal of Pediatric Ophthalmology and Strabismus*, 39: 90

Sugawara M, Awaya A & Majima A. (1982) General fibrosis syndrome. *Acta Societatis Ophthalmologicae Japonicae*, 86: 657

Villaseca A. (1959) Strabismus fixus. *American Journal of Ophthalmology*, 48: 51

von Noorden GK. (1992) Recession of both horizontal recti muscles in Duane's retraction syndrome with elevation and depression of the adducted eye. *American Journal of Ophthalmology*, 114: 311

Wachler BS & Holds JB. (1998) The missing muscle syndrome in blow out fractures – an indication for urgent surgery. *Ophthalmic Plastics Reconstruction Surgery*, 14: 17

Waddell E. (1983) Retinal detachment and orthoptics. *British Orthoptic Journal*, 40: 5

Waddell E, Fells P & Kornneef L. (1982) The natural and unnatural history of a blow-out fracture. *British Orthoptic Journal*, 39: 29

Werner SC. (1969) Classification of the eye changes in Graves' disease. *American Journal of Ophthalmology*, 68: 646

Werner SC. (1977) Modification of the classification of the eye changes in Graves' disease. *American Journal of Ophthalmology*, 83: 725

Wolff SM. (1983) Strabismus after retinal detachment surgery. *Transactions of the American Ophthalmic Society*, 81: 182

FURTHER READING

Apt L & Axelrod RN. (1978) Generalised fibrosis of the extraocular muscle. *American Journal of Ophthalmology*, 85: 822

Bagolini B, Tamburrelli C, Dickmann A & Colosimo C. (1990) Convergent strabismus fixus in high myopic patients. *Documenta Ophthalmologica*, 74: 309

Bahn RS & Heufelder AE. (1993) Pathogenesis of Grave's ophthalmopathy. *New England Journal of Medicine*, 329: 1468

Beck SR, Freitag SL & Singer N. (1996) Ocular injuries in battered women. *Ophthalmology*, 103: 997

Blodi FC, van Allen MW & Yarbrough JC. (1964) Duane's syndrome: a brain stem lesion. *Archives of Ophthalmology*. 72: 171

Bloom JN, Graviss ER & Mardelli PG. (1991) A magnetic resonance imaging study of the upshoot–downshoot phenomenon of Duane's retraction syndrome. *American Journal of Ophthalmology*, 111: 548

Brown HW. (1950) Congenital structural muscle anomalies. In: Allen JH (ed) *Strabismus Ophthalmic Symposium*. Mosby, St Louis, p. 205

Crawford JS. (1976) Surgical treatment of true Brown's syndrome. *American Journal of Ophthalmology*, 81: 289

Cross HE & Pfaffenbach DD. (1972) Duane's retraction syndrome and associated congenital malformations. *American Journal of Ophthalmology*, 73: 442

Demer JL & von Noorden GK. (1989) High myopia as an unusual cause of restrictive motility disturbance. *Survey of Ophthalmology*, 33: 281

Dodick JM, Galin MA & Kwitko M. (1969) Medial wall fracture of the orbit. *Canadian Journal of Ophthalmology*, 4: 377

Duane A. (1905) Congenital deficiency of abduction associated with impairment of adduction, retraction movements, contraction of the palpebral fissure and oblique movements of the eye. *Archives of Ophthalmology*, 34: 133

Dunlap EA. (1967) Plastic implants in muscle surgery: a study of the possible use of plastic material in the management of extraocular motility restrictions. *Transactions of the American Ophthalmological Society*, 65: 393

Emery JM, von Noorden GK & Schlernitzauer DA. (1972) Management of orbital floor fractures. *American Journal of Ophthalmology*, 74: 299

Eustis HS, O'Reilly C & Crawford JS. (1987) Management of superior oblique palsy after surgery for true Brown's syndrome. *Journal of Pediatric Ophthalmology and Strabismus*, 24: 10

Fells P & McCarry B. (1986) Diplopia in dysthyroid eye disease. *Transactions of the Ophthalmological Society of the United Kingdom*, 105: 413

Fells P, Rosen P, Pickard B & Plowman N. (1989) Radiotherapy or surgery for orbital decompression in dysthyroid eye disease? In: Kauffman H (ed) *Transactions of the Eighteenth European Strabismological Association*. Krakow, p. 239

Feric-Seiwerth F & Celic M. (1972) Contribution to the knowledge of the superior oblique tendon sheath syndrome (Brown's syndrome). In: Mein J, Bierlaagh JJM & Brummelkamp-Dons TEA (eds) *Orthoptics*. Excerpta Medica, Amsterdam, p. 354

Gregerson E & Rindziunski E. (1993) Brown's syndrome – a longitudinal long-term study of spontaneous course. *Acta Ophthalmologica*, 71: 371

Grootendorst RJ, Verhoeff K, Wijngaarde R & de Man K. (1995) Surgical repair of orbital fracture: at what time? *Transactions of the 22nd European Strabismological Association*. Cambridge, UK, p. 255

Hamed LM, Helveston EM & Ellis FD. (1987) Persistent binocular diplopia after cataract surgery. *American Journal of Ophthalmology*, 103: 741

Hansen E. (1968) Congenital general fibrosis of the extraocular muscles. *Acta Ophthalmologica*, 46: 469

Helveston EM. (1971) Muscle transposition procedures. *Survey of Ophthalmology*, 16: 92

Helveston EM. (1993) Brown's syndrome: anatomic considerations and pathophysiology. *American Orthoptic Journal*, 43: 31

Huber A. (1984) Duane's retraction syndrome. Considerations on pathophysiology and aetiology. In: Ravault AP & Lenk M (eds) *Transactions of the Fifth International Orthoptic Congress*. LIPS, Lyon, p. 119

Isenberg S & Urist MJ. (1977) Clinical observations in 101 consecutive patients with Duane's retraction syndrome. *American Journal of Ophthalmology*, 84: 419

Kendall-Taylor P, Atkinson S & Holcombe M. (1984) A specific IgG in Graves ophthalmopathy and its relation to retro-orbital and thyroid autoimmunity. *British Medical Journal (Clinical Research)*, 288: 1183

Khodadoust AA & von Noorden GK. (1967) Bilateral vertical retraction syndrome. *Archives of Ophthalmology*, 78: 606

Kushner BJ. (1995) Fixation switch diplopia. *Archives of Ophthalmology*, 113: 896

Lawton N, Ekins RP & Nabarro JD. (1971) Failure of pituitary response to TRH in euthyroid Grave's disease. *Lancet*, 2: 14

Leone CR & Leone RT. (1986) Spontaneous cure of congenital Brown's syndrome. *American Journal of Ophthalmology*, 102: 542

Lyons CJ, Vicker SF & Lee JP. (1990) Botulinum toxin therapy in dysthyroid strabismus. *Eye*, 4: 538

Mein J. (1971) Superior oblique sheath syndrome. *British Orthoptic Journal*, 28: 70

Mourits RW, Prummel MF, Wiersinga WM & Koornneef L. (1994) Measuring eye movements in Graves ophthalmopathy. *Ophthalmology*, 101: 1341

Munoz M & Parrish R. (1992) Hypertropia after implantation of a Molteno drainage device (letter). *American Journal of Ophthalmology*, 113: 98

Munoz M & Parish RK. (1993) Strabismus following implantation of Baerveldt drainage devices. *Archives of Ophthalmology*, 111: 1096

Nutt AB. (1955) Observations on the aetiology and treatment of the vertical congenital ocular palsies. *British Orthoptic Journal*, 12: 4

Pacheco EM, Guyton DL & Repka MX. (1992) Changes in eyelid position accompanying vertical rectus muscle surgery and prevention of lower lid retraction with adjustable surgery. *Journal of Pediatric Ophthalmology and Strabismus*, 29: 265

Parks MM & Eustis HS. (1987) Simultaneous superior oblique tenectomy and inferior oblique recession in Brown's syndrome. *Ophthalmology*, 94: 1043

Pfaffenbach DD, Cross HE & Kearns TP. (1972) Congenital anomalies in Duane's retraction syndrome. *Archives of Ophthalmology*, 88: 635

Pratt-Johnson JA & Tillson G. (1989) Intractable diplopia after vision restoration in unilateral cataract. *American Journal of Ophthalmology*, 107: 23

Pressman SH & Scott W. (1986) Surgical treatment of Duane's syndrome. *Ophthalmology*, 93: 29

Rainin EA & Carlson BM. (1985) Postoperative diplopia and ptosis: a clinical hypothesis based on the myotoxicity of local anaesthetics. *Archives of Ophthalmology*, 103: 1337

Roper-Hall G & Burde RM. (1987) Management of A pattern exotropia as a complication of thyroid ophthalmopathy. In: Lenk-Schafer M, Calcutt C, Doyle M & Moore S (eds) *Transactions of the Sixth International Orthoptic Congress*. British Orthoptic Society, London, p. 361

Saed N, Freeman B & Lee J. (1994) The pathogenesis of Duane's syndrome. *Strabismus*, 2: 137

Sandford-Smith JH. (1969) Intermittent superior oblique tendon sheath syndrome. *British Journal of Ophthalmology*, 53: 412

Sandford-Smith JH. (1975) Superior oblique tendon sheath syndrome and its relationship to stenosing tenosynovitis. *British Journal of Ophthalmology*, 59: 385

Scott AB. (1977) The faden operation: mechanical effects. *American Orthoptic Journal*, 27: 44

Sharkey JA & Sellar PW. (1994) Acquired central fusion disruption following cataract extraction. *Journal of Pediatric Ophthalmology and Strabismus*, 31: 391

Stager D, Stager DR & Parks MM. (1999) Long term results of silicone expander for moderate and severe Brown's syndrome (Brown's syndrome plus). *Journal of the American Association for Pediatric Ophthalmology and Strabismus*, 3: 328

Stephens KF & Reinecke RD. (1967) Quantitative forced duction. *Transactions of the American Academy of Ophthalmology and Otolaryngology*, 71: 324

Strachan IM & Brown BH. (1972) Electromyography of extraocular muscles in Duane's syndrome. *British Journal of Ophthalmology*, 56: 594

Trimble RB. (1988) An alternative management of Brown's syndrome. In: Murabe J (ed) *Transactions of the Seventeenth European Strabismological Association*. Madrid, p. 181

Trimble RB, Kelly V & Mitchell M. (1984) Acquired Brown's syndrome. In: RavaultAP & Lenk M (eds) *Transactions of the Fifth International Orthoptic Congress*. LIPS, Lyon, p. 267

Verhoeff K, Grootendorst RJ, Wijngaarde R & de Man K. (1998) Surgical repair of orbital fractures: how soon after trauma? *Strabismus*, 6: 77

von Noorden GK & Murray E. (1986) Upshoot and downshoot in Duane's syndrome. *Journal of Pediatric Ophthalmology and Strabismus*, 23: 212

von Noorden GK & Oliver P. (1982) Superior oblique tenectomy in Brown's syndrome. *Ophthalmology*, 89: 303

Waddell E. (1982) Brown's syndrome revisited. *British Orthoptic Journal*, 39: 17

Whyte DK. (1968) Blowout fractures of the orbit. *British Journal of Ophthalmology*, 52: 721

Wilson-Holt N, Franks W, Nourredin B & Hitchings R. (1992) Hypertropia following insertion of inferiorly sited double-path Molteno tubes. *Eye*, 6: 515

Wojno TH. (1987) The incidence of extraocular muscle and cranial nerve palsy in orbital floor blowout fractures. *Ophthalmology*, 94: 682

Wright KW. (1991) Superior oblique silicone expander for Brown's syndrome and superior oblique overaction. *Journal of Pediatric Ophthalmology and Strabismus*, 28: 101

Chapter 16
Myogenic disorders

Myogenic conditions may involve individual extraocular muscles or a combination and are often bilateral.

Classification

- Thyroid eye disease
- Chronic progressive external ophthalmoplegia
- Myasthenia gravis
- Myotonic dystrophy
- Ocular myositis
- Kearns–Sayre ophthalmoplegia

THYROID EYE DISEASE

The wet phase of the thyroid ocular condition is a myogenic disorder which progresses to a mechanical condition. This has been discussed in Chapter 15.

CHRONIC PROGRESSIVE EXTERNAL OPHTHALMOPLEGIA

This is a relatively benign progressive ocular disorder which can occur as an isolated condition or as part of a more widespread clinical picture. There may be long static periods but it often progresses to a complete external ophthalmoplegia with no remissions. It occurs before the age of 30 years and is usually hereditary. In some cases it begins in early childhood when there is a more rapid deterioration which may be complete by the age of five years.

Aetiology

The condition is due to primary myopathy of the extraocular muscles.

Investigation

Case history   This condition is associated with pharyngeal weakness, cerebellar ataxia, deafness, peripheral neuropathy, optic atrophy and dementia. There is often a familial tendency.

The patient is frequently symptom free, probably due to the gradual onset and symmetrical involvement of both eyes.

Cover test   The deviation noted is usually hypotropia and exotropia.

Abnormal head posture	A chin elevation is adopted where there is bilateral ptosis and there is often frontalis muscle overaction. A face turn to aid fixation is adopted if a large deviation is present.
Ocular motility	Limitation of movement is demonstrated, usually the elevators first and horizontally acting muscles last. Convergence is affected last of all. There is no ocular response to caloric or vestibular stimulation.

Ptosis may be unilateral initially, but becomes bilateral and eventually is complete with no levator function. The pupil is unaffected and there is an absent Bell's phenomenon. |
| *Forced duction test* | Positive. |
| *Associated clinical signs* | The condition may also affect facial muscles and muscles of mastication and occasionally the neck and shoulder muscles. |

Management

Ptosis props on spectacles may be useful in cases of complete bilateral ptosis. The poor Bell's phenomenon must be taken into consideration. Anterior levator advancement or brow suspension may be undertaken (Lane & Collins 1987). Ptosis surgery is often unsuccessful and adequate corneal cover must be ensured to prevent exposure keratitis.

Diplopia rarely occurs but prisms or occlusion may be used if indicated. Surgery is usually contraindicated as the condition is progressive and results are often unsuccessful. If considered, the aim is for a cosmetic result and to reduce an abnormal head posture. An attempt is made to move eyes from the depressed position. The procedure may involve an inferior rectus recession and superior rectus resection and use of stay sutures. Large lateral rectus recessions and medial rectus resections may also be considered.

MYASTHENIA GRAVIS

This is a relatively rare disease where the most prominent sign is weakness of single muscles. Myasthenia gravis takes two forms. There may be ocular involvement alone or the condition may be generalised with both ocular and non-ocular features. Certain muscles are affected more frequently and many patients present initially with weakness of the extraocular muscles, either of ptosis or diplopia or both.

Thyroid eye disease and myasthenia gravis are associated in approximately 5% of cases. Myasthenia gravis may occur at any age but is more frequently seen between the ages of 20 and 40 years. It may be neonatal in children born to myasthenic mothers but is of a remitting nature. It may be congenital with autosomal recessive inheritance. It may be juvenile which is similar to adults but affects girls more and there is good prognosis for remission (Davitt *et al.* 2000). It may be of adult onset and either ocular, mild generalised, moderate generalised, acute fulminant or late severe. Characteristically remissions occur which may last for days, weeks or years and different muscles may be affected each time.

Aetiology

This is an autoimmune disease where there is a disorder of neuromuscular transmission due to a reduction of acetylcholine receptor sites at the motor endplate. This reduction occurs as a result of the patient producing antibodies to these receptor sites which in turn prevent acetylcholine from being taken up by the motor endplate. The effectiveness of transmission is reduced and early muscle fatigue occurs as stores of acetylcholine become depleted from continued release.

Investigation

Case history

There is often a history of fatigue involving the limbs or eyes. In particular, there is easy fatigability of legs climbing stairs, arms on combing hair, weakness of jaw, difficulty in swallowing and speech and weakness of muscles of respiration. The patient may appreciate diplopia or be aware of intermittent ptosis.

Ocular motility

Variable eye signs from visit to visit and at the same visit are characteristic of the condition. Variable ptosis may be evident which is unilateral or bilateral. An isolated single muscle paresis is common, classically an inferior rectus paresis. However, there may be multiple extraocular muscle involvement and occasionally it may mimic internuclear ophthalmoplegia. Pupil reactions are normal.

Other characteristics include Cogan's lid twitch and upper lid retraction. Investigation of ocular motility must include assessment of fatigue, saccadic velocity, ptosis and nystagmus.

Simpson test

Any fatigue on sustained lid and eye elevation is observed.

Cogan's lid twitch sign

Excess innervation to the lid occurs on rapid pursuit movement from a depressed position to the primary position. Transient eyelid retraction is seen during the refixation movement (Cogan 1965).

Hess chart

Variable responses, at the same visit or from visit to visit, are typical.

Tensilon test

A test dose of edrophonium is given intravenously followed by a brief interval and then the remainder is given in small increments. A positive response occurs within 10–60 seconds but only lasts a few minutes. A placebo can be given first to check for functional problems. Intravenous atropine should be available for systemic cholinergic effects.

False negatives are common, especially in ocular myasthenia.

Acetylcholine receptor antibody assay

If positive, this is diagnostic but results can also be negative.

Electromyography

Reduced muscle firing.

Imaging

For thymoma or thymic hyperplasia.

Management

Medical: the condition is treated medically with anticholinesterase drugs and corticosteroids, cyclosporin A and azathioprine (immunosuppressants).

Thymectomy is often indicated as there is an autoimmune deficit (Olanow *et al.* 1982).

Prisms or occlusion: where the patient is symptomatic, prisms or occlusion may be used to join or eliminate the diplopia.

Surgery may be considered where there is a residual deviation. The ocular condition must be static and stable for at least 12 months and the general condition stabilised with medical treatment (Acheson *et al.* 1991; Davidson *et al.* 1993).

Ptosis props on glasses, tape, tarsal resection and brow suspension can be used/instigated dependent on the severity of the ptosis (Kapetansky 1972).

MYOTONIC DYSTROPHY

There is a symmetrical external ophthalmoplegia. The myotonic muscles have abnormal membranes and are therefore unable to release their contractions.

Aetiology

Primary myopathy.

Investigation

Visual acuity   Visual acuity may be defective where there is development of cataracts.

Ocular motility   Progressive external ophthalmoplegia with eventual limitation of ocular motility in all directions of gaze is documented. Ptosis may be evident and there are sluggish pupils which dilate poorly with mydriatics.

Associated clinical signs   There may be face, neck and limb myopathy with atrophy and baldness.

Management

Ptosis props on spectacles may be of use where there is bilateral ptosis.

Surgery may be considered for the cosmetic position of eyes and ptosis but is often unsuccessful.

OCULAR MYOSITIS

Extraocular muscle inflammation occurs with resultant impairment of function (Slavin & Glaser 1982).

Investigation

Case history   The patient commonly complains of photophobia.

Visual acuity   There is reduced visual acuity. The chronic form of the condition results in raised intraocular pressure, culminating in optic atrophy.

Ocular motility   Exophthalmos and lid oedema are evident with multiple extraocular muscle paresis.

Management

Steroids are used in the medical management of the inflammation. Surgery may be required for residual restrictive strabismus (Bessant & Lee 1995).

KEARNS–SAYRE OPHTHALMOPLEGIA

Aetiology

There is a mitochondrial abnormality of ocular muscles.

Investigation

Case history   There is a childhood onset but no positive family history.

Visual acuity   Retinal pigment degeneration is responsible for reduced visual acuity.

Ocular motility   Progressive external ophthalmoplegia with eventual limitation of ocular motility in all positions of gaze is demonstrable.

Associated clinical signs   General signs include cardiac defects and an increased cerebrospinal fluid protein detectable on cerebrospinal fluid analysis (Petty *et al.* 1986).

Management

Prisms are of benefit where the patient appreciates diplopia. **Surgery** is indicated for the alignment of the eyes and also for ptosis but there are often unsuccessful results.

REFERENCES

Acheson JF, Elston JS, Lee JP & Fells P. (1991) Extraocular muscle surgery in myasthenia gravis. *British Journal of Ophthalmology*, 75: 232

Bessant DAR & Lee JP. (1995) Management of strabismus due to orbital myositis. *Eye*, 9: 558

Cogan D. (1965) Myasthenia gravis – a review of the disease and a description of lid twitch as characteristic clinical sign. *Archives of Ophthalmology*, 74: 217

Davidson JL, Rosenbaum AL & McCall LC. (1993) Strabismus surgery in patients with myasthenia gravis. *Journal of Pediatric Ophthalmology and Strabismus*, 30: 292

Davitt BV, Fenton GA & Cruz OA. (2000) Childhood myasthenia. *Journal of Pediatric Ophthalmology and Strabismus*, 37: 5

Kapetansky DI. (1972) Surgical correction of blepharoptosis in myasthenia gravis. *American Journal of Ophthalmology*, 74: 818

Lane CM & Collins JR. (1987) Treatment of ptosis in chronic progressive external ophthalmoplegia. *British Journal of Ophthalmology*, 71: 290

Olanow CW, Lane RJM & Roses AD. (1982) Thymectomy in late onset myasthenia gravis. *Archives of Neurology*, 39: 82

Petty RKH, Harding AE & Morgan-Hughes JA. (1986) The clinical features of mitochondrial myopathy. *Brain*, 109: 915

Slavin ML & Glaser JS. (1982) Idiopathic orbital myositis: a report of six cases. *Archives of Ophthalmology*, 100: 1261

FURTHER READING

Dunlap EA. (1967) Plastic implants in muscle surgery: a study of the possible use of plastic material in the management of extraocular motility restrictions. *Transactions of the American Ophthalmological Society*, 65: 393

Ing MR. (1991) Infection following strabismus surgery. *Ophthalmic Surgery*, 22: 41

Morris JE. (1982) Ocular presentation of juvenile myasthenia gravis. *American Orthoptic Journal*, 32: 51

Osserman KE. (1958) *Myasthenia Gravis*. Grune and Stratton, New York

Osserman KE. (1967) Ocular myasthenia gravis. *Investigative Ophthalmology*, 6: 277

Scadding GK & Harvard CWH. (1981) Pathogenesis and treatment of myasthenia gravis. *British Medical Journal*, 283: 1008

Chapter 17
Nystagmus

Nystagmus is a condition in which there are repetitive oscillatory movements of one or both eyes in a horizontal, vertical or rotary direction. It may be present in all positions of gaze or only in one position and is nearly always involuntary.

Nystagmus usually consists of a slow phase abnormality with a fast phase recovery and is due to a disruption of gaze holding mechanisms (vestibular system, neural integrator and pursuit systems).

Vestibular nystagmus shows a linear constant velocity slow phase. There is an imbalance in nerve input with a resultant slow phase to the side of the lesion. An impaired neural integrator can cause gaze evoked nystagmus with a decreasing exponential slow phase. Saccadic movements are generated by the pulse-step mechanism and failure of the step process can result in nystagmus. The step process maintains eye position and a fault in this results in a drift of the eyes (slow phase) back towards the midline. High gain instability of slow eye movement subsystems (pursuit system) may also cause nystagmus, with the nystagmus slow phase having an exponentially increasing slow phase.

Classification

Physiological

(1) Endpoint: this is present on extreme gaze, commonly lateral gaze.
(2) Optokinetic nystagmus: a combination of pursuit and saccadic eye movements to achieve fixation of consecutive target stimulus.
(3) Caloric nystagmus: vestibular response following stimulation or inhibition of one or more of the semicircular canals. Unilateral irrigation produces nystagmus that is horizontal, rotary or oblique, depending on the position of the head. Bilateral irrigation produces vertical nystagmus, e.g. cold: opposite, warm: same (COWS).
(4) Rotational nystagmus: there are fine oscillatory movements which occur during the maintenance of steady fixation.

Pathological early onset

(1) Congenital idiopathic nystagmus develops in early infancy. This is always bilateral, usually horizontal and jerky, with the fast phase to the right on right gaze and to the left on left gaze. There is often a null point between the two positions and vision improves on using the null point and on convergence. An abnormal head posture is

adopted to make use of the null point. The amplitude of nystagmus increases on occlusion. Nystagmus is abolished during sleep. Patients are unaware of oscillopsia.

(2) Latent and manifest latent nystagmus: jerky, horizontal fine nystagmus is seen when the light stimulus to one or other eye is diminished. There is an involuntary rhythmical oscillation of both eyes with the fast phase to the fixing eye. Latent nystagmus applies to patients with binocular single vision and with no nystagmus evident with both eyes open.

Manifest latent nystagmus is the term applied to patients exhibiting nystagmus of this latent type with both eyes open, but only one eye is actively used for vision due to manifest strabismus, amblyopia or ocular pathology. This is common in infantile esotropia. There may be a face turn to the side of the fixing eye.

(3) Acquired secondary to severely defective vision: pendular nystagmus is seen with a jerk element on versions. Monocular visual loss may produce monocular vertical nystagmus known as the Heimann–Bielchowsky phenomenon.

(4) Acquired secondary to central nervous system disease.

(5) Spasmus nutans: there is a combination of nystagmus, involuntary head nodding and abnormal head posture. Intermittent rapid small oscillations are seen with onset at 3–18 months, with resolution at 36 months. This is usually a benign condition (Gottlob *et al.* 1990). The jerky fine nystagmus may be horizontal, vertical, rotary or a combination. The head movements do not compensate for the nystagmus.

(6) Nystagmus block syndrome: the congenital nystagmus of these patients reduces or disappears on induced esotropia while fixing a distant target. During the esotropia the nystagmus may convert to manifest latent nystagmus.

Pathological later onset

(1) Acquired pendular (sinusoidal oscillation) nystagmus. This is commonly the result of cerebellar or brainstem lesions due to vascular or demyelinating disease. The nystagmus may have horizontal and vertical components. A frequency of 2–7 cycles per second is seen.

(2) Acquired jerk (slow and fast phase) nystagmus. This may be horizontal, vertical or rotary and is usually due to a supranuclear defect.

(3) Vestibular nystagmus. With peripheral disease, horizontal, jerky nystagmus is seen often with a rotary element. There may also be a vertical element in central disease. This is due to acquired destruction of the inner ear, vestibular nerves or the cerebellar flocculus and vestibular nuclei.

(4)   Gaze evoked nystagmus. There is an inability to maintain the eyes in a lateral or vertical gaze position. The eyes drift back to the primary position then make a correction saccade to look in the position of defective gaze. It is commonly seen during recovery of a supranuclear gaze palsy, neuromuscular fatigue or muscle weakness.

(5)   Dissociated nystagmus. Oscillatory movements of the eyes are noted which are dissimilar in direction, amplitude and/or speed. This may be seen where there is damage to the medial longitudinal fasciculus as in internuclear ophthalmoplegia.

(6)   See-saw nystagmus. There is alternation of the eyes where one eye elevates and intorts while the other depresses and extorts. The pattern is then repeated in the opposite direction. A frequency of one cycle per second is usual. This is most commonly seen in patients with bitemporal hemianopia due to large pituitary tumours or suprasellar tumours, head trauma or midbrain infarctions.

(7)   Convergence retraction nystagmus. This is classically seen in Parinaud's syndrome. On attempted upgaze, the eyes are seen to converge and retract in nystagmoid type jerk movements.

(8)   Downbeat nystagmus. This is due to central nervous system lesion, often of the posterior fossa and craniocervical junction. Jerky vertical nystagmus is seen with the fast phase beating in a downward direction and with increased amplitude on downgaze. The eyes drift up and beat down again.

(9)   Upbeat nystagmus. This is due to lesions of the anterior vermis of the cerebellum or medulla. Jerky vertical nystagmus is seen with the fast phase beating in an upward direction and with increased amplitude on upgaze. The eyes drift down and beat up again.

(10)   Periodic alternating nystagmus. Jerk nystagmus is seen which alters in direction approximately every two minutes with a period of oscillation of 4–5 minutes (Shallo-Hoffman et al. 1999). Smooth pursuit movements are commonly impaired. This may be due to pathology of the craniocervical junction or cerebellum, drugs or multiple sclerosis.

(11)   Brun's nystagmus. This is due to tumours at the cerebellopontine angle. There is ipsilateral large amplitude low frequency nystagmus and contralateral small amplitude high frequency nystagmus.

(12)   Drug induced nystagmus. This is often in the form of gaze evoked nystagmus, most commonly upbeating jerky vertical nystagmus.

(13)   Alcohol induced nystagmus. This occurs with chronic disease with degenerative brain changes. There is often associated vertigo.

(14)   Voluntary nystagmus. This purposive self-induced nystagmus with intermittent rapid oscillations usually lasts for periods of ten seconds. The lid flutters in association with the eye movement.

Ocular flutter/opsoclonus

This is a series of to and fro saccades. If the movement is horizontal, this is termed ocular flutter. If both horizontal and vertical, it is termed opsoclonus. A brief intermittent binocular oscillation occurs during straight ahead fixation.

Square-wave jerks

Small amplitude saccades of 0.5–5 degrees move the eyes away from fixation and back with a 200 msec intersaccadic interval. These can occur in normal subjects and increase in darkness and with age. They are also common in cerebellar disease, Parkinson's disease and progressive supranuclear palsy.

Bobbing/dipping

There are fast downward jerks of both eyes followed by a slow drift to the midline. The jerks may be disconjugate in the two eyes and often the eyes remain deviated for several seconds before returning to the midline. Usually occurs in comatose patients with extensive destruction of the pons.

Investigation

Case history

The age of onset, family history of nystagmus and associated symptoms should be ascertained. The medical history should be determined in regard to drug therapy, previous head injury and diseases causing central nervous system disorders.

The patient is questioned as to whether the nystagmus is present constantly or intermittently or whether it increases on direction of gaze.

Associated signs/symptoms include oscillopsia, vertigo, gait and loss of acuity.

Visual acuity

Visual acuity may be normal or reduced. Visual acuity may improve with use of a null point on lateral gaze or on convergence. Latent nystagmus will result in reduced monocular acuity but with good binocular visual acuity (Spierer 1991).

Abnormal head posture

Patients often have a face turn to make use of a null point to dampen the amplitude of nystagmus.

Cover test

The pattern of nystagmus is noted. The direction of nystagmus may be horizontal, vertical, rotary or retractory and the amplitude may be gross, coarse or fine. The frequency of nystagmus may be fast or slow and the waveform may be jerky or pendular.

Jerky nystagmus involves oscillatory movements showing a fast phase in one direction and slow phase in the opposite direction. Pendular nystagmus involves oscillatory movements which do not show a slow or fast phase. Velocity is equal in opposing directions.

The presence of a null zone should be ascertained along with the use of an abnormal head posture.

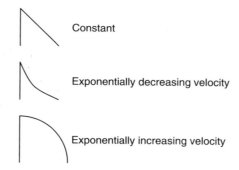

Figure 17.1   Nystagmus velocity.

Velocity	See Fig. 17.1.
Ocular motility	The pattern of nystagmus in each position of gaze is noted, recording the direction, amplitude and waveform. The direction and amplitude of nystagmus are often seen to vary on changing fixation and direction of gaze. Alexander's law states that gaze in the direction of the fast component increases the frequency and amplitude of nystagmus while gaze in the opposite direction has the reverse effect.
Convergence	The amplitude may decrease on convergence and therefore may indicate the use of a null point (Dickinson 1986).
Optokinetic nystagmus	Inversion of the optokinetic nystagmus response is seen with congenital nystagmus.

Management

Acquired cases

Drugs
Baclofen is usually effective in treating acquired periodic alternating nystagmus and acetazolamide is effective in treating some cases of familial ataxia with nystagmus.

Carbamazepine has been successful in cases of superior oblique myokymia.

Prisms
These may be useful in moving eyes away from a position of nystagmus. Base-down prisms are used for upbeat nystagmus on elevation.

Botulinum toxin
Botulinum toxin is useful for non-ambulant patients whereby one eye is stopped from moving by injecting retrobulbar botulinum toxin and the other eye is occluded.

Congenital cases

Aims
- Improve acuity
- Reduce abnormal head posture

Amblyopia
Part time total occlusion is attempted unless there is marked nystagmus. If marked, there may be an indication for use of atropine occlusion and/or penalisation. Use of a high plus lens to fog the vision will allow partial occlusion without increasing the amplitude of nystagmus (Calcutt & Crook 1972).

Non-surgical methods
Where the child sits in the classroom is important. The teacher should allow the child to use their abnormal head posture comfortably. Low vision aids may be beneficial occasionally. Hold print close to make use of a reduced amplitude on convergence.

Strabismus
Surgery should be undertaken as indicated for the strabismus.

Nystagmus
Contact lenses may be used for correction of moderate to high refractive errors to obtain the best possible visual acuity as the lenses will move with the oscillatory eye movements. The contact lenses may also dampen some of the nystagmoid movements.

Biofeedback has been used to treat patients with congenital nystagmus. It may reduce but does not eliminate the oscillation (Stahl *et al.* 2000).

Prisms may be used diagnostically prior to surgery or therapeutically for constant wear to determine the effectiveness of a null point. In cases with a null point on lateral gaze and abnormal head posture, prisms are placed before either eye with the apex towards the null point. In cases with reduction of nystagmus on convergence, prisms are placed before either eye base out to induce convergence. The strength of prism is decided by checking the visual acuity level while increasing the strength of prisms.

Surgery is indicated if there is a marked face turn and demonstrable improvement in visual acuity with the face turn. The principle of surgery is to move the eyes conjugately and symmetrically towards the side of the face turn and away from the null point. When the patient receives the stimulus to place the eyes straight ahead, he is in fact moving into the direction of the null point and, as a result, nystagmus decreases (Lee 1988; Helveston *et al.* 1991).

Commonly the initial improvement is not maintained but reverts to approximately half way. However, patients are symptomatically improved with a broadened null zone.

Surgery is undertaken after the age of five years to allow for consistent abnormal head posture and other measurements.

The Kestenbaum procedure is often the procedure of choice. All four horizontal recti are moved by equal amounts: right lateral rectus resection, right medial rectus recession, left medial rectus resection and left lateral rectus recession. A variation on Kestenbaum's procedure is Parks' procedure (Parks 1973) where the four horizontal recti are moved by differing amounts (13 mm per eye: 5 and 8 mm; 6 and 7 mm). In both procedures the amounts can be altered to include the correction of strabismus. Further variations include Anderson's and Goto procedures in which two muscle are moved by recession and resections respectively, e.g. null zone to the left and abnormal head posture to the right.

- Anderson's: right medial rectus recession and left lateral rectus recession.
- Goto: right lateral rectus resection and left medial rectus resection.

REFERENCES

Calcutt C & Crook W. (1972) The treatment of amblyopia in patients with latent nystagmus. *British Orthoptic Journal*, 29: 70

Dickinson CM. (1986) The elucidation and use of the effect of near fixation in congenital nystagmus. *Ophthalmic and Physiological Optics*, 6: 303

Gottlob I, Zubcov A, Catalano RA, Reinecke RD, Koller HP, Calhoun JM & Manley DR. (1990) Signs distinguishing spasmus nutans (with and without central nervous system lesions) from infantile nystagmus. *Ophthalmology*, 97: 1166

Helveston EM, Ellis FD & Plager DA. (1991) Large recession of the horizontal rectus muscles for treatment of nystagmus. *Ophthalmology*, 98: 1302

Lee JP. (1988) Surgical management of nystagmus. *Eye*, 2: 44

Parks MM. (1973) Congenital nystagmus surgery. *American Orthoptic Journal*, 23: 35

Shallo-Hoffman J, Faldon M & Tusa RJ. (1999) The incidence and waveform characteristics of periodic alternating nystagmus in congenital nystagmus. *Investigative Ophthalmology and Visual Science*, 40: 2546

Spierer A. (1991) Etiology of reduced visual acuity in congenital nystagmus. *Annals of Ophthalmology*, 23: 393

Stahl JS, Lehmkuhle M, Wu K, Burke B, Saghafi D & Pesh-Iman S. (2000) Prospects for treating acquired pendular nystagmus with servo-controlled optics. *Investigative Ophthalmology and Visual Science*, 41: 1084

FURTHER READING

Abadi RV & Pascal E. (1994) Periodic alternating nystagmus in humans with albinism. *Investigative Ophthalmology and Visual Science*, 35: 4080

Abadi RV & Whittle J. (1992) Surgery and compensatory head postures in congenital nystagmus. *Archives of Ophthalmology*, 110: 632

Abel LA. (1984) Square wave oscillations. The relationship of saccadic intrusions and oscillations. *NeuroOphthalmology*, 4: 21

Allen ED & Davies PD. (1983) Role of contact lenses in the management of congenital nystagmus. *British Journal of Ophthalmology*, 67: 834

Antony JH, Ouvrier RA & Wise G. (1980) Spasmus nutans – a mistaken identity. *Archives of Neurology*, 37: 373

Averbuch-Heller L, Zivotofsky AZ, Das VE, DiScenna AO & Leigh RJ. (1995) Investigations of the pathogenesis of acquired pendular nystagmus. *Brain*, 118: 369

Baloh RW, Honrubia V & Konrad HR. (1976) Periodic alternating nystagmus. *Brain*, 99: 11

Baloh RW & Spooner JW. (1981) Downbeat nystagmus; a type of central vestibular nystagmus. *Neurology*, 31: 304

Barton JJS. (1995) Blink and saccade induced see saw nystagmus. *Neurology*, 45: 831

Bellur SN. (1975) Opsoclonus. Its clinical value. *Neurology*, 25: 502

Bleik J & von Noorden GK. (1992) Surgical treatment of compensatory head posture in asymmetrical gaze nystagmus. *Saudi Journal of Ophthalmology*, 6: 15

Calhoun JH & Harley RD. (1973) Surgery for abnormal head position in congenital nystagmus. *Transactions of the American Ophthalmological Society*, 71: 70

Cogan DG. (1967) Congenital nystagmus. *Canadian Journal of Ophthalmology*, 2: 4

Crone RA. (1971) The operative treatment of nystagmus. *Ophthalmologica*, 163: 15

Daroff RB. (1965) See-saw nystagmus. *Neurology*, 15: 874

Dell'Osso LF & Daroff RB. (1975) Congenital nystagmus waveforms and foveation strategy. *Documenta Ophthalmologica*, 39: 155

Dell'Osso LF & Leigh RJ. (1992) Ocular motor stability of foveation periods. *NeuroOphthalmology*, 12: 303

Dell'Osso LF, Schmidt D & Daroff R. (1979) Latent, manifest latent and congenital nystagmus. *Archives of Ophthalmology*, 97: 1877

Gilman N, Baloh RW & Tomiyasu U. (1977) Primary position upbeat nystagmus. *Neurology*, 27: 294

King RA, Nelson LB & Wagner RS. (1986) Spasmus nutans. *Archives of Ophthalmology*, 104: 1501

Pratt-Johnson JA. (1991) Results of surgery to modify the null-zone position in congenital nystagmus. *Canadian Journal of Ophthalmology*, 26: 219

Raab-Sternberg A. (1963) Anderson-Kestenbaum operation for asymmetrical gaze nystagmus. *British Journal of Ophthalmology*, 47: 339

Ruben ST, Lee JP, O'Neill D, Dunlop I & Elston JS. (1994) The use of botulinum toxin for treatment of acquired nystagmus and oscillopsia. *Ophthalmology*, 101: 783

Spielmann A. (1993) Nystagmus and strabismus. *Current Opinions in Ophthalmology*, 4: 25

von Noorden GK & LaRoche R. (1983) Visual acuity and motor characteristics in congenital nystagmus. *American Journal of Ophthalmology*, 95: 748

von Noorden GK, Munoz M & Wong S. (1987) Compensatory mechanisms in congenital nystagmus. *American Journal of Ophthalmology*, 104: 387

von Noorden GK & Sprunger DT. (1991) Large rectus muscle recession for the treatment of congenital nystagmus. *Archives of Ophthalmology*, 109: 221

Yee RD, Wong EK, Baloh RW & Honrubia V. (1976) A study of congenital nystagmus waveforms. *Neurology*, 26: 326

Chapter 18
Internuclear and supranuclear disorders

INTERNUCLEAR DISORDERS

Classification

Internuclear disorders include:

- internuclear ophthalmoplegia
- WEBINO syndrome
- INO of Lutz
- one and a half syndrome
- brainstem syndromes.

Internuclear ophthalmoplegia

Internuclear ophthalmoplegia (INO) occurs when there is a lesion of the medial longitudinal fasciculus between the III and IV nerve nuclei. This causes a disjugate deviation on conjugate gaze to the unaffected side with an ataxic nystagmus of the abducted eye.

Aetiology

- Multiple sclerosis
- Vascular lesions involving the basilar artery or brainstem infarction
- Space occupying lesions of the brainstem and fourth ventricle
- Infection, viral and other forms of encephalitis
- Head trauma

Bilateral INO is most commonly caused by multiple sclerosis. Unilateral INO is most commonly caused by vascular lesions due to the midline separation of the blood supply to the two halves of the brainstem. It is important to note that myasthenia gravis can mimic INO (Glaser 1966).

Investigation

Case history   Symptoms include diplopia and oscillopsia. Signs may include numbness and pins and needles. Previous signs include diplopia, visual loss and retrobulbar neuritis. The patient may have a history of multiple sclerosis or hypertension.

Visual acuity   This may be reduced if there has been a previous episode of retrobulbar neuritis.

Cover test	A divergent deviation is expected which may be manifest at near fixation with crossed diplopia. There may be an associated skew deviation.
Ocular motility	There is a limitation of adduction with abducting jerky nystagmus of the other eye (Zee *et al.* 1987). In bilateral cases, the limitations may or may not be symmetrical. Slight limited adduction may only be apparent on repeated testing of saccades which shows dysmetric undershooting of the adducted eye and overshooting of the abducted eye. Oscillopsia may be noted. Vertical nystagmus is frequently noted in bilateral INO. Vertical vestibular and smooth pursuit eye movements may be impaired in bilateral cases.
Optokinetic nystagmus	With unilateral INO, optokinetic nystagmus is defective when the stripes are rotated to the side of the lesion and normal when rotated in the opposite direction.
Convergence	This may or may not be present, depending on the site of the lesion. Retention of convergence is noted if the lesion is posterior to the III nerve nucleus. Convergence is absent if the lesion is anterior to the III nerve nucleus and therefore interferes with that pathway. Rostral (upper) lesions are more likely to affect descending tracts that initiate convergence or the subnucleus of the medial rectus itself, resulting in absent convergence. Discrete caudal (lower) lesions are more likely to spare the subnucleus of the medial rectus and descending tracts for convergence, resulting in intact convergence.
Asymmetric convergence	The eyes are positioned so that the abducting nystagmus is barely perceptible. The target is brought toward the abducted eye along its visual axis. The position of the eye remains constant whereas there is the stimulation to converge in the affected eye. As the target is brought closer, the amplitude of nystagmus increases.
Stroud prism test	This test is used to induce abducting nystagmus. A base-out prism (10–20 prism dioptres) is placed before the affected eye. This stimulates the eye to adduct, producing abducting nystagmus in the other eye.
Hess chart	Limited adduction will be recorded.

WEBINO syndrome

Wall-eyed bilateral INO syndrome with a marked exotropic manifest deviation.

INO of Lutz

INO with partial III nerve palsy. The medial longitudinal fasciculus is involved in the midbrain and abduction is impaired.

Management

Occlusion may be used to eliminate the symptoms of diplopia and oscillopsia in the eye with the abducting nystagmus.

Prisms are often unsuccessful due to the incomitance of the deviation. The cause is treated where possible.

One and a half syndrome

This syndrome is produced where there is a unilateral pontine lesion which affects both the horizontal gaze centre in the VI nerve nucleus, the paramedian pontine reticular formation and the ipsilateral medial longitudinal fasciculus (Fig. 18.1), causing a combined ipsilateral horizontal gaze palsy and ipsilateral INO.

Aetiology

- Multiple sclerosis
- Basilar artery branch occlusion
- Pontine metastases of malignant tumours
- Brainstem ischaemia/infarction
- Trauma
- Pontine glioma
- Haemorrhage

Investigation

Ocular motility There is limited adduction of either eye with limited abduction to the side of the lesion and abducting nystagmus of the other eye (Fig. 18.1).

Diplopia is often not appreciated on lateral gaze to the side of the lesion due to symmetrical horizontal gaze palsy. Diplopia and oscillopsia are appreciated to the side opposite the lesion due to limited contralateral adduction and ipsilateral abducting nystagmus.

Cover test Exotropia in primary position – the eye opposite the side of the lesion is exotropic.

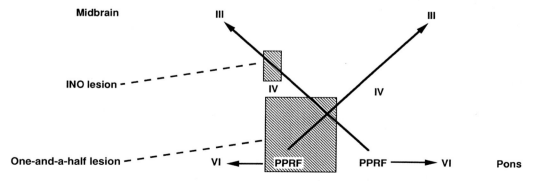

Figure 18.1   Internuclear ophthalmoplegia and one and a half syndrome – site of lesions.

Management

Occlusion may be used to eliminate the symptoms of diplopia and oscillopsia.

Prisms are often unsuccessful due to the incomitance of the deviation. The cause is treated where possible.

Brainstem syndromes

Discrete lesion of paramedian pontine reticular formation

The paramedian pontine reticular formation contains the nucleus pontis centralis caudalis and is responsible for saccadic generation via burst neurons. There is loss of saccadic and quick phase nystagmus to the side of the lesion. Vertical saccades are misdirected obliquely away from the side of lesion.

Nuclear VI nerve

An ipsilateral horizontal gaze palsy occurs as the VI nucleus controls horizontal gaze. This is rare as usually larger lesions occur, affecting medial longitudinal fasciculus and paramedian pontine reticular formation also.

Fascicular VI nerve

This results in ipsilateral abduction paralysis, facial palsy, Horner's syndrome, facial analgesia and peripheral deafness. Commonly this is due to vascular episodes. The following syndromes are caused by damage to this area.

- Millard–Gubler syndrome: this consists of VI nerve palsy, ipsilateral VII nerve palsy and contralateral hemiparesis.
- Raymond's syndrome: this consists of VI nerve palsy and contralateral hemiparesis.
- Foville's syndrome: this consists of horizontal gaze palsy, V, VII and VIII nerve palsies and ipsilateral Horner's syndrome.

Nuclear III nerve

The following subtypes may occur:

- unilateral III with contralateral superior rectus palsy and bilateral ptosis
- bilateral III with spared levator function
- bilateral total III
- bilateral ptosis
- bilateral medial rectus palsy
- isolated medial rectus, inferior oblique and inferior rectus palsy

Commonly due to infarction, demyelination and/or metastatic tumour.

Fascicular III nerve

This syndrome consists of III nerve palsy with contralateral hemiplegia with involvement of corticospinal tracts, contralateral ataxia and intention tremor with involvement of red nucleus. It is due to vascular episodes. The following syndromes are caused by damage to this area.

- Nothnagel's syndrome: there is a lesion in the superior cerebellar peduncle producing an ipsilateral III nerve palsy and cerebellar ataxia.
- Benedikt's syndrome: there is a lesion in the region of the red nucleus resulting in an ipsilateral III nerve palsy and contralateral hemitremor.
- Weber's syndrome: there is a lesion in the area of the cerebral peduncle resulting in ipsilateral III nerve palsy and contralateral hemiparesis.
- Claude's syndrome: this consists of features of Benedikt's and Nothnagel's syndrome.

Nuclear/fascicular IV nerve

This may be due to nuclear aplasia, arteriovenous malformation, demyelination, haemorrhage, ischemia/infarction or trauma.

Differential diagnosis of nuclear and fascicular aetiology is almost impossible. It may be associated with central Horner's syndrome and relative afferent papillary defect.

Medulla lesions

Disease affecting vestibular nuclei and nucleus prepositus hypoglossi results in vertical imbalance such as nystagmus (upbeat, torsional and sometimes horizontal with gaze evoked component), vertigo or skew deviation and impairment of gaze holding for all conjugate eye movements.

It can occur with lateral medullary infarction (Wallenberg syndrome; skew deviation with ipsilateral hypotropia, cyclodeviation (lower eye more excyclo) and ipsilateral head tilt (ocular tilt reaction), ipsilateral facial pain, Horner's syndrome, limb ataxia, dysarthria, dysphagia, contralateral trunk and limb pain).

SUPRANUCLEAR DISORDERS

Classification

Disorders involving supranuclear control pathways include:

- disorders of saccadic movements
- disorders of smooth pursuit movements
- disorders of the vergence system

- gaze palsy
- optokinetic movement disorders
- vestibular movement disorders
- skew deviation.

The lesions causing these disorders are a level higher than the ocular motor nerve nuclei including lesions of the cortical centres, pathways, subcortical centres, midbrain and cerebellum.

Saccadic movement disorders

Such disorders can be produced by lesions anywhere from the frontal lobe to the paramedian pontine reticular formation (Steiner & Melamed 1984; Kernan *et al.* 1993; Shawkat *et al.* 1996).

Disorders of saccades result in abnormalities of initiation, velocity, accuracy and inappropriate saccadic intrusions. Saccadic disorders can be classified according to whether the pulse, step or the pulse-step match is inappropriate. For example, hypometric saccades relate to a deficient pulse-step signal. Where burst neurons activate too much (excessive pulse) with a normal response from inhibitory neurons (normal step), an overshoot of the target results which then requires a drift of the eyes (glissade) back to the target. Dysfunction of specific cell types within the brainstem reticular formation may account for various types of saccadic disorders. Slow saccades may be noted with nerve palsies or drug use. Accuracy disorders may be noted with brainstem or cerebellar disease. Disturbance of saccadic initiation with prolonged latencies and inaccuracy can be seen in degenerative and demyelinating conditions such as Huntington's chorea and multiple sclerosis (Rowe 2003).

Unilateral saccadic deficit

There is loss of voluntary movement to the contralateral side. Binocular single vision is normally maintained in the primary position but diplopia is not commonly appreciated, even looking to the affected side, as the defect is conjugate. Doll's head movement is usually intact. An object may be followed slowly if foveal fixation is maintained into the affected field. Gaze paretic nystagmus may be seen to the affected side (jerky nystagmus with fast phase to the opposite side of the lesion). There may be facial and/or upper limb paralysis on the ipsilateral side. Destructive unilateral lesions result in a unilateral contralateral saccadic deficit which may be due to vascular or space occupying lesions or trauma. Vascular lesions are most common such as an acute cerebrovascular accident.

Bilateral saccadic deficit

There is a complete saccadic palsy with absent horizontal and vertical saccades and no voluntary movement. Bilateral cortical lesions, which may result in a complete saccadic palsy, are often associated with decreased levels of consciousness.

Ocular motor apraxia

This is a congenital condition in which there is an inability to make voluntary horizontal saccades when the head is immobilised. The patient makes use of head thrusts to induce compensatory movements of the vestibular system. Typically the eye lids are closed at the onset of the head movement in order to help break fixation. The head is thrust in the direction of and past the position of the target to be fixated. Due to the vestibulo-ocular reflex, the eyes deviate in the opposite direction. The head is moved until the eyes come in line with the target to be fixated. Once fixation is obtained, the head is moved back to a straight position, making use of the normal smooth pursuit movements to maintain fixation on the target. The thrusts become less apparent with age (Rowe 1995; Harris *et al.* 1996).

The condition may also be acquired, e.g. secondary to inflammation and with extensive bilateral cerebral disease. Balint's syndrome is an acquired condition of saccadic palsy. There may be impaired reading and simultanagnosia which is an inability to perceive more than one object at a time.

Huntington's chorea

This is an autosomal dominant defect with insidious onset, usually from 30 years onwards. Marked loss of saccadic velocity is noted and the patients develop dysarthria and choreic movements (most noticeable in the face and distal extremities). There is progressive mental deterioration in later stages.

Dementia

There is abnormal fixation with saccadic interruptions. Increased latency, hypometria and slowing of saccades are noted. Vertical saccades are affected more than horizontal saccades. There may be abnormalities of smooth pursuits with decreased gain. Saccadic deficits are due to frontal lobe dysfunction but there may also be some parietal lobe involvement. Conditions such as Alzheimer's disease may exhibit the above.

Multiple sclerosis

As a result of demyelination of nerve fibres large saccades may show velocity changes such as increased latency and inaccuracy. Smooth pursuit gain can be decreased. Other ocular motility disorders may be recorded including VI nerve palsy, INO and gaze palsies.

Pseudoabducens palsy

During horizontal saccades, the abducting eye may move more slowly and may reflect an excess of convergence tone. This is an early symptom of posterior commissure lesions such as pineal tumours, hydrocephalus, vascular lesions, metabolic disorders and MS. Reading difficulties are caused by poor tracking and focus.

Smooth pursuit movement disorders

Smooth pursuit disorders are caused by lesions involving the occipitoparietal lobe and pathways to the paramedian pontine reticular formation (Leigh & Tusa 1985; Lekwuwa & Barnes 1996; Morrow & Sharpe 1995). Normal smooth pursuit movements are replaced by series of small saccades termed 'cog wheeling'.

Unilateral smooth pursuit deficit

Unilateral disorders are most often caused by lesions in the posterior cortical hemisphere or in the hemisphere of the cerebellum. Cortical lesions produce loss of smooth pursuit to the ipsilateral side. This is accompanied by Cogan's sign and the patient may also have homonymous contralateral visual field defects. Hemisphere lesions produce ipsilateral smooth pursuit defects without producing the other signs found in cortical disease.

Cogan's sign is a tonic deviation of the eye occurring on forced lid closure and associated with lesions in the cerebral hemispheres.

Bilateral smooth pursuit deficit

Bilateral disorders are produced by diffuse posterior hemispheric, cerebellar or brainstem disease. A true smooth pursuit palsy with an absolute inability to track a moving target, in a patient with normal fixational saccades, is extremely rare.

Vergence movement disorders

Convergence paralysis, divergence paralysis and spasm of the near reflex may result from disorders of the vergence eye movement system. In certain brainstem conditions, such as INO, convergence may be absent due to involvement of the convergence fibres in the pathological lesion.

Convergence paralysis

This has been previously discussed under convergence defects in Chapter 12.

Convergence paralysis may be secondary to various organic processes such as encephalitis, diphtheria, multiple sclerosis and occlusive vascular disease involving the rostral midbrain (Guiloff et al. 1980; Ohtsuka et al. 2002). It may also occur in isolation as a sequela of a flu syndrome. Patients usually present with exotropia and diplopia for near. They will have normal adduction of either eye. The deviation can be said to be concomitant across the field of gaze.

Divergence paralysis

This may be associated with encephalitis, demyelinating disease, neurosyphilis, trauma and space occupying lesions in and around the cerebellum (Chamlin & Davidoff 1951; Krohel *et al.* 1982; Roper-Hall & Burde 1987). The patients appreciate diplopia on distance fixation and there is an esotropia demonstrable on cover test for distance. There is normal abduction of either eye which differentiates the condition from lateral rectus paresis (Cunningham 1972). If there are no other associated neurological factors, it is considered benign and self-limiting.

Divergence insufficiency

There is intermittent or constant esotropia at distance fixation with diplopia. A reduced fusional divergence is noted (Rutkowsky & Burian 1972; Jacobsohn 2000). Prisms are usually beneficial and may be reduced with time. Bilateral lateral rectus resection may be considered in cases where surgery is required (Lyle 1954).

Spasm of near reflex

This involves convergence, accommodation and miosis and may be psychogenic. It is rarely due to organic disease such as trauma, dorsal midbrain syndrome, intoxication and Wernicke's encephalopathy (Dagi *et al.* 1987). This has been previously discussed in Chapter 12.

Gaze palsy

There is an inability to move the eyes either by saccades or smooth pursuit in a given direction. It may be caused by lesions anywhere from the cerebral cortex (where they must be profuse, involving both the frontal and occipitoparietal centres) to the paramedian pontine reticular formation.

Horizontal gaze palsies (involving both saccadic and smooth pursuit movements) result from lesions involving the VI nerve nucleus such as vascular or space occupying pathology or multiple sclerosis (Pierrot-Deseilligny & Goasguen 1984; Bronstein *et al.* 1990). There is often VII nerve involvement because of its close proximity to the VI nerve but it can occur without VII nerve involvement (Miller *et al.* 2002). An isolated lesion of the paramedian pontine reticular formation will not result in a complete horizontal gaze palsy but a horizontal saccadic gaze palsy due to involvement of burst neurons required for saccadic generation.

Isolated horizontal gaze palsy

- **Congenital**. This is a familial congenital paralysis of horizontal gaze. All horizontal conjugate eye movements, optokinetic nystagmus and convergence are affected to a variable extent.
- **Acquired**. Lesions in the VI nerve nucleus produce an ipsilateral gaze paresis. Bilateral lesions are associated with paralysis of all voluntary and reflex horizontal eye movements.

Vertical gaze palsy

Vertical gaze palsies, whether saccadic or smooth pursuit only, or combined (more usual), commonly result from lesions in the brainstem as bilateral input is required to generate vertical gaze. The nuclei responsible for generating vertical gaze movements are connected via the medial longitudinal fasciculus and posterior commissure and vertical gaze palsies result from lesions to the rostral interstitial nucleus of the medial longitudinal fasciculus (riMLF) and rostral midbrain (Bender 1980; Green *et al.* 1993; Lagreze *et al.* 1996). Saccadic innervation from the riMLF is unilateral to depressor extraocular muscles but bilateral to elevator muscles. Therefore a unilateral lesion will result in a downward saccadic palsy.

Downgaze

An isolated paralysis of downgaze has been reported in a number of cases with pretectal disease.

Tonic downward gaze lesion
A chronic downward deviation is seen associated with failure of elevation. This is associated with recent bilateral thalamic infarcts or unrelieved hydrocephalus. If associated with upper lid retraction, this is termed the setting sun sign.

Double depressor palsy
This is extremely rare, usually congenital and sporadic (von Noorden & Hansell 1991). Causes can include inferior rectus palsy, supranuclear or secondary superior rectus contracture. Because bilateral riMLF lesions are less common than unilateral lesions, downgaze disorders are much less common than upgaze disorders.

Depression is limited in both adduction and abduction and hypertropia is seen in the affected eye. There is upper lid retraction with fixation of the unaffected eye. Differential diagnosis includes vertical retraction syndrome, congenital superior rectus fibrosis, congenital inferior rectus absence, III nerve palsy, orbital floor fracture, thyroid eye disease and surgically induced limitation.

Surgical treatment options include superior rectus recession or Knapp's procedure.

Inverse Parinaud's dorsal midbrain syndrome

An extremely rare condition in which there is an upper midbrain lesion affecting fibres mediating downgaze only. This is usually due to a discrete vascular lesion.

Upgaze

Parinaud's syndrome

This is an acquired palsy due to pineal gland tumour, midbrain infarction, congenital aqueductal stenosis, multiple sclerosis, arteriovenous malformation, midbrain haemorrhage, encephalitis, midbrain or third ventricle tumour, herniation of the uncus and lesions due to stereotactic surgery. There is bilateral upgaze paresis and when the patient attempts to look up, both eyes are seen to converge and retract into the orbit (convergence retraction nystagmus). The patient may appreciate diplopia if there is an associated III or IV nerve palsy, or skew deviation. The patient may also appreciate intermittent blurred vision due to papilloedema (Parinaud 1883; Lee *et al.* 1996).

The pupils may be mid dilated with light-near dissociation (pseudo Argyll Robertson pupil) and there may be lid retraction on downgaze (Collier's sign). Midbrain lid retraction is usually bilateral and symmetrical, but is occasionally unilateral. There is no lid lag on downgaze as in thyroid eye disease. With light-near dissociation, there is an absent pupil response to a light stimulus but normal pupil constriction occurs to an accommodative target. (When Collier's sign is associated with hydrocephalus in children, this is termed the setting sun syndrome.)

Double elevator syndrome

This is a rare acquired disorder in which there is an interruption of supranuclear input from the presumed vertical upgaze centre in the pretectum (Jampel & Fells 1968; Lessel 1975). It may be secondary to a vascular lesion. It is usually congenital but may be acquired. There is an acute onset and the patient may appreciate diplopia on upgaze due to limitation of elevation of one eye. Impaired elevation can be caused by inferior rectus restriction (Metz 1979) and supranuclear disorders (Barsoum-Homsy 1983; Thames *et al.* 1984; Ziffer *et al.* 1992).

Elevation is limited in both abduction and adduction. Abnormal head posture is usually that of a chin elevation if binocular function is present. There is usually no head posture if no binocular function. There may or may not be a manifest deviation (hypotropia) in the primary position. Rarely, fixation is with the affected eye, resulting in a large secondary hypertropia. Ptosis is evident and additionally pseudoptosis if hypotropic in the primary position. Bell's phenomenon may be reduced and there may be associated pupil abnormalities including anisocoria, sluggish light reaction and light-near dissociation.

Differential diagnosis is with forced duction test, presence or absence of Bell's phenomenon, saccadic velocity, laboratory tests (e.g. for thyroid eye disease) and neuro-imaging (e.g. for fractures).

Surgical correction is generally recommended only when a vertical deviation is present in the primary position. A Knapp procedure, transposing the horizontal recti to the borders of the superior rectus insertion, is the procedure of choice (Knapp 1969). This procedure corrects up to 20–35 prism dioptres of hypotropia in the primary position but with little improvement in elevation. Where there is less hypotropia there may be benefit from superior rectus resection only. An inferior rectus recession may also be considered (Metz 1981).

Upgaze and downgaze

Progressive supranuclear palsy

This is due to basal ganglia disease. It is a degenerative disease of the central nervous system with onset from 60 years. There is atrophy of the midbrain and dilation of the quadrigeminal cisterns, aqueduct, third and fourth ventricles. Neuronal loss, degeneration and gliosis principally affect the brainstem reticular formation and ocular motor nuclei.

The condition is characterised by defective downgaze initially. Saccades are normally defective first, followed by smooth pursuit movements. The condition deteriorates to complete ophthalmoplegia with absent Bell's phenomenon and eventual convergence. There are usually no ocular symptoms as the limitations of ocular movements are symmetrical. There is difficulty with swallowing and disturbance of posture and tone. The patient demonstrates mental slowing and death occurs within five years (Collins *et al.* 1995).

Parkinson's disease

This is a degenerative disease which is characterised by the triad of tremor, rigidity and akinesia. Early in the course of the disease, conjugate saccades are hypometric. Steady fixation is often disrupted by saccadic intrusions and square-wave jerks. Vertical gaze is decreased. Masked facial appearance, involuntary laughing, drooling and difficulty swallowing indicate the progression of the disease (Repka *et al.* 1996).

Whipple's disease

This is a rare multisystem disorder with resulting weight loss, diarrhoea, arthritis, lymphadenopathy and fever. It causes a defect of ocular motility that mimics progressive supranuclear palsy. Vertical saccades are involved initially, progressing to loss of all eye movements. The characteristic findings include pendular vergence oscillations and concurrent contractions of the masticatory muscles (oculomasticatory myorhythms). Treatment is with antibiotics.

Oculogyric crisis
A tonic vertical or horizontal deviation occurs. This can be overcome with the smooth pursuit vestibular reflex but the eyes then return to the tonically deviated position. It is seen with post-encephalitic parkinsonism and neuroleptic toxicity. There may be obsessional fixation of individual thoughts.

Roth–Bielchowsky phenomenon
Loss of saccadic and pursuit movements occur and this sometimes includes vertical movements. Eventually total paralysis of eye movement develops. The condition is due to disruption of occipital and frontal systems with bilateral hemispherical and brainstem defects involving both the saccadic and smooth pursuit pathways. The vestibular system may remain intact.

Optokinetic movement disorders

Optokinetic nystagmus (OKN) is impaired by any lesion involving the saccadic or smooth pursuit pathways and may also be impaired by any disruption of the neural integrators such as with cerebellar disease.

Vestibular movement disorders

The vestibulo-ocular reflex (VOR) and OKN may be affected by vestibular system lesions. Peripheral vestibular disorders due to imbalance of semicircular canal inputs may cause nystagmus, dynamic imbalance with lower gain for horizontal head rotation, loss of velocity determination with reduced VOR and OKN, and skew deviation. There may be head tilts due to perceived tilts of the environment. Cerebellar lesions may also affect the VOR gain but impair smooth tracking and gaze holding (neural integrator function). Symptoms of vertigo and oscillopsia may be noted. The VOR may be involved in pontine lesions but often remains intact in rostral brainstem lesions as ascending fibres from the cerebellum are below the level of the lesion (Rowe 2003).

Skew deviation

This is an acquired vertical misalignment of the visual axes caused by a disturbance of supranuclear function (Keane 1975; Brandt & Dieterich 1993). Disease of the vestibular organ, its nuclei or nerve can cause a skew deviation, as can cerebellar and brainstem disease.

The deviation is more common in unilateral lesions than bilateral lesions and the eye ipsilateral to the lesion is usually the hypotropic one. A disturbance of tonic vestibulo-ocular co-ordination is considered to be a primary factor in the aetiology of skew deviations. Diplopia is often present but no particular extraocular muscle is involved. The deviation may be constant in all positions of gaze or variable, when the vertical height reverses on laevo- and dextroversion. When incomitant, the deviation can only be differentially diagnosed from a vertical extraocular muscle palsy by the co-existence of signs of central neurological dysfunction.

INVESTIGATION OF INTERNUCLEAR AND SUPRANUCLEAR DISORDERS

Case history   General observations should include gait, paralysis or weakening of function, the level of patient's consciousness and mental alertness, and speech. Many patients may be disorientated and may feel generally unwell. Symptoms can include vertigo, pain, loss of sensation or tingling, reading difficulties, diplopia and oscillopsia.

Observations may be made while taking the case history, such as the presence of a head posture, pupil size, lid position and ocular posture.

Visual acuity   This may be reduced if papilloedema or any lesion of the optic nerve affecting the macular fibres in particular is present. Optic neuritis may be present in cases of multiple sclerosis.

Cover test   Usually binocular single vision is present with a latent deviation in the primary position. However, exotropia or esotropia may be seen with convergence or divergence paralysis. There may be a skew deviation or vertical misalignment in some unilateral conditions such as INO, one and a half syndrome and double elevator syndrome.

Ocular movements   All eye movement systems should be assessed.

Ocular dysmetria may be noted with defective saccades. Dysmetria indicates overshooting of saccades, hypometria indicates undershooting. Ocular flutter is a disturbance of position maintenance system with unsteady movement on fixation. Smooth pursuit movements should be assessed for conjugacy and smoothness of movement as these can be replaced by a series of cog-wheel movements.

When assessing the integrity of vergence movements, the convergence and divergence mechanisms should be included. Full gaze should be assessed along with the presence of gaze palsies, whether unilateral or bilateral.

Nystagmus is common in many lesions, particularly if the vestibular apparatus is involved. Note speed, amplitude and position of greatest and least amplitude, whether movements are jerky and, if so, the direction of the fast phase. Nystagmus may only be present on versions.

Testing OKN assesses the integrity of both saccadic and smooth pursuit pathways. It is tested in both directions plus horizontally and vertically. Responses are compared on each occasion. Any difference in response tested in either direction is indicative of abnormality.

Doll's head/head rotation may be used to assess the integrity of the vestibular pathway. Caloric stimulation may be used for some, particularly semi- or unconscious patients. Instillation of cold water into one ear results in eye movements in the opposite direction. Instillation of warm water into one ear results in eye movement towards the same direction (COWS).

Binocular function These patients usually demonstrate normal binocular single vision except in cases of prior existing strabismus. In conjugate deviations, diplopia is rarely appreciated as these deviations are symmetrical. Diplopia will be appreciated in asymmetrical deviations.

Angle of deviation In line with routine orthoptic evaluation, the angle of deviation must be measured with the appropriate test. Defective ocular movements may be recorded on a Hess chart and areas of diplopia recorded on a field of binocular single vision.

Ophthalmic investigation

Visual fields Post-chiasm lesions result in homonymous hemianopia or quadrantanopia. Pituitary lesions may lead to bitemporal hemianopia. Fusion is difficult due to this as there is no overlap of the visual fields. Field defects may cause difficulty in testing refixation movements. If the target to be fixed falls within a scotoma there may be an apparent defect of the saccadic system as no refixation movement will take place. However, on OKN testing the saccadic system may be intact. The type of field defect is a good localising sign for many lesions affecting the visual pathway at any point along its course.

Forced lid closure This can help in the diagnosis of vertical gaze anomalies. In dorsal midbrain syndrome, there is no upgaze movement but elevation is present on lid closure, indicating the integrity of the superior recti muscles and infranuclear pathway. In some parieto-occipital lesions, the eyes may deviate to one side. This is known as Cogan's sign.

MANAGEMENT OF INTERNUCLEAR AND SUPRANUCLEAR DISORDERS

As evident from the discussion of these disorders, the prognosis for many conditions is poor. The primary aim following orthoptic investigation is to render the patient asymptomatic. Many conditions will have conjugate deviations and as a result will not appreciate diplopia. For those with asymmetrical deviations, diplopia is a frequently appreciated symptom. Prisms may be tried but the incomitance of the deviation often makes the use of prisms difficult. Occlusion may then be considered. Occlusion is also useful where there is dissociated nystagmus and oscillation. Convex lenses or miotics may be prescribed for those with associated pupil and accommodative anomalies.

Surgery, as for other forms of strabismus, may only be considered in a stable deviation. Concomitant deviations associated with congenital supranuclear disorders may be performed in line with normal indications, e.g. infantile esotropia with ocular motor apraxia. For incomitant deviations, transposition surgery may often be considered to improve movement of the affected eye, e.g. Knapp procedure for double elevator palsy.

REFERENCES

Barsoum-Homsy M. (1983) Congenital double elevator palsy. *Journal of Pediatric Ophthalmology and Strabismus*, 20: 185

Bender MB. (1980) Brain control of conjugate horizontal and vertical eye movements; a survey of the structural and functional correlates. *Brain*, 103: 23

Brandt T & Dieterich M. (1993) Skew deviation with ocular torsion: a vestibular brainstem sign of topographic diagnostic value. *Annals of Neurology*, 33: 528

Bronstein AM, Rudge P, Gresty MA, DuBoulay G & Morris J. (1990) Abnormalities of horizontal gaze. Clinical, oculographic and MRI findings. II Gaze palsy and INO. *Journal of Neurology, Neurosurgery and Psychiatry*, 53: 200

Chamlin M & Davidoff L. (1951) Divergence paralysis with increased intracranial pressures (further observations). *Archives of Ophthalmology*, 46: 195

Collins SJ, Ahlskog JE, Parisi JE & Maraganor DM. (1995) Progressive supranuclear palsy: neuropathologically based diagnostic clinical criteria. *Journal of Neurology, Neurosurgery and Psychiatry*, 58: 167

Cunningham RD. (1972) Divergence paralysis. *American Journal of Ophthalmology*, 74: 630

Dagi LR, Chrousos GA & Cogan DG. (1987) Spasm of the near reflex associated with organic disease. *American Journal of Ophthalmology*, 103: 582

Glaser J. (1966) Myasthenic pseudo-internuclear ophthalmoplegia. *Archives of Ophthalmology*, 75: 363

Green JP, Newman NJ & Winterkorn JS. (1993) Paralysis of downgaze in two patients with clinical-radiologic correlation. *Archives of Ophthalmology*, 111: 219

Guiloff RJ, Whiteley A & Kelly RE. (1980) Organic convergence spasm. *Acta Neurologica Scandinavica*, 61: 252

Harris CM, Shawkat F, Russell-Eggitt I, Wilson J & Taylor D. (1996) Intermittent horizontal saccadic failure (ocular motor apraxia) in children. *British Journal of Ophthalmology*, 80: 151

Jacobsohn DM. (2000) Divergence insufficiency revisited: natural history of idiopathic cases and neurological associations. *Archives of Ophthalmology*, 118: 1237

Jampel RS & Fells P. (1968) Monocular elevation paresis caused by a central nervous system lesion. *Archives of Ophthalmology*, 80: 45

Keane JR. (1975) Ocular skew deviation. *Archives of Neurology*, 32: 185

Kernan JC, Devinsky O, Luciano DJ, Vazquez B & Perrine K. (1993) Lateralising significance of head and eye deviation in secondary generation tonic-clonic seizures. *Neurology*, 43: 1308

Knapp P. (1969) The surgical treatment of double elevator paralysis. *Transactions of the American Ophthalmology Society*, 67: 304

Krohel GB, Tobin DR, Hartnett ME & Barrows NA. (1982) Divergence paralysis. *American Journal of Ophthalmology*, 94: 506

Lagreze W-D, Warner JEA, Zamani AA, Gouras GK, Koralnik IJ & Bienfang DC. (1996) Mesencephalic clefts associated with eye movement disorders. *Archives of Ophthalmology*, 114: 429

Lee AG, Brown DG & Diaz PJ. (1996) Dorsal midbrain syndrome due to mesencephalic hemorrhage. Case report with serial imaging. *Journal of NeuroOphthalmology*, 16: 281

Lessel S. (1975) Supranuclear paralysis of monocular elevation. *Neurology*, 25: 1134

Lyle DJ. (1954) Divergence insufficiency. *Archives of Ophthalmology*, 52: 858

Metz HS. (1979) Double elevator palsy. *Archives of Ophthalmology*, 97: 901

Metz HS. (1981) Double elevator palsy. *Journal of Pediatric Ophthalmology and Strabismus*, 18: 31

Miller NR, Biousse V, Hwang T, Patel S, Newman NJ & Zee DS. (2002) Isolated acquired unilateral horizontal gaze paresis from a putative lesion of the abducens nucleus. *Journal of Neuro-Ophthalmology*, 22: 204

Ohtsuka K, Maeda S & Oguri N. (2002) Accommodation and convergence palsy caused by lesions in the bilateral rostral superior colliculus. *American Journal of Ophthalmology*, 133: 425

Parinaud H. (1883) Paralysie des movements associes des yeux. *Archives of Neurology*, 5: 145

Pierrot-Deseilligny C & Goasguen J. (1984) Isolated abducens nucleus damage due to histiocytosis X. Electro-oculographic analysis and physiological deductions. *Brain*, 107: 1019

Repka MX, Claro MS, Loupa DN & Reich SG. (1996) Ocular motility in Parkinson's disease. *Journal of Pediatric Ophthalmology and Strabismus*, 33: 144

Roper-Hall G & Burde RM. (1987) Diagnosis and management of divergence paralysis. *American Orthoptic Journal*, 37: 113

Rowe FJ. (1995) Developmental delay in congenital ocular motor apraxia. In: Louly M, Doyle M, Hirai T & Tomlinson E (eds) *Transactions of the Eighth International Orthoptic Congress*. Japan, p. 68

Rowe FJ. (2003) Supranuclear and internuclear control of eye movements. A review. *British Orthoptic Journal*, 60: 2

Rutkowsky PC & Burian HM. (1972) Divergence paralysis following head trauma. *American Journal of Ophthalmology*, 73: 660

Shawkat FS, Harris CM, Taylor DSI & Kriss A. (1996) The role of ERG/VEP and eye movement recordings in children with ocular motor apraxia. *Eye*, 10: 53

Steiner I & Melamed E. (1984) Conjugate eye deviation after acute hemispheric stroke: delayed recovery after previous contralateral frontol lobe damage. *Annals of Neurology*, 16: 509

Thames PB, Trobe JD & Ballinger WE. (1984) Upgaze paralysis caused by lesion of the periaqueductal gray matter. *Archives of Neurology*, 41: 437

von Noorden GK & Hansell R. (1991) Clinical characteristics and treatment of isolated inferior rectus paralysis. *Ophthalmology*, 98: 253

Zee D, Hain TC & Carl JR. (1987) Abduction nystagmus in internuclear ophthalmoplegia. *Annals of Neurology*, 21: 383

Ziffer AJ, Rosenbaum AL, Demer JL & Yee RD. (1992) Congenital double elevator palsy: vertical saccadic velocity utilizing the scleral search coil technique. *Journal of Pediatric Ophthalmology and Strabismus*, 29: 142

FURTHER READING

Boeder P. (1961) The co-operation of extra ocular muscles. *American Journal of Ophthalmology*, 51: 469

Bruce GM. (1935) Ocular divergence: its physiology and pathology. *Archives of Ophthalmology*, 13: 639

Burian HM, van Allen MW, Sexton RR & Baller RS. (1965) Substitution phenomena in congenital and acquired supranuclear disorders of eye movement. *Transactions of the American Academy of Ophthalmology and Otolaryngology*, 69: 1105

Dunphy EB. (1968) Paralysis of divergence. *American Journal of Ophthalmology*, 11: 298

Ficker LA, Collin JRO & Lee JP. (1986) Management of ipsilateral ptosis with hypotropia. *British Journal of Ophthalmology*, 70: 732

Goldstein JH & Schneekloth BB. (1996) Spasm of the near reflex: a spectrum of anomalies. *Survey of Ophthalmology*, 40: 269

Hoyt CS. (1978) Acquired double elevator palsy and polycythemia vera. *Journal of Pediatric Ophthalmology and Strabismus*, 15: 362

Kirkham TH, Bird AC & Sanders MD. (1972) Divergence paralysis with increased intracranial pressure: an electro-oculographic study. *British Journal of Ophthalmology*, 56: 776

Leigh RJ & Tusa RJ. (1985) Disturbances of smooth pursuit caused by infarction of occipito-parietal cortex. *Annals of Neurology*, 17: 185

Lekwuwa GU & Barnes GR. (1996) Cerebral control of eye movements. I The relationship between cerebral lesion sites and smooth pursuit deficits. *Brain*, 119: 473

Moore S, Harbison JW & Stockbridge L. (1971) Divergence insufficiency. *American Orthoptic Journal*, 21: 59

Morrow MJ & Sharpe JA. (1995) Deficits in smooth pursuit eye movements after unilateral frontal lobe lesions. *Annals of Neurology*, 37: 443

Rambold H, Churchland A, Selig Y, Jasmin L & Lisberger SG. (2002) Partial ablations of the flocculus and ventral paraflocculus in monkeys cause linked deficits in smooth pursuit eye movements and adaptive modification of the VOR. *Journal of Neurophysiology*, 87: 912

Scott WE & Jackson OB. (1977) Double elevator palsy: the significance of inferior rectus restriction. *American Orthoptic Journal*, 27: 5

Strachan IM & Innes JR. (1987) Congenital paralysis of vertical gaze. In: Lenk-Schafer M, Calcutt C, Doyle M & Moore S (eds) *Transactions of the Sixth International Orthoptic Congress*. British Orthoptic Society, London, p. 140

SECTION IV
APPENDICES

Diagnostic aids

COVER TEST POINTERS

- Compare near and distance fixation
- Compare with and without abnormal head posture; why has the patient developed a head posture?
- Latent deviation, intermittent manifest or constantly manifest
- Eso- , exo- , hyper- or hypodeviation (watch lids to help detect vertical deviation)
- Primary and secondary deviation
- Diplopia: type; is it relevant to the deviation seen?
- Nystagmus, pupil anomalies

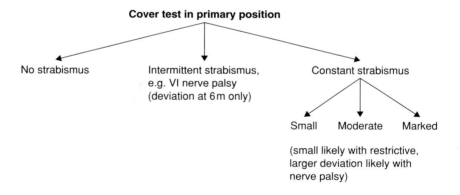

OCULAR MOVEMENT POINTERS

Smooth pursuit assessment from primary position into eight cardinal positions.

- Are the movements symmetrical and smooth in either eye?
- Underactions, overactions, restrictions – compare ductions and versions
- A or V patterns
- Nystagmus, lid or pupil changes
- Enophthalmos or exophthalmos
- Diplopia: type; is it relevant to the deviation seen in each position of gaze?

Saccadic assessment

- Compare horizontal and vertical saccades
- Compare eyes for symmetrical movement
- Hypo- or hypermetric movements, under- or overshooting

Vergence assessment

- Convergence to nose: do both eyes move symmetrically?
- Divergence: do both eyes relax out from converged position to distance fixation?

MAINTENANCE OF BINOCULAR VISION/ALLEVIATION OF DIPLOPIA

Conservative

- Abnormal head posture
- Prisms
- Occlusion
- Bangerter filters

Intervention

- Botulinum toxin
- Surgery

ANGLE OF DEVIATION POINTERS

- Measure angle of deviation at near and distance fixation, with and without abnormal head posture.
- Is there a primary and secondary angle of deviation? If yes, could indicate restrictive condition or recent onset cranial nerve palsy.
- Measure angle of deviation in cardinal positions of gaze.
- Where is the maximum angle of deviation?
- Does this coincide with the patient's perception of maximum symptoms?

DIAGNOSTIC CONSIDERATIONS

Always consider whether the ocular motor problem could fit a category of motility impairment. Remember to look for associated signs such as lid and pupil changes.

- Neurogenic: III, IV or VI cranial nerve palsy or combination
- Mechanical: Brown's syndrome, Duane's retraction syndrome, thyroid eye disease, orbital fractures

- Myogenic: myasthenia gravis, chronic progressive external ophthalmoplegia, extraocular muscle inflammation
- Nystagmus: check direction, waveform, amplitude, frequency and velocity
- Internuclear: internuclear ophthalmoplegia, one and a half syndrome
- Supranuclear: saccadic deficit, smooth pursuit deficit, vergence paralysis, gaze palsy, skew deviation

Remember to work through the most likely diagnoses first.

COVER TEST RESULTS

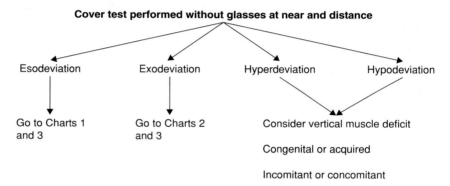

Cover test performed without glasses at near and distance

Esodeviation

Go to Charts 1
and 3

Exodeviation

Go to Charts 2
and 3

Hyperdeviation

Hypodeviation

Consider vertical muscle deficit

Congenital or acquired

Incomitant or concomitant

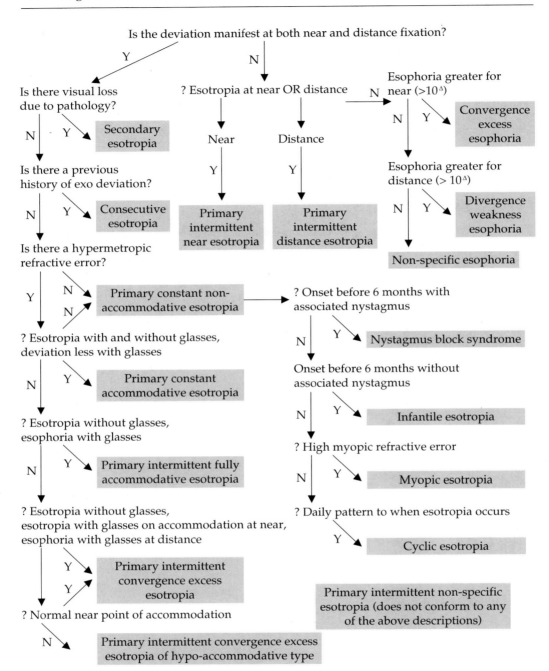

Chart 1   Esodeviations. (Reprinted with permission from: Rowe FJ. (2003) Diagnosis of concomitant strabismus. *Eye News*, 9: 18.)

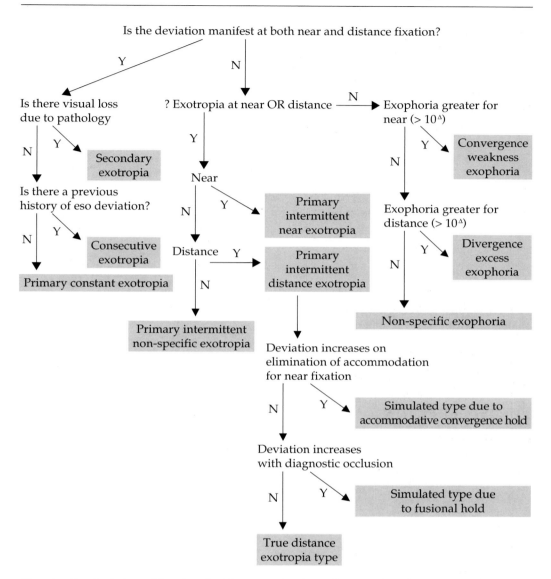

Chart 2 Exodeviations. (Reprinted with permission from: Rowe FJ. (2003) Diagnosis of concomitant strabismus. *Eye News*, 9: 18.)

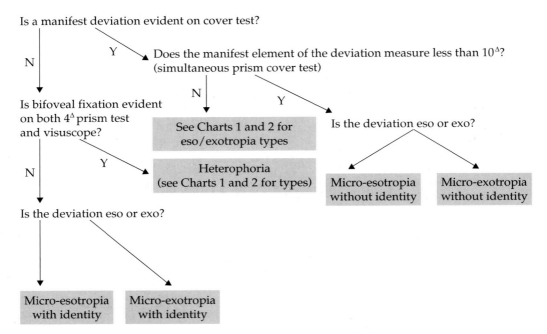

Chart 3   Microtropia. (Reprinted with permission from: Rowe FJ. (2003) Diagnosis of concomitant strabismus. *Eye News*, 9: 18.)

FURTHER READING

Rowe FJ. (2002) Use of orthoptic investigations in the assessment of incomitant strabismus. *Eye News*, 9: 7

Rowe FJ. (2003) Diagnosis of concomitant strabismus. *Eye News*, 9: 18

Abbreviations of orthoptic terms

Accom	Accommodation.
AC/A	Accommodative convergence/accommodation ratio.
ACS	Alternating convergent strabismus.
ADS	Alternating divergent strabismus.
AHP	Abnormal head posture.
ARC	Abnormal retinal correspondence.
A Eso	A pattern esotropia/esophoria.
A Exo	A pattern exotropia/exophoria.
bd/bid	Twice daily (bis die/bis in die).
Bag. gls.	Bagolini glasses.
BD	Base-down prism.
BE	Both eyes.
BEO	Both eyes open.
BF	Binocular function.
BHTT	Bielchowsky head tilt test.
BI	Base-in prism.
BO	Base-out prism.
BO#	Blow-out fracture.
BSV	Binocular single vision.
BTXA	Botulinum toxin A.
BVA	Binocular visual acuity.
BU	Base-up prism.
CC	Cardiff cards (vanishing optotypes).
CF	Counting fingers.
CH	Case history.
CHP	Compensatory head posture.
CI	Convergence insufficiency.
c/o	Complains of.
Conv.	Convergence.
CSM	Central steady maintained (fixation).
CT	Cover test.
Cyl	Cylinder.
D	Dioptre.
Del. rec.	Delayed recovery.
Dep.	Depression.
Dip	Diplopia.
DistET/DET	Distance esotropia.
DistXT/DXT	Distance exotropia.

Div	Divergence.
DS	Dioptre sphere.
DV/DVA	Distance vision.
DVD	Dissociated vertical deviation.
DVM	Delayed visual maturation.
Ecc. fix.	Eccentric fixation.
EE	Either eye.
Elev.	Elevation.
EP	Esophoria.
Eso	Esodeviation.
ET	Esotropia.
E(T)	Intermittent esotropia.
Exo	Exodeviation.
FCPL	Forced choice preferential looking.
FEE	Fixing either eye.
FLE	Fixing left eye.
FRE	Fixing right eye.
FTTO	Full time total occlusion.
Gd. rec.	Good recovery.
H/A	Headache.
H&T	Hundreds and thousands.
HP	Hyperphoria.
HT	Hypertropia.
HM	Hand movements.
IO	Inferior oblique.
IPD	Interpupillary distance.
IR	Inferior rectus.
ISQ	In status quo (in the former state).
KP	Kay's pictures (single optotypes).
L	Left.
LCS	Left convergent strabismus.
LDS	Left divergent strabismus.
LE	Left eye.
LN	Latent nystagmus.
LogMAR	Logarithm of the minimal angle of resolution.
LP	Light perception.
LPS	Levator palpebrae superioris.
LR	Lateral rectus.
L/R	Left hyper/right hypodeviation.
LVA	Low vision aid.
LVA/LV	Low visual acuity.
MA	Major amblyoscope.
MBWNL	Muscle balance within normal limits.
MLN	Manifest latent nystagmus.
MR	Medial rectus.

N	Near test type size/near/nerve.
NAD	Nil abnormal detected/no apparent deviation.
N&D	Near and distance.
NP	Near point.
NPA	Near point of accommodation.
NPC	Near point of convergence.
NPL	No perception of light.
Nr	Near
NRC	Normal retinal correspondence.
o/a	Overaction.
Obj	Objective.
Occl	Occlusion.
OD	Right eye.
OKN	Optokinetic nystagmus.
OM	Ocular motility.
OS	Left eye.
OU	Both eyes.
PBD	Prism base down.
PBI	Prism base in.
PBO	Prism base out.
PBU	Prism base up.
PCT	Prism cover test.
PD	Pupillary distance.
PERLA	Pupils equal and reactive to light and accommodation.
PF	Palpebral fissure.
PFR	Prism fusion range.
PH	Pinhole.
PL	Preferential looking.
PL	Perception of light.
PRT	Prism reflection test.
PTTO	Part time total occlusion.
RAF	Royal Air Force (rule).
Rap. rec.	Rapid recovery.
RAPD	Relative afferent pupillary defect.
RC	Retinal correspondence.
RCS	Right convergent strabismus.
RDS	Right divergent strabismus.
RE	Right eye.
RET	Right esotropia.
Rec	Recovery.
ROP	Retinopathy of prematurity.
R/L	Right hyper/left hypodeviation.
rr	Rapid recovery.
RVA	Right visual acuity.
RXT	Right exotropia.

Rec/recess	Recession.
Res/resect	Resection.
SA	Stereoacuity.
SFP	Simultaneous foveal perception.
SG/SSG	Sheridan Gardiner (singles).
Sl. rec.	Slight recovery.
SMP	Simultaneous macular perception.
Sn	Snellen's.
SO	Superior oblique.
SP	Simultaneous perception.
Sph	Sphere.
sr	Slow recovery.
SR	Superior rectus.
Subj	Subjective.
Supp	Suppression.
SV	Stereo vision.
tid/td	Three times daily (ter in die/ter die).
u/a	Underaction.
VA	Visual acuity.
VEP	Visual evoked potential.
VER	Visual evoked response.
V 'eso'	V pattern esotropia/esophoria.
V 'exo'	V pattern exotropia/exophoria.
VF	Visual field.
VFA	Visual field assessment.
VOR	Vestibulo-ocular reflex.
X pattern	X pattern.
XP	Exophoria.
XT	Exotropia.
X(T)	Intermittent exotropia.
'	Minute of arc.
"	Second of arc.
Δ	Prism dioptre.
$\oplus$	No deviation.
ϕ	No horizontal deviation.
$\ominus$	No vertical deviation.
°	Degree.
1/3 m	One-third metre testing distance.
3 m	Three metre testing distance.
6 m	Six metre testing distance.
$\bar{c}$	With.
$\bar{s}$	Without.
>	Greater than.
<	Less than.

1/7	One day.
1/52	One week.
1/12	One month.
Rx	Prescription.
Sx	Surgery.
#	Fracture.

DIAGRAMMATIC ABBREVIATIONS

E	Esophoria.
RET	Right esotropia.
R(E)T	Intermittent right esotropia predominantly controlled.
RE(T)	Intermittent right esotropia predominantly manifest.
RH	Right hyperphoria.
RHT	Right hypertropia.
R(H)T	Intermittent right hypertropia predominantly controlled.
RH(T)	Intermittent right hypertropia predominantly manifest.
Rhypo	Right hypophoria.
RhypoT	Right hypotropia.
R(Hypo)T	Intermittent right hypotropia predominantly controlled.
Rhypo(T)	Intermittent right hypotropia predominantly manifest.
RXT	Right exotropia.
R(X)T	Intermittent right exotropia predominantly controlled.
RX(T)	Intermittent right exotropia predominantly manifest.
X	Exophoria.

Replace R (right) with L (left) or A (alternating).

Glossary

Abduction

Uniocular eye movement where the eye is rotated outwards from the midline.

Abnormal binocular single vision

A form of binocular vision which occurs in the absence of bifoveal fixation, usually with abnormal retinal correspondence in everyday sight.

Abnormal head posture

An abnormal position of the head due to ocular or non-ocular causes. This may consist of:

- chin elevation
- face turn to the right or left
- head tilt to the right or left shoulder.

These components may exist together or singly.

Abnormal retinal correspondence

A binocular condition in which there is a change in visual projection such that the fovea of the fixing eye has a common visual direction with an area other than the fovea of the deviating eye. The pairing of all retinal elements is similarly changed. It may occur whichever eye is used for fixation.

Accommodation

The ability of the eye to increase its dioptric power (the convexity of the crystalline lens) in order to obtain a clear image of a near object.

Accommodative convergence/accommodation (AC/A) ratio

Ratio of accommodative convergence in prism dioptres in relation to one dioptre sphere of accommodation.

Accommodative esotropia

The convergent deviation is affected by the state of accommodation and this is a significant factor in the aetiology of the squint.

Accommodative facility

A measure of how fast clarity is restored following a rapid change of focus.

Adduction

Uniocular eye movement to describe rotation inwards towards the midline.

Alexander's law

     Relating to nystagmus where gaze in the direction of the fast component increases the frequency and amplitude while gaze in the opposite direction has the reverse effect.

Alternating strabismus

     Either eye may be used for fixation.

Amblyopia

     A condition of diminished visual form sense which is not the result of any clinically demonstrable anomaly of the visual pathway and which is not relieved by the elimination of any defect which constitutes a dioptric obstacle to the formation of the foveal image.

Amblyopic (amblyogenic) factors

     Factors which are thought to cause amblyopia. (1) Form deprivation at the fovea. (2) Abnormal binocular interaction. (3) Light deprivation of the entire retina.

Amplitude of accommodation

     The difference in dioptres between the near and far points of accommodation (between the minimum and maximum amount of accommodation).

Angle kappa

     The angle between the mid-pupillary line and the visual axis.

Angle of anomaly

     The difference between the objective and subjective angles of deviation.

Aniseikonia

     A difference in size and/or shape of the retinal images of the two eyes.

Anisometropia

     A difference in refractive error between the two eyes.

Antagonist

     Extraocular muscle whose action opposes that of the contracting muscle.

Aphakia

     Absence of the crystalline lens from the pupillary line.

Asthenopia

     The collective term for various ocular symptoms, including sore and aching eyes, blurred vision and ocular fatigue.

Bell's phenomenon

     Elevation of both eyes with divergence when the eyelids are closed.

Bifoveal fixation

     Imaging of an object on both foveae at the same time.

Binocular convergence

Convergence associated with binocular single vision.

Binocular diplopia

This results from the presence of a manifest ocular deviation and is the simultaneous appreciation of two separate images caused by the stimulation on non-corresponding points by one object. This separation may be horizontal, vertical or torsional, or any combination.

Binocular function

The ability of the two eyes to co-ordinate binocularly either in free space, using prisms, or instrumentally, using a haploscope. It may be normal or abnormal.

Binocular single vision

The ability to use both eyes simultaneously so that each eye contributes to a common single perception and may be bifoveal or monofoveal.

Binocular visual acuity

The maximum visual acuity obtainable while maintaining binocular single vision (as distinct from visual acuity with both eyes open).

Central fixation

The reception of the image of the fixation object by the fovea, the fixation object lying in the principal visual direction.

Cogan's lid twitch

Transient eyelid retraction during refixation from down to straight ahead seen in myasthenia gravis.

Cogan's sign

A tonic deviation of the eye occurring on forced eyelid closure and associated with lesions in the cerebral hemispheres.

Cog-wheel movements

Episodic rotations with pursuit movements.

Collier's sign

Unilateral or bilateral lid retraction due to a lesion in the midbrain.

Coloboma

A fissure or gap in the eyeball or one of its parts, e.g. iris.

Concomitant strabismus

Strabismus in which the angle of deviation remains the same in all directions of gaze, whichever eye is fixing.

Confusion

The simultaneous appreciation of two superimposed images due to the stimulation of corresponding retinal points by two different images.

Conjugate movements

Movements of the two eyes in the same direction.

Contracture

The inability of a contracted muscle to relax fully.

Contrast sensitivity

The ability of the eye to detect objects of varying contrast which can be tested using sinusoidal gratings of varying spatial frequency and varying luminance intensity.

Convergence

Simultaneous rotation of the eyes inwards.

Convergence accommodation/convergence ratio (CA/C ratio)

Ratio of convergence initiated accommodation per prism dioptre of convergence.

Crossed fixation

Patient uses right eye to fix in left field and left eye to fix in right field; seen in early onset esotropia, strabismus fixus and VI nerve palsy.

Crowding phenomenon (separation difficulty)

The phenomenon in which a line of letters or symbols of the same size on a test type are identified less easily than single optotypes.

Depression

Rotation of the eye downwards.

Dioptre

A unit of measurement of the power of a lens equal to the inverse of the focal length in metres. A 1 dioptre lens brings parallel light in focus at 1 metre.

Diplopia

The simultaneous appreciation of two images of one object.

Disjugate movements

Movements of the two eyes in which the visual axes do not remain parallel but move in opposite relative directions.

Divergence

Simultaneous rotation of the eyes outwards.

Donder's law

To each position of the line of sight belongs a definite orientation of the horizontal and vertical retinal meridians relative to the co-ordinates of space irrespective of the route taken.

Duction

Rotary movement of one eye from the primary position.

Eccentric fixation

> A uniocular condition in which there is fixation of an object by a point other than the fovea. This point adopts the principal visual direction. The degree of the eccentric fixation is defined by its distance from the fovea in degrees.

Eccentric viewing

> A uniocular condition in which there is fixation of an object by a retinal point other than the fovea without change in the principal visual direction.

Ecchymosis

> A bruise: an effusion of blood under the skin.

Elevation

> Rotation of the eye upwards.

Enophthalmos

> Recession of the eyeball into the orbit.

Epicanthus

> Skinfolds between the medial canthi and the nose causing pseudostrabismus.

Epiphora

> An excessive flow of tears.

Epistaxis

> Bleeding from the nose.

Esophoria

> On dissociation of the two eyes, the occluded eye deviates nasally.

Esotropia

> One or other eye deviates nasally when both eyes are open.

Exophoria

> On dissociation of the two eyes, the occluded eye deviates temporally.

Exophthalmos

> Protrusion of the eyeball.

Exotropia

> One or other eye deviates temporally when both eyes are open.

Faden

> A surgical procedure where the muscle is stitched to the globe, as far as possible behind the insertion, to further weaken its action in its field of gaze.

False localisation

> The incorrect uniocular subjective localisation of the fixation object.

Far point of accommodation

The furthest point at which an object can be seen clearly.

Field of binocular single vision

The extent to which binocular single vision is maintained by movement of the eyes whilst the head is kept still.

Field of uniocular fixation

The extent to which each eye can maintain foveal fixation whilst the head is kept still.

Fixation disparity

A phenomenon which occurs in binocular single vision in which the image is seen singly despite a slight under- or overconvergence of the visual axes, provided the disparate retinal points are within Panum's area. It generally increases if BSV is under stress and can be demonstrated instrumentally when fusion occurs for identical features of two targets but any dissimilar features are displaced in the direction of the heterophoria.

Fresnel lenses/prisms

Plastic lenses or prisms which can be adhered temporarily to spectacles.

Functional

(1) A deviation which has the ability, at least potentially, for binocular single vision.

(2) Patient shows signs or symptoms of a disorder but careful examination fails to reveal any evidence of structural or physiological abnormalities.

Fusional vergence

The range of convergence and divergence of the eyes whilst maintaining clear binocular single vision.

Gait

Manner of walking.

Glissade

A small corrective movement slower than a saccade, used to fixate an object after a hypo- or hypermetric saccade.

Grades of binocular vision

These are the aspects of binocular function which indicate the degree of binocular vision present, i.e. simultaneous perception, superimposition, fusion and stereopsis.

Harmonious abnormal retinal correspondence

The angle of anomaly is equal to the objective angle.

Hering's law

A law of ocular motor innervation. Whenever an impulse for the performance of an eye movement is sent out, corresponding muscles of each eye receive equal innervations to contract or relax.

Heteronymous (crossed) diplopia

Binocular diplopia associated with exotropia in which the image of the fixation object is received on the temporal area of the retina of the deviating eye and is projected nasally.

Homonymous (uncrossed) diplopia

Binocular diplopia associated with esotropia in which the image of the fixation object is received on the nasal area of the retina of the deviating eye and is projected temporally.

Horopter

The locus of all points in space that are imaged on corresponding retinal points.

Iatrogenic

A disorder resulting from treatment.

Idiopathic

Without apparent cause.

Incomitant strabismus

Strabismus in which the angle of deviation differs depending upon the direction of gaze or according to which eye is fixing, associated with:

(1)   defective movement of the eye
(2)   asymmetrical accommodative effort.

Infantile

Occurring in the first months of life.

Intermittent strabismus

A manifest deviation which is only present under certain conditions.

Interpupillary distance

The distance between the two pupillary centres. The average for an adult is 65 mm when the eyes are fixing in the distance.

Ipsilateral

Referring to the same side.

Lid lag

A condition occurring in thyroid eye disease where the upper lid does not follow the eye fully when changing fixation from upgaze to downgaze. An area of white sclera will be exposed (von Graefe's sign).

Lid retraction

Raised upper lid due to overaction of Muller's muscle.

Linear optotype

Letters, symbols or pictures presented in evenly spaced rows with separation between the letters equal to the size of the letter.

Linear visual acuity

Visual acuity tested using a line of optotype.

Listing's law

A law elaborating Donder's law of combined actions of the extraocular muscles: each movement of the eye from the primary position to any other position involves a rotation around a single axis lying in the equatorial plane called Listing's plane.

LogMAR

The logarithm of the minimum angle of resolution.

Macropsia

Objects appear larger than their natural size.

Mechanical strabismus

A squint caused by obstruction to movement of the extraocular muscles.

Micropsia

Objects appear smaller than their natural size.

Miosis

Constriction of the pupil.

Monocular diplopia

Double vision attributable to one eye.

Motor fusion

The ability to maintain sensory fusion through a range of vergence, which may be horizontal, vertical or cyclovergence.

Muscle sequelae

Sequence of extraocular muscle adaptation following muscle weakness or limitation. Relates to Hering's and Sherrington's laws of innervation.

Mydriasis

Dilation of the pupil.

Myectomy

Removal of a portion of a muscle.

Myopathy

A primary disease of the muscle, causing it to underact.

Myositis

Inflammation of a muscle.

Myotomy

Incision into the muscle.

Near point of accommodation

The nearest point at which an object can be seen clearly.

Near point of convergence

The nearest point at which convergence can be achieved.

Near triad

Association between convergence, accommodation and pupil reflexes.

Negative fusional range/vergence

Motor fusion maintained with base-in prisms or with the eye diverging.

Negative relative convergence

Exerting less convergence in association with the required accommodation.

Neuropathy

A disorder affecting the structure and function of the nervous system.

Normal retinal correspondence

A binocular condition in which the fovea and areas on the nasal and temporal side of one retina correspond to and have a common visual direction with the fovea and temporal and nasal areas of the retina of the other eye.

Null position of nystagmus

Position of the eyes in which nystagmus is least.

Objective

Responses observed by the examiner.

Objective angle

The angle of misalignment of the visual axes as measured by the observer.

Occluder

A device for obscuring the vision of one eye, either totally or partially, so as to ensure the use of the other eye.

Occlusion

The reduction or elimination of retinal image in order to prevent or reduce visual stimulation.

Ocular adnexa

Term applied to eye lids, lacrimal glands, accessory nasal sinuses, etc.

Optokinetic nystagmus

Normal oscillatory eye movements which occur with movement of the visual environment.

Optotype

Letter, symbol or picture used to test visual acuity.

Oscillopsia

An illusion of oscillatory movement of the environment experienced in patients with nystagmus.

Overaction

Excessive action of a muscle caused by increased innervation as a consequence of palsy or limitation to the ipsilateral antagonist or contralateral synergist.

Palpebral fissure

The distance/gap between the upper and lower lids.

Palsy

Partial or complete loss of function of a muscle.

Panoramic vision

The awareness of an enlarged field of vision due to the separation of visual fields occurring in exotropia.

Panum's area

The area surrounding corresponding retinal points within which disparity of correspondence may occur whilst maintaining binocular single vision.

Panum's space

A band around the horopter in space within which object points give rise to binocular single vision.

Paradoxical diplopia

Pathological binocular diplopia in which heteronymous (crossed) diplopia occurs in esotropia or homonymous (uncrossed) diplopia occurs in exotropia.

Paralysis

Complete inability of a muscle to act.

Paresis

Partial paralysis or defective action in a muscle.

Penalisation

The treatment of amblyopia and/or eccentric fixation by optical reduction of form vision of the non-amblyopic eye at one or all fixation distances. The effect may be achieved by the alteration of the spectacle correction and/or use of a cycloplegic drug.

Photophobia

An intolerance of light.

Physiological diplopia

A type of diplopia which exists in the presence of binocular single vision. It consists of the appreciation that a near object appears double when a distant object is fixated (heteronymous or crossed diplopia) and a distant object appears double when a near object is fixated (homonymous or uncrossed diplopia).

Positive fusional range/vergence

Motor fusion maintained with base-out prisms or with the eyes converging.

Positive relative convergence

Exerting more convergence in association with the required accommodation.

Primary angle of deviation

The deviation when fixing with the unaffected eye in paralytic incomitant strabismus.

Principal visual direction

The line of projection in subjective space of images stimulating the fovea or eccentric point used for fixation.

Prism

A wedge shaped refracting medium which deflects traversing rays of light towards the base.

Prism dioptre

A unit of measurement of the strength of a prism. A prism of 1 dioptre displaces the image of the object through 1 cm for each metre of distance between the object and the prism.

Projection

The subjective interpretation of the direction of an object.

Proptosis

Protrusion of one or both eyeballs.

Recession

A surgical procedure which weakens the action of the muscle by moving the insertion towards the origin.

Resection

A surgical procedure which strengthens the action of the muscle by removing a portion close to the insertion. The muscle is then reattached to the original insertion.

Retinal correspondence

Retinal areas of each eye have the same visual direction during binocular vision.

Retinal rivalry

Occurs in binocular vision when non-fusible images are presented to corresponding retinal points. The images are alternately suppressed, 'shimmer' or form a changing mosaic.

Saccade

Rapid eye movement to obtain fixation on an object.

Sagittalisation

A surgical procedure where the insertion of the oblique muscle is moved more anteriorly which enhances the torsional action.

Scotoma

An area of partial or complete blindness surrounded by normal or relatively normal visual field.

Secondary angle of deviation

The deviation when fixing with the affected eye in paralytic incomitant strabismus.

Sensory fusion

The ability to perceive two similar images, one formed on each retina, and interpret them as one.

Sherrington's law

A law of reciprocal innervation: whenever an agonist receives an impulse to contract, an equivalent inhibitory impulse is sent to its antagonist which relaxes.

Simultaneous perception

The ability to perceive simultaneously two images, one formed on each retina.

Smooth pursuit movement

Movement of the eyes to maintain fixation on a moving object.

Stereoacuity

An angular measurement of the minimum resolvable binocular disparity necessary for the appreciation of stereopsis.

Stereoscopic vision

The perception of relative depth of objects on the basis of binocular disparity.

Strabismus

A manifest or latent ocular deviation.

Subjective

Response from the patient or subject.

Subjective angle

The angle between the visual direction of the retinal element in each eye receiving images of the fixation object. It is shown by the subjective separation of diplopia in heterotropia or dissociated heterophoria.

Superimposition

The simultaneous perception of two images formed on corresponding areas, with the projection of these images to the same position in space. This may occur whether the correspondence is normal or abnormal. If fusion is absent two similar images are seen as separate but superimposed and no fusion range is demonstrable.

Suppression

The mental inhibition of visual sensations on one eye in favour of the other eye, when both eyes are open. This may occur in binocular single vision and in manifest strabismus. It may vary in area and density. A defined area is known as suppression scotoma.

Synergists

Contralateral muscles which normally work together.

Tenectomy

A surgical procedure which removes a portion of the tendon, thereby weakening its action (usually the superior oblique).

Tenotomy

A surgical procedure which cuts into the tendon, thereby weakening its action (usually the superior oblique).

Transposition

A surgical procedure which moves the insertion of the muscle to alter its action.

Tuck (plication)

A surgical procedure which shortens the tendon and thereby strengthens its action (usually performed on superior oblique).

Underaction

Reduced ocular rotation which improves on testing ductions, often associated with neurogenic palsy.

Unharmonious abnormal retinal correspondence

The angle of anomaly is less than the angle of deviation.

Version

Movement of the two eyes in the same direction.

Visual direction

The line of projection in subjective space associated with a given retinal point.

Visual impairment

Any loss or abnormality of visual function.

Yoke muscle

See Synergists.

Case reports

CONCOMITANT STRABISMUS
Case report 1

Case history   A child was referred by his GP at the age of six months with a history of a convergent deviation from the age of one month. There was no significant family history.

Refraction   There was no significant refractive error.

Fundus and media   Normal.

Cover test   Marked angle alternating esotropia.

Ocular motility   The child used crossfixation on lateral gaze but ocular movements were full on testing.

Angle of deviation   60 prism dioptres.

Diagnosis   A diagnosis of infantile esotropia was made.

Management   The child was reviewed over the following eight months and surgery of bilateral medial rectus recessions was performed at the age of 14 months. Post-operatively, the eyes appeared aligned although it was not possible to demonstrate evidence of binocular function due to the young age.

    Orthoptic examination at the age of four years demonstrated a minimal left microtropia with good binocular function.

Case report 2

Case history   A seven year old girl attended for a follow-up appointment at the orthoptic clinic. An intermittent alternating convergent deviation had been noted from the age of four years with no symptoms of diplopia.

Refraction   She had a hypermetropic refractive error and was currently wearing +3.50 DS before either eye.

Visual acuity   Equal and normal visual acuities of 6/6 right and left.

Cover test   Slight angle esophoria with good recovery with the spectacles and a moderate angle right esotropia without the spectacles.

Binocular function   Normal with the spectacles with a prism fusion range of 45 prism dioptres convergent range and 12 prism dioptres divergent range. Binocular visual acuity was to the level of visual acuity with the spectacles and there was bifoveal fixation evident with the 4 prism dioptre test.

Diagnosis	A diagnosis of intermittent accommodative esotropia of the fully accommodative type was made.
Management	The spectacles were reviewed on a yearly basis and no further management was required.

Case report 3

Case history	A four year old girl was referred by her GP with a history of intermittent convergent squint over the past year. There was a history of hypermetropic refractive error in the immediate family.
Refraction	Retinoscopy revealed a hypermetropic refractive error and spectacles of +2.0 DS right and left were ordered.
Visual acuity	Equal.
Cover test	Small angle esophoria to a light target for near fixation becoming a moderate angle right esotropia to a detailed target. There was a slight angle esophoria in the distance. Without the spectacles, there was a moderate angle right esotropia on near fixation and a moderate angle esophoria for distance which was easily dissociated to a right esotropia.
Binocular function	Poor responses at near fixation. However, a normal motor fusion range and stereopsis were demonstrable using the synoptophore.
Angle of deviation	The angle of deviation measured 40 prism dioptres for near fixation and 14 prism dioptres for made.
+3.0 DS lenses	The deviation was again measured with additional +3.0 DS lenses for near fixation and the angle of deviation decreased to 16 prism dioptres.
AC/A ratio	An AC/A ratio of 8:1 was calculated by the gradient method.
Diagnosis	A diagnosis of intermittent accommodative exotropia of the convergence excess type was made.
Management	The angle of deviation was found to increase on testing at follow-up visits and binocular function deteriorated. Surgery was planned and bilateral medial rectus recessions were done at the age of five years.
	Post-operatively, there was a small residual manifest angle of deviation on near fixation with a latent deviation in the distance. This persisted and two months post-operatively, the child was given miotic drops. The manifest deviation was controlled for near fixation with good binocular function while using these drops. After two months of full control of the deviation, the drops were gradually withdrawn over a further two month period. The child has retained good binocular function and a small angle esophoria is present on cover test.

Case report 4

Case history	A five year old boy was referred with a history of sore eyes when watching TV. His father also noted that the eyes appeared to lack co-ordination at times.

Refraction	There was no significant refractive error on retinoscopy.
Visual acuity	Equal in either eye.
Cover test	Small angle exophoria was present for near fixation with delayed recovery. On distance fixation, a moderate angle exophoria decompensated easily to a left exotropia. This was more evident on far distance fixation.
Ocular motility	Ocular motility revealed a V exo pattern with underactions of the superior rectus of either eye.
Convergence	Binocular convergence was reduced at 14 cm.
Binocular function	Reduced with a low convergent motor fusion range of 18 prism dioptres.
Angle of deviation	The angle of deviation measured 12 prism dioptres for near fixation and 30 prism dioptres for distance.
+3.0 DS lenses	The angle was measured with additional +3.0 DS lenses and noted to be 30 prism dioptres.
AC/A ratio	An AC/A ratio of 6:1 was calculated using the gradient method.
Diagnosis	A diagnosis of intermittent exotropia of the simulated distance exotropia type was made.
Management	Although young, the child was very co-operative and convergence exercises were commenced to improve his level of binocular convergence. Pen convergence exercises were advised initially, and after three weeks his convergence level had improved to 8 cm with improvement in his convergent motor fusion range also. He continued with pen convergence exercises and was given a dotcard to use as well. Binocular convergence improved to the normal level of 6 cm at follow-up and exercises were stopped. He maintained good binocular function with control of the latent deviation for near fixation. As the deviation was not cosmetically unacceptable for distance, further management was not planned and the child remained under observation.

Case report 5

Case history	A 21 year old male presented with a cosmetically unacceptable left exotropia. There was a history of a penetrating injury to the left eye at the age of seven years. A traumatic cataract was removed six months later and an intraocular lens implanted. He also had left corneal scarring related to the penetrating injury.
Visual acuity	6/6 in the right eye and perception of light in the left eye.
Cover test	Moderate angle left exotropia by corneal reflections with poor left fixation.
Angle of deviation	Estimated to be 35 prism dioptres by corneal reflections using the prism reflection test.
Suppression	A post-operative diplopia test elicited no diplopia responses at the corrected angle or when under- or overcorrected by prisms.
Diagnosis	A diagnosis of secondary exotropia was made.

Management Surgery was planned for a cosmetic result, aiming to leave the left eye in a slight convergent position.

Case report 6

Case history A three year old girl presented with a one year history of intermittent esotropia. The parents had noted an alternate day tendency to squint and had documented this over a six week period.

Visual acuity Equal in either eye.

Cover test Marked left esotropia at near and distance fixation.

Binocular function Absent with suppression responses on testing in free space and on the synoptophore.

Angle of deviation 50 prism dioptres at near and distant fixation.

Observation In view of the parents' observations of the frequency of the deviation, appointments were arranged for consecutive day assessments. On day 1, the marked left esotropia was evident. On day 2, the child was orthophoric with excellent binocular function.

Diagnosis A diagnosis of cyclic esotropia was made.

Management A squint chart was documented daily over the follow-up period which showed a break in the pattern with the squint more frequent. A left medial rectus recession and lateral rectus resection procedure was performed at this stage, and post-operatively a minimal esophoria with excellent binocular function was demonstrated. This latent deviation has remained well controlled over a four year follow-up period with no return of the cyclic pattern.

Case report 7

Case history A girl aged six years was referred by her optician having failed a school vision test. There had been no previous ocular history and no significant family history.

Refraction Spectacles of +1.0 DS for the right eye and +3.75 DS for the left eye.

Visual acuity 6/5 in the right eye and 6/36 in the left eye.

Cover test A minimal left esotropia was noted which increased slightly on dissociation but recovered to the minimal manifest angle.

Binocular function Demonstrable with a motor fusion range of 30 prism dioptres convergent range and 12 prism dioptres divergent range. Stereopsis was reduced at 400 seconds of arc. Fixation was central and steady in the right eye but was unsteady and nasal to foveal fixation in the left eye.

Angle of deviation 12 prism dioptres by prism cover test and 6 prism dioptres by simultaneous cover test.

Diagnosis A diagnosis of microesotropia without identity was made.

Management Occlusion therapy was commenced with occlusion for a minimum of six hours daily initially. The visual acuity improved over the follow-up period but did not improve beyond the 6/9 level. Occlusion was discontinued at this stage. No further management was required.

Case report 8

Case history   A five year old boy was referred having moved into the area. He had previously been under the care of another hospital. Treatment had included one operation for a convergent deviation which had been present from infancy. This had been successful in aligning the eyes. Visual acuity had been found to be slightly reduced and the child had had one year of part time occlusion treatment.

Visual acuity   6/9 in the right eye and 6/6 in the left eye.

Cover test   Slight right exotropia with DVD and latent nystagmus.

Binocular function   Suppression responses were obtained.

Diagnosis   A diagnosis of consecutive exotropia with DVD and latent nystagmus was made.

Management   The strabismus was cosmetically good and no further management was indicated.

Case report 9

Case history   A 15 year old girl was referred by her GP with general asthenopic symptoms of intermittent headache, blurred vision and jumbling of print when reading. Her general health was good and there was no significant family history.

Refraction   She had a mild myopic refractive error and had been wearing spectacles for the past nine months.

Visual acuity   Equal visual acuities in either eye.

Cover test   A small angle exophoria was noted at near fixation and a minimal exophoria for distance.

Ocular motility   Full.

Convergence   Reduced to 25 cm and fatigue was noted on repeated testing.

Accommodation   Slightly defective for the patient's age.

Binocular function   Reduced convergent range of the prism fusion range.

Diagnosis   A diagnosis of exophoria of the convergence weakness type and convergence insufficiency was made.

Management   She was given pen convergence exercises to practise daily and reviewed after two weeks at which time the level of binocular convergence had improved to 12 cm. She was then given a dotcard in addition to the pen convergence exercises. The level of binocular convergence continued to improve and cat stereograms were given. At the next follow-up visit, binocular convergence was to a normal level of 6 cm. She was given detailed stereograms at this stage. Binocular convergence remained at

6 cm and was well maintained at this level. The convergence range of the prism fusion range had also improved to normal and the patient was asymptomatic. Exercises were discontinued, and at follow-up two months later she remained asymptomatic with a normal orthoptic assessment, and was discharged.

INCOMITANT STRABISMUS

Case report 10

Case history	A 58 year old male presented with a sudden onset of horizontal diplopia two days previously. The diplopia was worse on right gaze and there were no other associated symptoms. He had a history of diabetes for the past 15 years.
Cover test	Right esotropia for near fixation which increased in angle at distance. With a small abnormal head posture of face turn to the right, the deviation was controlled for near fixation but readily decompensated in the distance.
Ocular motility	Small right lateral rectus (VI nerve) palsy.
Angle of deviation	18 prism dioptres at near fixation and 25 prism dioptres at distance.
Binocular function	Diplopia could be joined with 16 prism dioptres for both fixation distances.
General investigation	Neurological assessment, including a CT brain scan, was normal. However, the diabetes was found to be poorly controlled and the patient's treatment was altered.
Diagnosis	A diagnosis of right VI nerve palsy due to a probable microvascular episode was made.
Management	A 15 prism dioptre fresnel lens was fitted to the patient's spectacles. The lateral rectus palsy gradually improved over the following four months. During this time, the fresnel prism was reduced in strength and eventually discarded.

Case report 11

Case history	A 26 year old male was seen on the neurology ward. He had been involved in a road traffic accident and had suffered a closed head injury.
Cover test	Complete left ptosis with no lid crease. The patient did not complain of diplopia as the ptosis covered the visual axis. On lifting the lid, the left eye was in a depressed and divergent position. The pupil was semi-dilated.
Ocular motility	Complete left III nerve palsy with limited elevation, adduction and depression of the left eye.
Diagnosis	A diagnosis of traumatic III nerve palsy was made.

Management   An outpatient appointment was arranged for a three month follow-up visit. At that time, the ocular movements were seen to be recovering. At his six month follow-up, there was a slight limitation of adduction with a residual left exotropia. Elevation and depression of the left eye had recovered. The left exotropic angle of deviation remained static over a further nine month period and surgery of a left lateral rectus recession was performed. Thereafter, the patient regained binocular single vision in the primary position.

Case report 12

Case history   A 42 year old female was referred by her GP with a six month history of intermittent diplopia and grittiness of her eyes. She was aware of a puffy appearance around her eyes. She had had a thyroidectomy three years previously and was currently on thyroxine and clinically euthyroid.

Visual acuity   Reduced at 6/18 in the right eye and 6/12 in the left eye.

Cover test   A slight exophoria with a small right hyperphoria was seen.

Ocular motility   Slight limitation of either eye on abduction. There was a moderate limitation of either eye on elevation with the left eye slightly more limited than the right. The right eye was slightly limited on depression, maximum in an abducted position. Bilateral lid retraction and proptosis were noted.

Binocular function   A good motor fusion range was demonstrable, including an extended vertical fusion range consistent with a gradual increase in the vertical deviation.

Hess chart   Confirmed restricted ocular movements.

General investigation   An MRI orbital scan demonstrated enlarged extraocular muscles, particularly near the orbital apex. An MRI stir sequence showed increased signal from the extraocular muscles, confirming active thyroid eye disease.

Diagnosis   A diagnosis of thyroid eye disease was made. In view of the enlarged extraocular muscles at the orbital apex and the reduced visual acuity, optic compression was diagnosed.

Management   The patient was admitted and commenced on pulsed IV methylprednisolone for immediate medical decompression. She then had a course of oral prednisolone and azathioprine. Visual function was monitored by automated visual field assessment and acuities improved to normal at 6/6. The ocular motility limitations were also noted to improve and MRI demonstrated a reduction of the extraocular muscle bulk. The plan was to reduce the medical treatment very gradually.

The patient did not require further treatment for her ocular motility limitations as she was only aware of intermittent diplopia on extreme elevation and she avoided looking in this position of gaze. She had a good field of binocular single vision in the primary and reading positions.

Case report 13

Case history   A three year child was referred for a second opinion regarding her esotropia and marked abnormal head posture. Her parents were concerned about the degree of head turn and the cosmesis.

Visual acuity   Equal.

Abnormal head posture   The head posture was of a marked face turn to the left.

Cover test   With the head posture, there was a slight esophoria. Without the head posture, cover testing revealed a marked left esotropia with some left enophthalmos.

Ocular motility   Marked limitation of left abduction with widening of the palpebral fissure and slight limitation of left adduction with moderate retraction of the globe and narrowing of the palpebral fissure. The left eye was seen to upshoot on elevation in adduction. There was slight limitation of right abduction with widening of the palpebral fissure but no obvious limitation or retraction on right adduction.

Binocular function   With the head posture there was demonstrable binocular function.

Diagnosis   A diagnosis of Duane's retraction syndrome was made.

Management   The child was reviewed during the following six months. The binocular function while adopting the abnormal head posture deteriorated and the latent deviation was noted to decompensate at times. In view of this decompensation and the very marked abnormal head posture, it was decided to list the child for surgery. Bilateral medial rectus recessions and a left lateral rectus recession were performed to reduce the convergent angle of deviation and the globe retraction.

Post-operatively, a small abnormal head posture was still adopted but to a much reduced degree. The convergent deviation was well controlled with the abnormal head posture with good binocular function and the manifest deviation without the abnormal head posture was reduced in measurement.

Case report 14

Case history   A 74 year old male presented with a three day history of sudden onset vertical diplopia. This was worse when reading. He had had a mild left CVA (cerebral vascular accident) one week previously, resulting in hand weakness which later resolved.

Visual acuity   Equal.

Cover test   Small right hypertropia with a slight right exotropia on near fixation with diplopia. At distance, there was a slight right hypertropia with diplopia.

Ocular motility   Small underaction of the right eye on depression in adduction and an overaction of the right eye on elevation in adduction consistent with a right superior oblique (IV nerve) palsy with secondary inferior oblique overaction.

Angle of deviation   5 prism dioptres R/L at near fixation and 3 prism dioptres R/L at distant fixation.

Hess chart   Confirmation of ocular motility findings.

Diagnosis   A diagnosis of IV nerve palsy due to cerebrovascular accident was made.

Management   The patient was mainly troubled by the diplopia in the near position and a 5 dioptre fresnel prism was placed on his reading spectacles which joined the diplopia comfortably. The prism was reduced to a 3 dioptre strength at subsequent follow-up. As the deviation did not recover any further, this prism was incorporated into the spectacle correction eight months later.

Case report 15

Case history   A 53 year old male presented with diplopia on upgaze. He had been assaulted two weeks previously, resulting in a facial injury. A CT scan showed a right orbital floor fracture with entrapment of tissue.

Abnormal head posture   Small abnormal head posture of chin elevation.

Cover test   Minimal esophoria with slight right hypophoria with this head posture. Without the head posture, the deviation became a manifest left hypertropia with diplopia.

Ocular motility   Slight limitation of the right eye on abduction and adduction and a moderate limitation of the right eye on all elevated positions. There was slight enophthalmos with some tingling over his upper lip.

Management   The patient was reviewed by the maxillofacial team and underwent orbital surgery which freed the entrapped tissue and a Silastic plate was inserted over the fracture site.

Post-operatively, the patient still had a small limitation of the right eye on elevation with diplopia. However, he was not bothered by this diplopia and was happy to continue using a small abnormal head posture. No further management was indicated.

Case report 16

Case history   A three year old child was seen in a community vision screening clinic and was referred with limited elevation of the right eye.

Refraction   The child was unco-operative on attempts to check refraction and his fundus and media. He was therefore admitted for an examination under anaesthetic. There was no significant refractive error and his fundus and media were normal and clear.

Visual acuity   Equal in either eye.

Cover test   Slight exophoria with a minimal right hypophoria.

Ocular motility   Moderate limitation of right elevation which was marked in adduction. On left gaze, a downdrift of the right eye was noted. Motility of either eye was normal on depression.

Binocular function   Excellent with a normal motor fusion range.

Forced duction test   Performed under anaesthetic and positive on elevation in adduction.

Diagnosis   A diagnosis of right Brown's syndrome was made.

Case report 17

Case history   An 11 year old child was seen in the ophthalmology casualty clinic. She complained of intermittent blurred vision and diplopia. She had been seen by an optician regarding the blurred vision and was now wearing spectacles with a mild myopic prescription.

Refraction   A cycloplegic refraction revealed a slight hypermetropic refractive error which was not significant. The myopic spectacles were discarded.

Fundus and media   Normal.

Visual acuity   Reduced in both eyes but improved with additional minus lenses.

Cover test   Small esophoria was demonstrated. This increased on dissociation and intermittently became a marked alternating esotropia with diplopia. The pupils were noted to be constricted with the manifest deviation.

Diagnosis   A diagnosis of accommodative convergence spasm was made.

Management   An MRI brain scan was arranged to exclude any organic cause for the condition. This scan was normal in appearance. The child was commenced on atropine drops 1% daily and given +3.0 DS spectacles for close work. In the interim, she was referred to a child psychologist. On questioning, a history of bullying at school was revealed. The school was contacted and this problem addressed. The child was weaned off the atropine over a period of four months and has remained asymptomatic.

Case report 18

Case history   A 45 year old male presented to ophthalmology casualty complaining of difficulties in reading and headaches.

Investigation   Orthoptic assessment was normal with full ocular movements and a well compensated exophoria.

Observation   In view of the symptoms, a one week follow-up appointment was arranged.

Ocular motility   Upgaze palsy with convergence retraction nystagmus on elevation.

General investigation   A CT brain scan revealed increased signal in the upper midbrain with scattered signal areas in the cortex.

Diagnosis A diagnosis of disseminating disease causing Parinaud's (dorsal midbrain) syndrome was made.

Management There was complete recovery of the ocular motility signs during the following three months. No treatment other than observation was required.

Case report 19

Case history A 42 year old female presented with a ten day history of right eye pain and diplopia on right gaze which was both horizontal and vertical. She had a medical history of Parkinson's syndrome and medication included antidepressants and sedatives.

Cover test Slight exophoria with good recovery.

Ocular motility Slight limitation of the right eye on adduction and moderate limitation of either eye on elevation consistent with an upgaze palsy. There was bilateral ptosis. Saccadic movements were tested which showed defective horizontal saccades and absent saccades on upgaze. Vertical saccades were full on depression.

Convergence Binocular convergence was reduced to 25 cm.

Diagnosis A diagnosis of supranuclear ocular motility deficit due to Parkinson's disease was made.

Case report 20

Case history A 32 year old male presented complaining of a gradual onset of intermittent blurring of vision and oblique diplopia (combined horizontal and vertical separation of images) for the past year. No other ocular symptoms. General health was good with no medication taken. Previous history of road traffic accident ten years ago with concussion. New job in the past year with increasing VDU work.

Abnormal head posture Small tilt and turn to left with chin depression.

Cover test Slight right hyperphoria and esophoria with abnormal head posture. Angle increases with fair recovery without abnormal head posture, with near angle greater than distance fixation.

Ocular motility

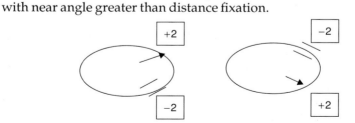

Convergence Normal.

Binocular function Normal values with abnormal head posture.

Angle of
deviation
R/2 prism dioptres and eso 4 prism dioptres at near fixation, R/1 prism dioptres and eso 4 prism dioptres at distance fixation with abnormal head posture. R/5 prism dioptres and eso 4 prism dioptres at near fixation, R/4 prism dioptres and eso 4 prism dioptres at distance fixation without abnormal head posture and fixing either eye.

Synoptophore

R/3ᐞ, +3°		R/7ᐞ, +2°
	R/4ᐞ, +2°, 1° excyclo	
R/3ᐞ, +2°, 4° excyclo		R/6ᐞ, +3°, 2° excyclo

Diagnosis
Diagnosis of right superior oblique paresis as abnormal head posture includes chin depression to move eyes away from position of maximum action of affected muscle, near measurements are greater than distance measurements, symptom of torsion is maximum on downgaze and is excyclo rather than incyclotorsion. Long-standing condition due to con-comitant ocular motility and measurements (no difference in primary or secondary angle of deviation), gradual onset of symptoms and not aware of torsion.

Case report 21

Case history
A 16 year old female complained of symptoms of horizontal diplopia for the past six months, particularly when looking to the right. Not very bothered by diplopia and no other symptoms. General health good and family history of brother with a squint.

Abnormal head
posture
Slight face turn to right.

Cover test
Slight esophoria with abnormal head posture. Slight right esotropia without abnormal head posture greater for distance than near fixation with intermittent diplopia.

Ocular motility

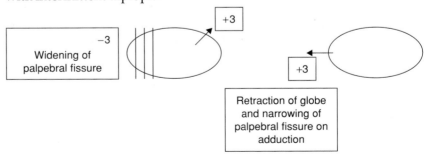

Convergence   Normal.
Binocular   Normal values with abnormal head posture. Intermittent suppression/
function   diplopia on right gaze.

| *Angle of deviation* | Eso 6 prism dioptres at near fixation, eso 8 prism dioptres at distance fixation with abnormal head posture. Eso 14 prism dioptres at near fixation, eso 18 prism dioptres at distance fixation without abnormal head posture fixing left eye. Eso 18 prism dioptres at near fixation, eso 25 prism dioptres at distance fixation without abnormal head posture fixing right eye. |

Synoptophore

+20°	+10°	+6°

| *Diagnosis* | Diagnosis of Duane's retraction syndrome due to palpebral fissure changes, globe retraction on adduction of the affected eye and upshoot of affected eye on elevation in adduction. Incomitant angle of deviation which increases fixing with the affected eye. Abnormal head posture is only slight and patient is unaware of this. Intermittent symptoms with intermittent suppression/diplopia responses on investigation can be expected in Duane's retraction syndrome. Constant diplopia would be expected more with VI nerve palsy without suppression responses. |

Case report 22

Case history	A three year old boy was referred by his GP as the family had noticed a squint when the child looked up at them. General health was good with no family history of eye problems and a normal birth history.
Cover test	Slight exophoria for near and distance fixation.
Convergence	Normal.
Binocular function	Normal values in primary position.
Ocular motility	

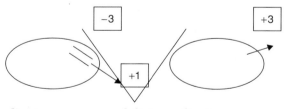

| *Angle of deviation* | Exo 4 prism dioptres on near and distance fixation. |

Synoptophore

L/6$^\Delta$,−4°	L/8$^\Delta$,−3°	L/10$^\Delta$,−3°
	−2°	L/2$^\Delta$,−3°
−2°		−1°

Diagnosis   Diagnosis of Brown's syndrome as muscle sequelae is limited to over-action of the left superior rectus. There is minimal deviation in the primary position with no abnormal head posture and no abnormalities of ocular movement in any depressed position of gaze. A V pattern is present on ocular movements rather than an A pattern.

Index